PLAGUE HO

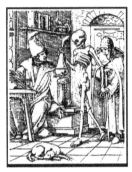

The History of Medicine in Context

Series Editors: Andrew Cunningham and Ole Peter Grell

Department of History and Philosophy of Science
University of Cambridge

Department of History
Open University

Titles in this series include

Plague Hospitals

Public Health for the City in Early Modern Venice

JANE L. STEVENS CRAWSHAW

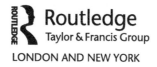
Routledge
Taylor & Francis Group

LONDON AND NEW YORK

First published 2012 by Ashgate Publishing

Published 2016 by Taylor & Francis
2 Park Square, Milton Park, Abingdon, Oxfordshire OX14 4RN
711 Third Avenue, New York, NY 10017, USA

First issued in paperback 2016

Routledge is an imprint of the Taylor & Francis Group, an informa business

British Library Cataloguing in Publication Data
Crawshaw, Jane L. Stevens.
  Plague hospitals : public health for the city in early modern Venice. — (The history of medicine in context)
  1. Plague—Italy—Venice—History—16th century. 2. Plague—Italy—Venice—History—17th century. 3. Plague—Treatment—Italy—Venice—History. 4. Social medicine—Italy—Venice—History. 5. Public hospitals—Italy—Venice—History--16th century. 6. Public hospitals—Italy—Venice—History—17th century. 7. Public health—Italy—Venice—History—16th century. 8. Public health—Italy—Venice—History—17th century. 9. Venice (Italy)—Social conditions—16th century. 10. Venice (Italy)—Social conditions—17th century.
  I. Title II. Series
  362.1'969232'00945311–dc23

Library of Congress Cataloging in Publication Data
Crawshaw, Jane L. Stevens.
  Plague hospitals : public health for the city in early modern Venice / by Jane L. Stevens Crawshaw.
    pages cm. — (The history of medicine in context)
  Includes bibliographical references and index.
  ISBN 978-0-7546-6958-6 (hardback : alkaline paper)
  1. Plague—Italy—Venice—History—16th century. 2. Plague—Italy—Venice—History—17th century. 3. Plague—Treatment—Italy—Venice—History. 4. Social medicine—Italy—Venice—History. 5. Public hospitals—Italy—Venice—History—16th century. 6. Public hospitals—Italy—Venice—History—17th century. 7. Public health—Italy—Venice—History—16th century. 8. Public health—Italy—Venice—History—17th century. 9. Venice (Italy)—Social conditions—16th century. 10. Venice (Italy)—Social conditions—17th century. I. Title.
  RC178.I92V463 2012
  616.9'23200945311—dc23

2011944550

ISBN 13: 978-1-138-24589-1 (pbk)
ISBN 13: 978-0-7546-6958-6 (hbk)

For Daphne and Stan Parker

and Elizabeth and Bill Stevens

Contents

List of Illustrations and Plates

List of Abbreviations

ACA	The *Archivio civico antico* in the Paduan and Veronese State Archives
Arsenal	The archive of the Venetian *Provveditori et patroni all'Arsenale*
ASV	*Archivio di Stato*, Venice
ASVer	*Archivio di Stato*, Verona
ASP	*Archivio di Stato*, Padua
Beni inculti	The archive of the Venetian *Provveditori sopra i beni inculti*, responsible for land reclamation and uncultivated land within Venetian territory
b.	*busta* (bundle)
BMC	The *Biblioteca del Museo Correr*, Venice
BMV	The *Biblioteca Marciana*, Venice
Cini	*Fondazione Giorgio Cini*, Venice
Collegio	The archive of the Venetian College, the part of the Senate which controlled proposals made and topics discussed
Consiglio dei Dieci	The archive of the Venetian Council of Ten, the executive council which had particular responsibility for the security of the state
Cucino	The letterbook of Ludovico Cucino, doctor to the Venetian Health Office held at the Wellcome library for the History and Understanding of Medicine
filza	file
Ingrassia	The account by Giovan Filippo Ingrassia published in an edited volume by Luigi Ingaliso, *Informatione del pestifero et contagioso morbo / Giovan Filippo Ingrassia* (Milan, 2005).
ms.	manuscript
NT	The Bible, New Testament
OT	The Bible, Old Testament
PSMc	The archive of the Venetian *Procuratia de San Marco de Citra* (Procurators of St Mark *de citra*)
reg.	*registro* (register)
Sal	The archive of the Venetian *Provveditori al Sal* (Salt Office)
Sanità	The archive of the *Ufficio della Sanità* in Verona and Padua or *Provveditori alla Sanità* in Venice (Health Office)

SEA	The archive of the Venetian *Savi ed esecutori alle acque*, responsible for the maintenance of waterways and bodies of water within and surrounding Venice
Secreta MMN	The series *Secreta, Materia miste notabili* in the Venetian State Archive
Senato Terra	Copies of the proposals put to vote in the Venetian Senate, the main decision-making council in Venice
SILT	The archive of the Veronese *Ospedale di San Giacomo e Lazzaro alla Tomba*
v.	verse within a chapter of the Bible
vol.	volume

A note on dates: The Venetian calendar traditionally started on 1 March. Instead of giving dates as they are stated in archive documents (denoted in the historiography by m.v. or *more veneto*), they are given in the text in their modern equivalent, unless otherwise stated.

Acknowledgements

Funding for this project was provided by the Wellcome Trust (in the form of a doctoral studentship) and the Society for Renaissance Studies (through a postdoctoral fellowship). Individual research trips were funded by Downing College, Cambridge and The Gladys Krieble Delmas Foundation. The latter also generously provided assistance towards the costs of publication of the book, which enabled the inclusion of the images in this volume. I would like to express my sincere thanks to each of these institutions.

In Italy, I am grateful to the staff of the research institutions in which I worked, particularly the Archivio di Stato in Venice, Verona and Padua. Dr Gerolamo Fazzini of the *lazaretto nuovo* has been extremely supportive of this research and generous with his time. I am also grateful to Dr Giampietro Mayerle and Dr Luigi Fozzati for granting me permission to visit the archaeological digs on the *lazaretto vecchio* and to Dr Luisa Gambaro for showing me round.

The History Department at Oxford Brookes has provided a stimulating context within which this book was finished. I am grateful to my colleagues for their support, particularly Alysa Levene who, amongst other things, took the time to look over one of the chapters and saved me from a number of embarrassing blunders in my handling of quantitative material. She is, of course, in no way responsible for those that remain. Andrew Spicer was very generous with his time and read the whole of the manuscript and provided a number of valuable comments and constructive criticisms.

There are many people who have influenced the development and my enjoyment of this project and I hope that they know who they are. It is a pleasure to single out the impact of the conversation and company of Vicky Avery, Alex Bamji, Ersie Burke, Georg Christ, Julia DeLancey, John-Paul Ghobrial, Deborah Howard, Jane Kromm, Andrea Mozzato, Courtney Quaintance, Rosa Salzberg, James Shaw, Kevin Siena, Nelli-Elena Vanzan Marchini and Paul Warde. It was fantastic fun developing a love of Venice and a friendship with Lydia Hamlett and Angela Roberts Christ. Their influence means that I have seen the inside of more sacristies and considered the placement of more medieval donor paintings than anyone could have imagined in a lifetime but it was worth it!

Tricia Allerston and Richard Mackenney both inspired me as an undergraduate and continue to do so today. Without their guidance and scholarship, I would not have conceived of this book, let alone written it. Tricia also very generously passed on a number of references to me, prominent amongst which were the Cucino letterbook at the Wellcome as well as those given to her by Dennis Romano for salary information in the Salt Office records in the Venetian *Archivio di Stato*. At Downing, Richard Smith acted as an advisor for my thesis and his breadth of knowledge added much to the project. John Henderson and Nick Davidson examined the thesis out of which this book developed and have provided tremendous insight and assistance both in that role and since. At St Andrews, where I held my first teaching job, Bruce Gordon and Andrew Pettegree taught me a great deal about model scholars and scholarship and their advice and encouragement has proven to be invaluable. Finally, Samuel Cohn has been extremely generous in sharing the fruits of his work. He read the manuscript of this book in its entirety and provided many helpful criticisms and questions.

Mary Laven supervised both my MPhil thesis and PhD. I have thanked her twice already (in the acknowledgements to those pieces) for her patience and good humour. She may not be surprised that I am going to show a characteristic lack of imagination and thank her for the same things here. Her tremendous insight meant that she identified, in our earliest supervisions, the elements of my work and this project which needed the most attention. She has looked on, patiently, as I have only slowly learned the lessons that she has taught me. I am sure that looking through this book in its published form, she will be twitching to pick up those infamous pastel pens to challenge ideas and improve my writing. I only hope that she knows how much I have learned, and continue to learn, from her and that she can see the transformative effect that she has had on this book.

It is a privilege to have the opportunity to express my thanks to friends and family who are a blessing and source of much joy. This book is dedicated to my four wonderful grandparents. I am only sorry that three of them did not get to see this book published: I think that they would have been amazed, if bemused! Unfailing love, encouragement and support came from my brother and my parents; in every way, this book could not have been written without them. It has taken me a number of years to fulfil their request to wrap my book for them and put it under the Christmas tree. I hope that they think that it has been worth the wait!

Of everyone, Brad Crawshaw must be the most relieved to see this book finished. He has amazed me with his goodness and patience, often coming home after a long day in his own, busy job, only to have the latest chapter thrust into his hand. He read every word and dealt kindly with the sometimes waspish responses that came back to his (absolutely correct) constructive criticism: further proof, if proof was needed, that he is the most extraordinary man I have ever known. For everything, from the countless cups of peppermint tea to making my life happier than I could have hoped or imagined, I thank him.

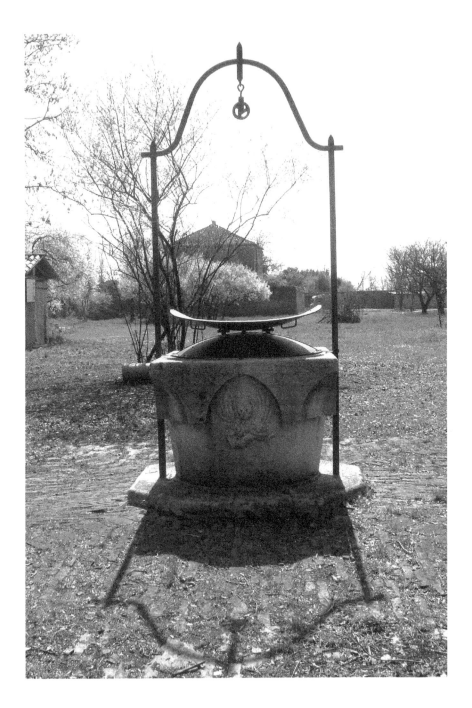

Figure I.1   Well in the *lazaretto nuovo*

Introduction

In one corner of the island of the *lazaretto nuovo*, in the Venetian lagoon, stands a beautiful, sixteenth-century well [Figure I.1]. From the fifteenth century, wells had become common features of squares, private courtyards and public institutions across Venice.[1] Drinking water was famously difficult to source: the proverb runs that Venice is in water, but it has no water (*Venezia è in aqua et non ha acqua*). Wells like this one, which were paid for by the Venetian Republic, displayed the lion of St Mark, the symbol of Venice, as a testament to the paternal care of the government towards the city's inhabitants in securing this indispensible resource. The lion on the well was shown *in moleca* (winged) and holding a book which contained the words, 'Peace be unto you, Mark my Evangelist' (*Pax Tibi Marce Evangelista Meus*). A lingering look at this well, which is replete with state iconography, can tell us much about Venice in the past. Above all, the well and its symbols illustrate how important the physical environment and perceived godly nature of the city were for shaping early modern Venice.[2]

The distinctive lagoon environment may have resembled the 'lifeblood of the city' because of its role in Venice's maritime trading empire but it also represented the Republic's most formidable and long-standing enemy.[3] The tidal lagoon

---

[1] There were 160 public wells in the city according to Robert C. Davis. See 'Venetian shipbuilders and the fountain of wine', *Past and Present*, 156 (1997), p. 62. A system had been developed for the construction of wells with an elaborate filtration system through layers of sand and stone. See Richard Goy, *Venetian vernacular architecture: traditional housing in the Venetian lagoon* (Cambridge, 1989), p. 86. For the wells on the *lazaretto nuovo* see Gerolamo Fazzini (ed.), *Venezia: isola del lazzaretto nuovo* (Venice, 2004) pp. 151–4. For an excellent, interdisciplinary study of housing, courtyards and squares see Giorgio Gianighian and Paola Pavarini, *Dietro i palazzo: tre secoli di architettura minore a Venezia 1492–1803* (Venice, 1984).

[2] A key work on the relationship between Venetian social, political and economic structures and the urban environment is Elizabeth Crouzet-Pavan's, *'Sopra le acque salse': espaces, pouvoir et société à Venise à la fin du Moyen Âge* (2 vols, Rome, 1992). See also Karl Appuhn, *A forest on the sea: environmental expertise in Renaissance Venice* (Baltimore MD, 2009).

[3] On Venice's maritime empire and on the crisis occasioned by the Portuguese discovery of a route around the Cape of Good Hope in 1497–99 see Robert Finlay, 'Crisis and crusade in the Mediterranean: Venice, Portugal and the Cape Route to India (1498–1509)', *Studi veneziani*, n.s. 28 (1994), pp. 45–91 and the seminal work by Frederic C. Lane collated in *Venice and history: the collected papers of Frederic C. Lane* (Baltimore MD, 1966). The diarist Gerolamo Priuli described the effect on Venice of the Portuguese discovery as akin to depriving a child of its milk and food. For an overview of the history

corrupted drinking water, attacked the physical structure of the city, created a damp environment with poor quality air and, through facilitating trade, was the path along which one of the most formidable adversaries of the early modern period could enter Venice: plague. This disease could devastate cities, killing up to a third of a population in a single outbreak, and was actively combated in the name of public health. The intricate nature of early modern disease causation meant that public health measures addressed issues of sin, pollution and infection in relation to entire societies as well as individuals. Accordingly, the authorities assumed responsibility for regulating morality, behaviour and the environment in the fight against epidemic disease.[4]

During the early modern period, the fight against disease was carried out, in part, in the celestial rather than the earthly realm; here, at least, Venice seemed to be well equipped. During his life, St Mark was said to have sought shelter in Venice. In a dream, an angel told the Evangelist 'Peace to you, Mark. Here is where your body will rest' (*Pax tibi, Marce. Hic requiescet corpus tuum*).[5] In 827 this dream became a reality, as the relics of St Mark were stolen from Alexandria and brought to Venice.[6] St Mark ousted St Theodore as the patron saint of the city and, through his permanent presence, confirmed divine blessing on and for Venice. The extraordinary nature of the city continued from the point of origin and the characteristics of the lagoon environment were thought to have seeped into the structures of the ideal, godly Republic, just as the salt water permeated the stones of the city. Liberty, stability, longevity, social tolerance and economic prosperity infused the history of Venice, and never more effectively than when the city was in hot water (so to speak) in times of crisis.[7]

---

of the Italian states more generally, including the episodes of invasion and warfare, during this period see John Najemy, *Italy in the age of the Renaissance* (Oxford, 2004) and John Marino, *Early modern Italy* (Oxford, 2002). For an introduction to Venice in the same period see David S. Chambers, *The Imperial age of Venice 1380-1580* (New York, 1970) and the introduction to Brian Pullan, *Rich and poor in Renaissance Venice: the social institutions of a Catholic state, to 1620* (Oxford, 1971).

[4]   For an introduction to Venetian public health measures see Paolo Preto, *Peste e società a Venezia, 1576* (Vicenza, 1978) and Richard J. Palmer, 'The control of plague in Venice and northern Italy 1348–1600' (unpublished PhD thesis, University of Kent, 1978). An unparalleled edition of primary sources, with secondary overview chapters, can be found in *Venezia e la peste 1348–1797* (Venice, 1980). Relevant material can also be found in Alberto Tenenti and Ugo Tucci (eds), *Storia di Venezia: vol. XII: Il mare* (Rome, 1991), particularly the contribution by Paolo Morachiello.

[5]   See Edward Muir, 'An escaped Trojan and a transported Evangelist: auspicious beginnings' in *Civic ritual in Renaissance Venice* (Princeton NJ, 1981), pp. 65–102.

[6]   See Patrick Geary, 'Translatio Sancti Marci' in *Furta sacra: thefts of relics in the central Middle Ages* (Princeton NJ, 1990), pp. 88–94.

[7]   These are elements which have been discussed as part of the historiographical 'myth of Venice'. For a discussion see James Grubb, 'When myths lose power: four decades of Venetian historiography', *Journal of modern history*, 58:1 (1986), pp. 43–94. On the anti-

On closer inspection of the well, we might notice that the lion is holding a closed rather than an open book. Someone once told me that this meant that the lagoon island of the *lazaretto nuovo* was on the margins of the city and that the iconography was designed to impart this sense of separation. Other depictions of the lion of St Mark on the island, however, are more conventional and show the lion with an open book. Examples of these closed books can be found in Venice too. Instead of emphasising a peripheral location, the imagery of the closed book is often interpreted by scholars to mean that the well-head was constructed when Venice was at war.[8] Even if division was not the message of the well-head iconography, the enduring perception of this island as being on the periphery of the city is important. For centuries, the island of the *lazaretto nuovo* accommodated one of Venice's two plague hospitals – the institutions at the heart of this book.

Although housed on small islands, the hospitals were two of the most powerful weapons in the fight against the plague between the fifteenth and seventeenth centuries and were central to Venice's public health strategy. The *lazaretto vecchio* (old *lazaretto*) was founded in 1423 as the first permanent plague hospital in the world. It was established to care for the plague sick by quarantining people and disinfecting goods. Venice's second plague hospital was termed the *lazaretto nuovo* (new *lazaretto*) to distinguish it from the *lazaretto vecchio*. It was established in 1456 and opened for business in 1471 as a site to which those suspected of having contracted the disease could be taken as a precaution; this often meant being part of the same household as someone who had died or shown signs of illness. Household quarantine within the city was used for those who had more limited contact with the disease. By the time of the plague outbreak of 1555, the *lazaretto nuovo* was also being used for those convalescing after a stay at the *lazaretto vecchio*.[9] These two *lazaretti* were state-funded hospitals, designed to protect the Venetian trade economy and make use of former monastic islands to

---

myth see David Wootton, 'Ulysses Bound? Venice and the idea of liberty from Howell to Hume' in David Wootton (ed.), *Republicanism, liberty, and commercial society, 1649–1776* (Stanford CA, 1994), pp. 341–67. On the counter-myth of the Venetian economy see Richard Mackenney, 'Letters from the Venetian archive', in Brian Pullan and Susan Reynolds (eds), *Towns and townspeople in Medieval and Renaissance Europe: essays in memory of J.K. Hyde, Bulletin of the John Rylands University Library of Manchester* 72:3 (1990), pp. 133–44 .

[8]   This is not always the case. Alberto Rizzi, *Vere da pozzo di Venezia: i puteali pubblici di Venezia e della sua laguna* (Venice, 1981) p. 23 makes the point that the book can be closed without necessarily having connortations of war. Rizzi also makes the point that the more usual style for a well constructed between the sixteenth and eighteenth centuries would be the *andante* lion, whereas here the Gothic *molecca* has been used (p. 22).

[9]   See the 'atto constitutivo del lazaretto vecchio' (28 August 1423) which is reprinted in *Venezia e la peste*, appendix seven, p. 365. For the *lazaretto nuovo* see the documents reprinted in Gerolamo Fazzini (ed.), *Venezia: isola del lazzaretto nuovo*. It is not clear precisely when the new policy regarding convalescing is introduced but regulations governing the practice can be found in the hospital statutes dating from this outbreak.

provide a breadth of care, which was in keeping with the nature of other early modern hospitals.

For over two hundred years, the *lazaretti* cared for Venetians and visitors alike, depending on whether or not the city itself was infected with plague. Beyond epidemics in the city, the social make up of patients could be quite narrow. At these times, the hospitals were used to treat incoming merchants and travellers. The hospitals operated very much as barriers on the outskirts of the city. The merchants and visitors who were sent to the hospitals beyond plague epidemics had to cover the costs of stays themselves. This is in contrast to the Venetians who were transported out to the islands from the city during epidemics, who were largely cared for at the expense of the state in the name of the godly Republic and the public good. These patients numbered in their thousands during the worst epidemics and were from across the social spectrum. From their foundation in the fifteenth century until the mid-seventeenth century, then, the *lazaretti* combined two functions: the care of inhabitants during epidemics and of entrants to the city beyond periods of infection. After the last outbreak of plague in Venice in 1630–31, the sites evolved into those solely providing quarantine for incomers – again, largely merchants. In the preceding period though – the focus for this study – the sites cared for a variety of patients, with the purpose of protecting as well as purifying the wider city in the context of epidemic disease.

Plague hospitals, although fascinating and important institutions, have received little sustained attention from historians working on Venice or beyond. The institution was developed in a number of other Italian and European cities during the fifteenth and sixteenth centuries. The lack of detailed study at the hands of historians, despite the geographical spread and importance of *lazaretti* within public health structures, relates in part to the wider historiography of plague, which tends to focus upon epidemics and periods of crisis rather than considering responses to the disease in their wider social and medical contexts.[10] The neglect may also be because, in some places, plague hospitals were founded as temporary, wooden structures for the duration of a plague outbreak or took over sites on a temporary basis and left little trace in archival material or cityscapes. Some permanent sites primarily consisted of open space for the disinfection of goods and have been thought to be, therefore, of little historical interest. In Venice, however, the city authorities developed permanent hospitals, which were elaborate

---

[10]   Key, early works on the plague in early modern Italy are the volumes by Carlo Cipolla on Tuscany: *Cristofano and the plague: a study in the history of public health in the age of Galileo* (Berkeley CA, 1973); *Public health and the medical profession in the Renaissance* (Cambridge, 1976); *Faith, reason and the plague: a Tuscan story of the seventeenth century* (trans.) M. Kittel (Ithaca NY, 1979); *Fighting the plague in seventeenth-century Italy* (Madison WI, 1981) and *Miasmi ed umori: ecologia e condizioni sanitarie in Toscana nel Seicento* (Bologna, 1989). These focused upon the crisis years of epidemics and provided an essential spark to early research but set out a methodology which, in many cases, continues to be adopted.

structures and offer an opportunity to make the first institutional study of plague hospitals, involving holistic consideration and wide-ranging contextualisation.[11]

A visit to the island of the *lazaretto nuovo*, or, indeed, to Venice itself during *acqua alta* (the seasonal high water which causes flooding in the city), can give the impression that, in the battle between the city and nature, nature eventually triumphed. Many of the buildings on the *lazaretto nuovo* have collapsed and the island combines the function of museum and nature reserve. However, all is not lost. The well with which we began is just one of the traces which remain of the two Venetian plague hospitals. In the archive, in literary sources, in maps and plans and *in situ* one can discover more about these early modern hospitals. Surviving fragments can be cast together to reveal the history of these sites and their significance. It is worth remembering that the distance between Venice and some of the lagoon islands is part of the reason that the decoration on the well survives at all on the *lazaretto nuovo*. Within the city, most of these symbolic lions on wells were removed after the fall of the Venetian Republic in 1797, when Venice succumbed to foreign invasion; the city was surrendered to Napoleonic troops and the 1,376 year-old Republic came to an end.[12] Over time, other carvings have been stolen and damaged.[13] On this largely deserted island, with its infected history, the lion has remained undisturbed. At the same time, the well is one of the few features of the island to survive virtually unscathed from the passages of time. The islands were used as *lazaretti* until the eighteenth century. Under Napoleonic and Austrian rule they became military sites.[14] By this time, the buildings had severely deteriorated and were largely rebuilt in line with their new purposes. Both islands were then abandoned, with the *lazaretto vecchio* becoming a home for stray dogs. In recent years, both locations have become sites of interest.[15] The *lazaretto vecchio* is due to open as an archaeological museum for the city. The

---

[11] A number of excellent examples could be cited reflecting the popularity of undertaking institutional studies. An early model, which effectively sets the institution in context, is Nicolai Rubinstein's study, *The palazzo vecchio, 1298–1532: government, architecture and imagery in the civic palace of the Florentine Republic* (Oxford, 1995).

[12] Alberto Rizzi, *Vere da pozzo*, p. 32 gives a number of examples of surviving lions on islands of the Venetian lagoon.

[13] On the issue of thefts from abandoned lagoon islands see Alberto Rizzi, *Scultura esterna a Venezia: corpus delle sculture erratiche all'aperto di Venezia della sua laguna* (Venice, 1987).

[14] For Venice under Austrian rule see David Laven, *Venice and Venetia under the Habsburgs, 1815–1835* (Oxford, 2002) which, although focused on the so-called Second Dominion, provides introductory material on the earlier period and ends by looking ahead to 1848.

[15] This was stimulated by the work of a number of Venetian writers, who called for restoration of elements of Venetian architecture including Giorgio and Maurizio Crovato in their *Isole abbandonate della Laguna: com'erano e come sono* (Padua, 1978) (which has recently been republished in a bilingual edition) and the publications of Alberto Rizzi cited in notes 12 and 13.

lazaretto nuovo is now a museum under the administration of the Venetian section of the *Archeoclub d'Italia*.[16] As we return to these neglected plague hospitals, it is worth remembering that their separation from the city has had both negative and positive effects on the fragments that survive.

In this study, the *lazaretti* will be situated in relation to Venetian history as well as early modern social and medical history. This book illustrates the ways in which illness was considered in the past and aligned with other social ills. It contends that the historiography has been anachronistically narrow in not aligning permanent plague hospitals with other medical and charitable institutions introduced in Renaissance and Catholic-Reformation Italian states.[17] Such an alignment is particularly important because diseases were conceptualised along a scale of infection rather than as individual entities by early modern contemporaries. There was a degree of fluidity, therefore, between diseases, as they threatened to develop into increasingly severe forms (with the most dangerous being plague). This was true of the causes of disease as well: sin and environmental pollution were dangerous not only because they were points of concern in their own right but also because the problems could escalate, causing epidemics. Public health policies were designed to prevent diseases as well as cure them; the wide-ranging policies addressed the threats of disease as well as diseases themselves and, therefore, crossed the boundaries between social, religious and medical concerns.

Public health addressed both epidemic and endemic diseases. The distinction between these two categories of disease has been overstated within the historiography and has particularly affected interpretations of the former. Epidemics are defined as diseases produced by causes not generally present in a locality and only prevalent at particular times. Endemic diseases are those regularly or constantly found in a particular place, prevalent due to permanent local causes.[18] Laura McGough, in a recent volume on the French disease in early modern Venice, described the pox as 'the disease that came to stay'.[19] The 'temporary' nature of epidemics can be overstated, however, and the plague in early modern Europe met many of the criteria listed by McGough for an endemic disease: its relatively common and widely distributed nature, its place in cultural myths and in a city's network of charitable and health care institutions.[20] Even if

---

[16]   Since the 1980s, this body has preserved and researched the use of the island as a medical site and carries out archaeological research on an ongoing basis. The findings of this body have been published in Gerolamo Fazzini (ed.), *Venezia: isola del lazzaretto nuovo*.

[17]   This contextualisation has been a key shift in the history of medicine over the past thirty years. Recent historians whose works have highlighted the importance of studying early modern history of medicine in context in Italy include William Eamon, John Henderson, David Gentilcore and Sandra Cavallo.

[18]   Oxford English Dictionary online (http://www.oed.com/) accessed 15/03/11.

[19]   Laura J. McGough, *Gender, sexuality and syphilis in early modern Venice: the disease that came to stay* (London, 2011).

[20]   Ibid., pp. 2–3.

a disease was not permanent within cities, public health responses and protection against the disease could be. As McGough writes, with reference to modern public health measures and the need for sustained attention to be directed towards endemics in the contemporary world, 'the commonness and seriousness of a disease is no guarantee that public attention and resources will be devoted to it'.[21] Across Europe, cities' responses to epidemic diseases varied enormously and were not dependent on levels of infection or the frequency of outbreaks of disease. Instead, the shape and form and timing of these responses were affected by a much broader context of concerns.

Responses to the plague did not simply develop in early modern Europe because the problem of epidemics worsened. Centralised government's developing responsibility for public health, social policies and urban space, and available investment, affected the form of the official policies. Although the divide between Christian and Muslim responses to plague may have been overstated (and the responses of the latter societies warrant further attention), there were some distinctive features of the European response to the disease – in particular the early introduction of institutions for quarantine on the boundary of towns and cities. In Europe, well-ordered cityscapes were thought to encourage well-ordered societies; the relationship between people and place was significant and intricate which led to a deep-rooted belief in the notion of 'safe space'. In Venice, this encouraged the 'isolation' of a number of groups on island-sites within the city and its unique lagoon environment. Although isolation is a familiar concept to the modern reader, the meaning of this idea was markedly different in the past. Venice provides an ideal location for illustrating that the use of islands did not always signify absolute division, nor were channels of water seen as impenetrable barriers. Contact between islands and the city endured and was considered essential in order to ensure good governance of groups resident on the sites, even when a degree of separation was thought to be necessary.

Like isolation, quarantine – the policy at the heart of public health for the plague – was a term which resonated differently in the past than in the present. The term developed from the Italian word for forty (*quaranta*) and was a symbolic and significant period for purification. The forty-day period regularly features in the Bible: it was the period of the flood in the Old Testament; Moses went to Mount Sinai for forty days before receiving the Ten Commandments; Jesus was tempted in the wilderness for a period of forty days; he appeared to the disciples forty days after the Crucifixion.[22] It was also the period set out for embalming in Genesis and was often the period for mourning or repentance as well as being the liturgically-sanctioned period for Lent and for purification through lying-in after childbirth.[23] Children were thought to be particularly vulnerable during their first forty days

---

[21]   Ibid., p. 149.

[22]   OT Genesis 7; Exodus 24 and 34; NT Luke 4 v.1–13 and Acts 1 v.3.

[23]   OT Genesis 50 v.2–4; Deuteronomy 9 v.25. For the forty-day period in relation to criminal cases see ASV, Senato Terra reg. 29 123r (26 May 1537).

of life.[24] Forty hours of devotion formed part of the Eucharist, whereby the host was displayed on the altar to commemorate the number of hours that Christ spent in the sepulchre.[25] The Jesuits reinvigorated this devotion during the Catholic Reformation and 'staged' dramatic forty-hours devotions during Carnival, which were designed to engage the whole of the community in a religious ritual in place of the 'unChristian' celebrations of Carnival.[26]

The resonance of the forty-day period of quarantine illustrates the way in which early modern responses to disease combined medical ideas with symbolic and religious ones. Charitable and pious acts during quarantine were encouraged in different ways by individuals or on behalf of society. In the case of the latter, in Venice, for example, monks and nuns were instructed to pray for the health of the city for eight days continuously whilst the city was under a general quarantine.[27] The religious significance of the period for quarantine was not simply coincidental – it was chosen in order to bring comfort to those in need and to encourage those undergoing quarantine to look on it as a period of purification to be spent in devotion.[28] As we will see in Chapter 2, these symbolic ideas combined with practical considerations to shape periods of quarantine that could last from eight to fifty days.

A combination of symbolic and practical ideas underpinned the introduction and development of the Venetian *lazaretti*. Initially conceived of as support structures for the Venetian trade economy, these hospitals developed a broader civic purpose and charitable function in the context of sixteenth- and seventeenth-century Venice, as the *lazaretti* came to be affected by the perceived responsibilities of the state to prevent and treat epidemics and developing attitudes to space and the environment.

The *Lazaretti* in Venice

Dealing with a disease which could kill up to a third of a city's population within a year was a challenge faced by most early modern European governments but their responses differed, and did not always include the introduction of a plague hospital. It may be useful to think of structures to protect against the plague as

---

[24]   Lyndal Roper, *Witch craze: terror and fantasy in Baroque Germany* (London, 2004) p. 150.

[25]   See Gaetano Moroni, 'Quarant'ore' in *Dizionario di erudizione storico-ecclesiastico* vol. LVI (Venice, 1852), pp. 113–21.

[26]   For the reinvigoration of this devotion during the Catholic Reformation see David Gentilcore, *From Bishop to Witch: the system of the sacred in early modern Terra d'Otranto* (Manchester, 1992), pp. 70–71 and 261. I am very grateful to Mary Laven for drawing this to my attention.

[27]   ASV, Senato Terra reg. 51 116v–119r (20 September 1576).

[28]   This idea is developed in more detail in Chapter 1, pp. 45–8.

falling into one of three classes: the third-class response involved temporarily requisitioning buildings or constructing wooden structures which would be burned after an outbreak; cities using second-class responses constructed permanent buildings which were used only during epidemics within cities; first-class measures consisted of permanent buildings in permanent use. The first-class responses were the most expensive but were also the easiest to administer during epidemics and guaranteed hospital space for those infected with the plague, since they had a permanent staff and permanent facilities.[29] Cities could also combine these approaches in their public health systems.

The reasons for the initial foundation of permanent *lazaretti* in Venice included the changing nature of early modern plague epidemics as well as developing ideas about the purpose of hospitals. After the large-scale episodes of the fourteenth century, epidemics during the fifteenth century hit, on average, once every decade.[30] Plague continued to change in its nature during the sixteenth and seventeenth centuries when epidemics hit cities less frequently but developed on a much larger scale.[31] During the eighteenth century, the threat of plague endured and outbreaks did occur in Europe (for example in Marseilles in 1721 and Moscow in 1771). Thereafter, protection against epidemic disease remained important and was used in response to diseases beyond plague.

Contemporaries believed that public health responses, effectively administered, could be beneficial in reducing the number of cases of plague as well as the number of deaths.[32] It is important to note, however, that Venice was badly affected by the outbreak of 1575–77 in comparison with Italian cities elsewhere on the peninsula despite its early introduction of mechanisms of disease prevention.[33] The city was

---

[29]   For an indication of the high costs of administering the Venetian *lazaretti* during an epidemic see ASV, Sal b. 10 reg. 13.

[30]   The plague is said to have affected Venice every seven or eight years until 1528 according to ASV, Sanità b. 2 5v (9 October 1528). A very useful annotated list of plague outbreaks between 1348 and 1631 in Venice is given in Richard J. Palmer, 'The control of plague', appendix 4, pp. 328–38. During the fourteenth and fifteenth centuries, Brian Pullan has recorded outbreaks in Venice in 1361, 1381–82, 1391, 1397, 1403, 1411, 1438, 1447, 1456, 1464, 1468, 1485, 1490 and 1498 in *Rich and poor in Renaissance Venice*, p. 219. Reinhold C. Mueller, 'Aspetti sociali ed economici della peste a Venezia nel Medioevo' in *Venezia e la peste*, pp. 71–92 considers these early outbreaks.

[31]   Information on the mortality rates of the largest outbreaks can be found in the works cited in note 30 as well as in Giulio Beloch, 'La popolazione di Venezia nei secoli 16 e 17', *Nuovo Archivio Veneto*, n.s.3 (1902), pp. 5–49 and Daniele Beltrami, *Storia della popolazione di Venezia dalla fine XVI alla caduta della Repubblica* (Padua, 1954).

[32]   See the comments by Giovan Filippo Ingrassia cited in Samuel K. Cohn Jr, *Cultures of plague: medical thought at the end of the Renaissance* (Oxford, 2010), p. 22.

[33]   Venice lost an estimated 50,721 people out of a total population of 170,000. ASV, Secreta, MMN 95 164r. For comparisons with elsewhere see ibid., pp. 20–21.

also badly affected by the plague outbreak of 1630–31.[34] It was only during the second half of the seventeenth century that Venice, along with a number of other cities in the north of the Italian peninsula, remained free from plague epidemics.[35] There is no sign that the *lazaretti* were effective at reducing the impact of plague over the first two centuries of their history, although that was certainly the intention which underpinned the development of the structures. In spite of this, the impact of the *lazaretti* on Venice's reputation in the sphere of public health was considerable within the city and beyond.

The early introductions made in Venice in the sphere of public health had ramifications beyond the city. Many of the cities on the Italian peninsula, which were at the forefront of developing systems of public health, were not only individual cities but also capitals of states.[36] Venice is no exception [see Map] and so, although an island, had important physical, economic and political associations with areas elsewhere. Venice controlled territories on the mainland (known as the *terraferma*), which stretched almost to Milan.[37] The Venetian maritime

---

[34]   46,490 people in Venice were said to have died during the outbreak of 1630–31 out of a population of *c.*141,625 (the statistic is that of the population size in 1624).

[35]   After 1631, Palermo and Florence were affected lightly by plague, Rome was affected moderately and Naples and Genoa suffered heavy losses during the outbreak of 1656.

[36]   For introductions see the volume by S. Bertelli, N. Rubinstein and C. Hugh Smyth (eds), *Florence and Venice: comparisons and relations vol. 2: Cinquecento* (Florence, 1980). Important work on Milan by Chittolini has considered Lombard territories. See his *Città, comunità e feudi negli stati dell'Italia centro-settentrionale (XIV–XVI sec.)* (Milan, 1996) and 'Cities, "City states" and regional states in North-central Italy' in Charles Tilly and Wim P. Blockmans, *Cities and the rise of states in Europe AD 1000-1800* (Oxford, 1994) pp. 28–43.

[37]   Classic studies of the *terraferma* are Marino Berengo, *La società veneta alla fine del Settecento: ricerche storiche* (Florence, 1956), Daniele Beltrami, *Forze di lavoro e proprietà fondiaria nella campagne venete dei sec XVII e XVIII: la penetrazione economica dei Veneziani in Terraferma* (Venice, 1961), Angelo Ventura, *Nobiltà e popolo nella società veneta del '400 e '500* (Bari, 1964), Amelio Tagliaferri (ed.), *Atti del convegno: 'Venezia e la Terraferma attraverso le relazioni dei rettori'* (Milan, 1981), Giorgio Borelli (ed.), *Mercanti e vita economica nella Repubblica Veneta sec XIII–XVIII* (2 vols, Verona, 1985), Gaetano Cozzi and Michael Knapton, *La Repubblica di Venezia nell'età moderna: dalla guerra di Chioggia al 1517* (Turin, 1986), Giuseppe del Torre, *Venezia e la terraferma dopo la guerra di Cambrai. Fiscalità e amministrazione 1515–1530* (Milan, 1986), Luciano Pezzolo, *L'oro dello stato: società, finanza e fisco nella Repubblica veneta del secondo '500* (Venice, 1990), Gaetano Cozzi, Michael Knapton and Giovanni Scarabello, *La Repubblica di Venezia nell'età moderna: dal 1517 alla fine della Repubblica* (Turin, 1992). See also the work of Claudio Povolo including 'Centro e perifera nella Repubblica di Venezia: un profilo' in Giorgio Chittolini, Anthony Molho and Pierangelo Shiera (eds), *Origini dello stato processi di formazione statale Italia fra medioevo ed età moderna* (Bologna, 1994), pp. 207–25. Useful studies on other cities of the Venetian *terraferma* include James S. Grubb, *Firstborn of Venice: Vicenza in the early Renaissance state* (London, 1988); Joanne Ferraro, *Family and public life in Brescia, 1580–1650* (Cambridge, 1992); Edward Muir, *'Mad blood stirring': Vendetta and factions in Friuli during the Renaissance* (London,

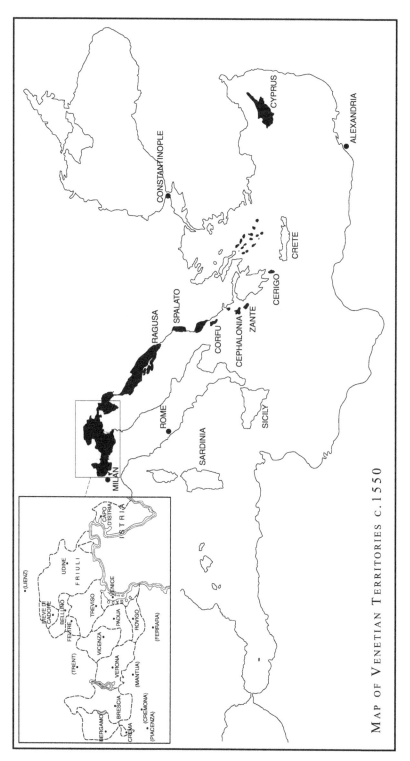

MAP OF VENETIAN TERRITORIES c.1550

Map of Venetian territories

territories (or *stato da mar*) occupied areas along the Adriatic Coast and into the Mediterranean.[38] The nature of the Venetian state was not defined precisely by contemporaries. Studies of the language used in interactions tend to reveal little other than the fluidity of usage of terms such as 'dominion' and 'imperium'.[39] The Venetians were careful not to push notions of empire too far, not least because part of the rhetoric of Venetian presence relied upon distinguishing Venetian rule from the 'tyrannical power' of other empires, such as that of Milan, on the *terraferma*. The two metaphors most commonly invoked to describe the relationships within the Venetian state were that of paternity and of the body and the Venetian political family was both sizeable and fragmented. In the governance of its political state, as in so many other matters, the Venetian authorities were forced to look both east and west.

As an economic fulcrum, Venice was one of the most important *entrepôts* of early modern Europe. Although overseas expansion by other European powers affected the trade economy of sixteenth-century Venice, the city experienced a relative rather than absolute decline through the century.[40] Trade and, therefore, protection against disease remained of paramount importance. Tommaso Porcacchi wrote that Venice was full of goods and commodities from all over the world. Large markets were held in many squares within the city; Porcacchi noted that the one at St Mark's Square, held every Saturday, resembled a trade fair.[41] The city was also a centre for the exchange of goods and for the transmission of ideas. It saw industrial success through shipbuilding in the Arsenal, glass production on Murano and the printing, wool and silk industries.[42] Its population throughout the sixteenth century was among the top ten in Europe, reaching the heights of 170,000 in the middle of the century and was international in character; Rocco Benedetti described Venice as a 'beautiful city, which was a gracious and constant

---

1993); John E. Law, *Venice and the Veneto in the early Renaissance* and Benjamin J. Kohl, *Culture and politics in early Renaissance Padua* (Aldershot, 2001).

[38]   On the *stato da mar* see Benjamin Arbel, 'Colonie d'oltremare' in Alberto Tenenti and Ugo Tucci (eds), *Storia di Venezia: dalle origini alla caduta della Serenissima* (12 vols, Rome, 1991) vol 5: Il Rinascimento: società ed economia, pp. 947–85.

[39]   James S. Grubb, *Firstborn of Venice,* pp. 15–23.

[40]   For particularly good overviews see Frederic C. Lane, *Venice and History* and Brian Pullan (ed.), *Crisis and change in the Venetian economy in the sixteenth and seventeenth centuries* (London, 1968). Richard Rapp, *Industry and economic decline in seventeenth-century Venice* (Cambridge MA, 1976) makes a useful assessment using the concepts of absolute and relative decline in Venice.

[41]   Tommaso Porcacchi, *L'isole piu famose del mondo* (Venice, 1572), pp. 2–3.

[42]   On the Arsenal see Robert C. Davis, *Shipbuilders of the Venetian Arsenal: workers and workplace in the pre-industrial city* (Baltimore MD, 1991). For the silk industry see Luca Molà, *The silk industry of Renaissance Venice* (London, 2000).

host to people from across the world'.[43] Porcacchi agreed with this complexion for the city: Venice, he said, was full of foreigners and many different languages were spoken in the streets.

In Venice, the city was less divided residentially along economic or social lines than others on the Italian peninsula: a cross section of individuals lived within most districts. There were occupational clusters: glass blowers on Murano, tanners on Giudecca, shipbuilders around the Arsenal and the deep sea fishermen of San Nicolò dei Mendicoli.[44] In general though, Venice was a city of residential mobility and architectural openness. It was against this backdrop that elements of society whose movements could pose a risk – Jews, Protestant or Turkish merchants, beggars or the sick – were, to a greater or lesser extent, enclosed during the early modern period. Venice's urban environment, naturally fragmented, offered unique opportunities to isolate groups. As part of these social and spatial policies, for example, the city can lay claim to the unfortunate accolade of being the site of the first Ghetto, established on an island within the city, to accommodate the city's Jews.[45]

The early modern period was an age of institution building, as centralised sites for charity and care were introduced to complement the structures already in place in the locality. These policies need to be considered beyond the shadow of Foucaultian interpretations. The closed institutions of the early modern city could have a variety of purposes. Architecture was used for protection as well as control, as can be seen when institutions for 'dangerous' groups are viewed alongside those for 'vulnerable' ones. All of these developments had a religious as well as a social impetus. For Italy, the establishment of institutions for a number of groups has been associated with Catholic-Reformation piety.[46] Institutions which were founded in Venice included the *Convertite* for reformed and aging prostitutes (1530–34), the *Catecumeni* for Jews, Turks and Moors who converted

---

[43]   'Dico adunque che questa gran bella Città, la quale fu sempre cortese e fedel albergo alle genti del Mondo' Rocco Benedetti, *Relatione d'alcuni casi occorsi in Venetia al tempo della peste l'anno 1576 et 1577 con le provisioni, rimedii et orationi fatte à Dio Benedetti per la sua liberatione* (Bologna, 1630), p. 17. For population statistics see Daniele Beltrami, *Storia della popolazione*, p. 57.

[44]   See Edward Muir and Ronald F.E. Weissman, 'Social and symbolic places in Renaissance Venice and Florence' in John A. Agnew and James S. Duncan (eds), *The power of place: bringing together geographical and social imaginations* (London, 1989), pp. 81–103. See Robert C. Davis, *The war of the fists: popular culture and public violence in late Renaissance Venice* (Oxford, 1994), pp. 19–28 for a discussion of the 'factional landscape' of the city. The deep sea fishermen of San Nicolò were distinguished from the lagoon fishermen who lived in Sant'Agnese and San Trovaso.

[45]   For works on the Venetian Ghetto see G. Cozzi (ed.), *Gli ebrei a Venezia secoli XIV–XVIII* (Milan, 1987); Ennio Concina, Ugo Camerino and Donatella Calabi, *La città degli Ebrei* and Robert C. Davis and Benjamin Ravid (eds), *The Jews of early modern Venice* (London, 2001).

[46]   A good overview is provided in Andrew Cunningham, Ole P. Grell and Jon Arrizabalaga, *Health care and poor relief in Counter-Reformation Europe* (London, 1999).

to Catholicism (1557), the *Zitelle* for young unmarried women (1559) and the *Soccorso* for adulterous women and prostitutes (1577).[47] Some confined sites were designed to protect the wider city, some to protect the elements or individuals they contained. Some institutions, like the *lazaretti*, combined these two functions. The use of confinement for the sick and those suspected of plague was used to deal with a social group which could be perceived as both dangerous and vulnerable, requiring control and worthy of charity. Considering the *lazaretti* in this context allows us to consider the influence that the plague hospitals had as early initiatives in shaping urban space in order to cleanse a city morally, physically and spiritually.

Idealised Renaissance attempts to order a cityscape so as to shape a society were disrupted by plague and the public health policies introduced to combat the disease. During epidemics, it was said that those who could fled the disease, abandoning cities for the fresh air of the countryside. In his account of Venice during 1576 and 1577, Rocco Benedetti described how the ambassadors, nobles, and citizens returned to villas in the *terraferma*. Merchants left, artisans shut up shop, lawyers, scribes and judges abandoned their work. The streets of the city, normally bustling and crowded, became deserted.[48] The option of flight from a city was not open to everyone during periods of crisis and, as a result, it is likely that the relative number of the poor within the city rose. For those who remained, many people were forced from their homes and sent to the plague hospitals. Familiar locations were transformed: who your neighbour was, where you could shop, who was making laws, who could pray for you were all altered by an epidemic. In his account of the plague outbreak in Venice of 1630–31, the Protomedico Cecilio Fuoli described some of these effects of the disease. Invoking the metaphor of a fire that ripped through the community, Fuoli observed that

> in a short time the city was left almost completely derelict, those who could escaped the blaze [of the disease] and the afflicted city remained diminished of inhabitants, emptied of courage and filled instead with unhappiness and misfortunes.[49]

Quarantine was an attempt to reintroduce order in times of plague, to shape urban space so as to deal with the difficult and disruptive context of epidemic disease. In Venice, at times, entire districts within cities were quarantined. Women and children were confined to their homes and a curfew was placed on everyone from

---

[47]   The seminal text is Brian Pullan, *Rich and poor in Renaissance Venice*. For information on the architecture see Bernard Aikema and Dulcia Meijers (eds), *Nel regno dei poveri: arte e storia dei grandi ospedali veneziani in età moderna 1474–1797* (Venice, 1989).

[48]   Rocco Benedetti, *Relatione d'alcuni casi*, p. 19.

[49]   'rimase in breve tempo la citta quasi del tutto derelitta, scappando chi potava l'incendio e restando l'aflitta citta scema d'habitanti vuota di coraggio e colma d'infelicita e miserie', BMC, Codice Cicogna 1509 17v.

two o'clock in the morning.[50] Women and children up to the age of eighteen were forbidden from leaving their parish.[51] Where possible, the sick were sent to the *lazaretti* in order to limit the number of people undergoing quarantine or treatment within the city and to avoid the issue expressed by a later Florentine health official when he said 'If I have to let the sick people here die in their own homes the whole of [the town] will be but a pesthouse..[52] The advantage of a plague hospital, as acknowledged by the Venetian Health Office, was that the sick could be separated: from one another, from their goods and from the city itself. Although many contemporary accounts emphasise abandonment in times of plague, early modern quarantine was, for the most part, a collective experience.[53] Ties with the locality were maintained. Patients received visitors, were often sent in groups and, indeed, carried out quarantine in groups or in wards – with separation being made between the sexes and sometimes between adults and children but not between all individuals. The hospitals continued to be tied to the city, like many early modern institutions, through networks of charity and developed alongside traditional forms of relief.[54]

This blend of civic purpose and piety can also be seen in the administration of the Venetian *lazaretti*. The responsibility for the day-to-day administration of the *lazaretti* was in the hands of a Prior and a Prioress. Despite the religious names given to these posts, they were staffed by citizens of the Republic – often a married couple.[55] Other members of staff in Venice were also Health Office employees, rather than members of the religious orders as they tended to be elsewhere in Europe. Religion played an important role in the Venetian plague hospitals: the hospitals were partly modelled on religious institutions and used the sites of religious buildings; the chaplain and his assistant carried out important work, which illustrated the emphasis placed on religious care alongside medical treatment. In Venice, however, attempts were made to develop a civic structure

---

[50] ASV, Secreta MMN 95 36r (3 July 1576). For restrictions on women and children in Palermo see Ingrassia, pp. 363–9.

[51] Ibid. 38r (7 July 1576).

[52] Father Dragoni cited in Carlo Cipolla, *Faith, reason and the plague: a Tuscan story of the seventeenth century* (London, 1979), p. 38.

[53] For a useful study which emphasises the endurance of the family unit in times of plague, taking issue with interpretations of societal breakdown, see Shona K. Wray, *Communities and crisis: Bologna during the Black Death* (Leiden, 2009). Giulia Calvi's *Histories of a plague year: the social and the imaginary in Baroque Florence* (Oxford, 1984) is an important work, which posits that plague time can be used as a filter through which society, social behaviour and ideas can be viewed.

[54] An overview of these institutions, their foundations and their architecture within a Venetian context can be found in Bernard Aikema and Dulcia Meijers (eds), *Nel regno dei poveri.*

[55] A detailed discussion of the roles of the Prior and Prioress is provided in Chapter 3 pp. 115–27.

which was influenced but not dominated by the religious ideas, which were essential in the sphere of early modern medicine. The effect of this was a plague hospital which was distinct from those of much of the rest of Europe.

During the sixteenth century, the development of systems of poor relief, founded on principles which cut across devotional lines, has been well-established.[56] The period saw a 'quest for civil harmony, civic decency and the triumph of Christian charity' in the commitment to social relief.[57] Sixteenth-century Christians were instructed to model themselves on Christ, who deliberately sought out the sick, the immoral, the lame and the blind and responded to them with love rather than revulsion. Brian Pullan's seminal work *Rich and Poor in Renaissance Venice* considered charity and social policy and what he termed 'the new philanthropy' between 1520–60, which led to a more rational and systematic form of charity on behalf of individuals and governments.[58] At the same time, population increase within cities during the sixteenth century had led to a concern with the increasingly visible and often demonised poor.[59] Unlike the early modern nobility or citizenry, the poor were not legally defined: membership was not restricted. Instead, poverty was a state which a number of individuals could pass through, hence the useful distinction made by economic historians between the structural and cyclical poor.[60] The structural poor were categorised by contemporaries into deserving and undeserving but the cyclical poor were less easily defined. Sandra Cavallo has described illness, along with 'status, gender and age, [as being] one of the components of contemporary definitions of poverty'.[61] During the sixteenth century, poverty was not assessed according to an overarching standard of subsistence. Instead, the term 'poor' could mean miserable and could be used to refer to anyone who could not afford the standard of living to which they had become accustomed. The *poveri vergognosi* (shamefaced poor), for example, were those who would not beg for alms because of their high social status.[62] The use of

---

[56]   See Brian Pullan, 'Catholics, Protestants and the poor in early modern Europe', *Journal of interdisciplinary history*, 35:3 (2005), 441–56; Ole P. Grell, 'Review: The religious duty of care and the social need for control in early modern Europe', *The Historical Journal*, 39 (1996), 257–63, for a discussion of the historiography.

[57]   Paul Slack, 'Social policy and the constraints of Government 1547–48' in Jennifer Loach and Robert Tittler (eds), *The mid-Tudor polity c. 1540–60* (London, 1980), p. 114.

[58]   Brian Pullan, *Rich and poor in Renaissance Venice.*

[59]   See the chapters in Thomas Riis (ed.), *Aspects of poverty in early modern Europe* (Alphen aan den Rijn, 1981) and Robert Jütte, *Poverty and deviance in early modern Europe* (Cambridge, 1994).

[60]   For an overview and recommendations of further reading see Robert Jütte, *Poverty and deviance*, chapter three, 'The causes of poverty', pp. 21–44.

[61]   Sandra Cavallo, *Charity and power in early modern Italy: benefactors and their motives in Turin 1541–1789* (Cambridge, 1995), p. 10.

[62]   See Richard Trexler, 'Charity and the defence of urban elites in Italian communes' in Frederic C. Janer (ed.), *The rich, the wellborn and the powerful: elites and upper classes*

the term 'sick poor' could simply refer to the economic hardships of periods of illness and the contemporary recognition of the plague sick as worthy recipients of charity.[63] Periods of disease, therefore, could transform the fortunes of people from across the social spectrum and charitable initiatives responded to the dual meaning of the term *povero* in Italian, caring for both the poor and miserable.

Early modern hospital structures ranged in their nature and could offer short-term hospitality for pilgrims or provide long-term care for the sick, often until death.[64] Unlike today, hospital treatment was not always intended to offer a cure for disease. In the past, historians highlighted this idea and the lack of medical structures of some sites in order to characterise early modern hospitals as charitable institutions to which individuals were sent, at best, to reside rather than to recover. This idea, however, reflects a misunderstanding of the different types of hospitals that existed and oversimplifies the care provided. Even in those hospitals which did not employ medical personnel, such as those of early Tudor England, medical care was provided through the regulation of diet and the environment.[65] John Henderson's monograph, *The Renaissance Hospital*, has illustrated the dual aims of care and cure, of religious and medical healing, for patients within these

---

in history (Urbana IL, 1975), pp. 64–110 and Amleto Spicciani, 'The "poveri vergognosi" in fifteenth-century Florence' in Thomas Riis (ed.), *Aspects of poverty*, pp. 119–82.

[63] For similar difficulties in translating the term 'poor' in the context of the early modern Ottoman empire see Miri Shefer-Mossensohn, *Ottoman medicine: healing and medical institutions, 1500–1700* (New York, 2009) p. 119.

[64] See Andrew T. Crislip, *From monastery to hospital: Christian monasticism and the transformation of health care in late Antiquity* (Ann Arbor MI, 2005). For a history of hospital development see Lindsay Granshaw and Roy Porter (eds), *The hospital in history* (London, 1989) and Günter B. Risse, *Mending bodies, saving souls: a history of hospitals* (Oxford, 1999). The wider context of the period is addressed in the series of volumes edited by Andrew Cunningham and Ole P. Grell including *Medicine in the Reformation* (London, 1993), *Health care and poor relief in Protestant Europe 1500–1700* (London, 1997), *Health care and poor relief in Counter-Reformation Europe*. For particular case-studies see Anne-Marie Kinzelbach, 'Hospitals, medicine and society: southern German imperial towns in the sixteenth century', *Renaissance studies*, 15:2 (2001), pp. 217–28; Paola Lanaro, 'Carità e assistenza, paure e segregazione: le istituzioni ospedaliere veronesi nel cinque e seicento verso la specializzazione' in Alessandro Pastore, Gian Maria Varanini, Paola Marini and Giorgio Marini (eds), *L'ospedale e la città: cinquecento anni d'arte a Verona* (Verona, 1996), pp. 43–57. See also the article by Colin Jones, 'The construction of the hospital patient in early modern France' in Norbert Finzsch and Robert Jütte (eds), *Institutions of confinement: hospitals, asylums and prisons in Western Europe and North America 1500–1950* (Cambridge, 1996), pp. 55–75.

[65] For an institutional study which illustrates the treatment provided by English hospitals without the service of doctors see Carole Rawcliffe, *Medicine for the soul: the life, death and resurrection of an English Medieval hospital* (Stroud, 1999). For the introduction of doctors into the Savoy hospital in London see John Henderson and Katherine Park, '"The first hospital among Christians": the Ospedale di Santa Maria Nuova in early sixteenth-century Florence', *Medical history*, 35 (1991), pp. 164–88.

early modern institutions.[66] The early modern *lazaretto*, however, has not received detailed, revisionist study and continues to be described as a 'prison-like house of death' to which the sick poor were cruelly abandoned, which, as this book will illustrate, does not reflect the elaborate nature of the care provided.[67]

The city of Venice offered various opportunities for charitable giving, including the *scuole grandi* and *piccole*, the convents and monasteries of the city, parish churches and hospitals.[68] Each of these bodies saw a particular intensity of charitable giving during times of crisis, such as outbreaks of disease, and the *lazaretti* were no exception.[69] Shortly after its foundation, the *lazaretto vecchio* became one of the *loci pii* (or pious institutions) of the city, for which it was compulsory for notaries to ask testators whether they would like to leave money in their wills.[70] The plague hospitals were a focus for pious bequests. An important branch of the Republic, the Procurators of St Mark *de citra*, invested bequests made to the *lazaretti* into government loan funds.[71] Financial administration on the part of the Procurators was just one of the ways in which the Republic assisted charitable institutions. The Arsenal, for example, gave wood from old ships to the building projects of hospitals and religious institutions.[72] Food and drink were given to institutions, particularly flour.[73] The charitable interests of individuals and the state bridged local structures and centralised institutions. In the context of care during times of plague, the parish was as important as the plague hospital and public health systems utilised both local and centralised systems.

---

[66] John Henderson, *The Renaissance hospital*.

[67] For descriptions of Italian *lazaretti* as sites of death see See Günter B. Risse, *Mending bodies, saving souls*, p. 190 and Grazia Benvenuto, *La peste nell'Italia nella prima età moderna: contagio, rimedi, profilassi* (Bologna, 1996) 'Lo spazio rivisitato', pp. 172–84. For an unusually balanced view of the *lazaretto* in Milan see A. Francesco La Cava, *La peste di S Carlo: note storico-mediche sulla peste 1576* (Milan, 1945).

[68] For the *scuole grandi* see Brian Pullan, *Rich and poor in Renaissance Venice*, part one, pp. 33–196; for the *scuole piccole* see Richard Mackenney, *Tradesmen and traders: the world of the guilds in Venice and Europe c.1250–c.1650* (London, 1987); for convents see Mary Laven, *Virgins of Venice: broken vows and cloistered lives in the Renaissance convent* (Harmondsworth, 2003), pp. 69–81.

[69] For charitable donations to the *lazaretti* see Chapter 5, pp. 203–4.

[70] This happened in 1431. See Richard J. Palmer, 'The control of plague', p. 185.

[71] Information on the loan funds can be found in Brian Pullan, *Rich and poor in Renaissance Venice*, particularly p. 138. The Procurators of St Mark had been divided into three sections in 1319: the Procurators *de supra* were responsible for the Basilica of St Mark (the Doge's private chapel until 1807). The Procurators *de citra* and *de ultra* administered estates and private bequests, dividing the task according to the geography of the city.

[72] Various examples can be found in ASV, Arsenal, capitolare 9 (1537–47) and 10 (1547–61).

[73] For example, the entry in the statutes in ASV, Provveditori alle Biave, b. 1 18v (1414).

The foundation of *lazaretti* to fight the plague is in keeping with a number of aspects of early modern Venetian history: the priority of protecting trade, the use of space for social and medical control and the development of charitable initiatives as a tie between the city's government and its people. Innovations in response to epidemic disease were made in Venice as a result of both the political will and available wealth. The institutions were deliberately discussed in ways which made links with the nature of the city explicit. It is important to recognise, however, that despite the Venetian claim of invention and associations with Venetian values, an earlier, temporary *lazaretto* had been established in fourteenth-century Ragusa. In Ragusa, quarantine was established for those arriving in the Republic from plague-infected areas and was carried out on the islet of Mrkan or in the monastery on the island of Mljet.[74] The legislation that founded the *lazaretto vecchio* in Venice in 1423 was a direct reaction to the early health policies of Milan and Ragusa and concurrently introduced a trade ban on infected states. Plague hospitals were developed across Europe, although a comprehensive study of the nature of quarantine structures remains lacking. In what follows, existing information on the widespread nature of these institutions both on the mainland and in port towns and cities will be provided.

The Development of Plague Hospitals

> LAZARETO, s.m. *Lazzaretto* A hospital for the plague-sick; also a site for the observation of people and goods suspected of infection with the plague.[75]

---

[74] Although Venice is often credited with the invention of the *lazaretti*, it is likely that the first *lazaretto* was established in Ragusa, on a temporary basis, at the end of the fourteenth century. This was done in 1377 and quarantine regulations were extended in 1397. I am grateful to Zlata Blažina Tomić for sharing her work on public health in Dubrovnik with me – particularly the text of the 1397 regulation. She is currently preparing an English version of her book *Kacamorti i kuga: utemeljenje i razvoj zdravstvene službe u Dubrovniku* (Dubrovnik, 2007). Currently, the most useful study of early Ragusan introductions in English is Bariša Krekić, *Dubrovnik in the fourteenth and fifteenth centuries: a city between East and West* (Norman OK, 1972), pp. 99–101; Krekić maintains that the Venetians invented quarantine in 1374 and that Dubrovnik followed suit in 1377 (p. 99) but the precise chronology has not been determined. See also Francis W. Carter, *Dubrovnik (Ragusa), A classic city-state* (London, 1972), p. 17 and Susan M. Stuard, 'A communal program of medical care: medieval Ragusa/Dubrovnik', *Journal of the history of medicine and allied sciences*, 28:2 (1973), 126–42.

[75] Giuseppe Boerio, *Dizionario del dialetto veneziano* (Venice, 1867), p. 504. Although the term used in the other early modern Italian states and in modern Italian for the institution is *lazzaretto*, the early modern Venetian term was *lazaretto;* it is the latter term which is adopted here. *Lazaretto* is also a noun which has been adopted in modern English.

The term *lazaretto* is a corruption of the name given to Venice's first plague hospital on the island of Santa Maria di Nazareth.[76] The etymology of the term *lazaretto* has led to some confusion in the historiography, with claims being made that the same word was used for leper hospitals and hospitals for the plague.[77] More common is the assertion that the later *lazaretti* grew out of the earlier leper hospitals.[78] In many cities, the same buildings were used for the two institutions.[79] In Venice, the island of San Lazaro was one of the islands to which the sick were sent when the *lazaretto vecchio* was full. The use of old leper hospitals, however, is likely to have been one of practical convenience rather than drawing on a conceptual link between the two diseases since there were important differences in understanding.[80]

The island of Santa Maria di Nazareth had previously been a monastic site.[81] In 1423 the four remaining brothers were moved elsewhere as the Senate, reputedly on the advice of St Bernardino of Siena, converted the island into a plague hospital for the sick. The island of the *lazaretto nuovo* was originally known as the *vigna murata* (or walled vineyard) and had been a possession of the monastery of San Giorgio Maggiore since 1107 and was chosen as the site for the city's second plague hospital in 1468.[82] The *lazaretti* were intended to respond to concerns about the importation of infection through both maritime and land-based trade.[83] Trade fairs

---

[76]   The name of the institution developed from a corruption of 'Nazareth', which can be traced through later documents in which the hospital is referred to as the 'Nazaretho'. The location of the *lazaretto vecchio* in close proximity to the island of San Lazaro, the site of the earlier leper hospital, may have contributed to the corruption of the term. The term 'Nazarīt' continues to be used in Arabic in seventeenth-century travel accounts. I am grateful to John-Paul Ghobrial for drawing this to my attention.

[77]   See A. Breda, 'Contributo alla storia dei lazaretti (leprosari) medioevali in Europa', *Atti del reale Istituto Veneto di scienze, lettere ed arti*, 68 (1908–1909), 133–94.

[78]   See Richard J. Palmer, 'The Church, leprosy and plague in medieval and early modern Europe', *Studies in Church History*, 19 (1982), pp. 79–101 and Günter B. Risse, *Mending bodies, saving souls*, chapter four 'Hospitals as segregation and confinement tools: leprosy and plague', pp. 167–229.

[79]   See Sandra Cavallo, *Charity and power*, p. 50 for the use of the old leper hospital as a *lazaretto* in 1590s Turin.

[80]   See the story of Miriam in OT Numbers 12 and 'The purity of the camp' in OT Numbers 5. It is important to recognise two ways of interpreting leprosy: see Carole Rawcliffe, *Leprosy in Medieval England* (Woodbridge, 2006) for the best study on the subject.

[81]   An account of the early history of the island is given in ASV, Sanità reg. 17 5r (undated).

[82]   For a discussion of the *vigna murata* see Gabriele Mazzucco, 'Una grangia del monastero di San Giorgio Maggiore di Venezia: l'isola della Vigna Murata poi Lazzaretto Nuovo' in Gerolamo Fazzini (ed.), *Venezia: isola del lazzaretto nuovo*, pp. 15–22.

[83]   For the idea of the importation of infection in literature see Jonathan Gil Harris, *Sick economies: drama, mercantilism and disease in Shakespeare's England* (Philadelphia PA, 2004).

were a particular source of concern regarding disease.[84] In Venice, investigations into the origins of outbreaks of plague often determined that infection had been carried into the city from the *terraferma* rather than by sea.[85] *Lazaretti* were established in cities of the Venetian *terraferma*: by 1437 for Padua, in 1438 in Brescia and 1473 for Verona, in Salò in 1484, in fifteenth-century Vicenza and Treviso and in Bergamo in 1503.[86] *Lazaretti* were also established to serve larger islands of the Venetian lagoon, including Chioggia in 1464, and throughout the Venetian *stato da mar*, such as in Corfu in 1517 and Spalato, Trau (Trogir) and Sebenico (Sibenik) by 1527.[87]

Lazaretti subsequently became features of a number of fifteenth- and sixteenth-century Italian states, which are widely recognised as having been proactive in their responses to epidemic disease.[88] Many Italian cities still contain a 'Via del Lazzaretto'.[89] *Lazaretti* were introduced in Milan and Florence (on a temporary basis) in 1448, Naples in 1464 and Genoa in 1467.[90] *Lazaretti* were established in

[84]   See, for example, ASP, Sanità b. 295 (6 August 1575) regarding the fair in Trent and ASVer, Sanità reg. 33 271r (3 November 1592) and the letters in ASV, Sanità b. 3 (various dates) for the fair in Bolzano. This fair is also mentioned by the contemporary chronicler Alessandro Canobbio, *Il successo della peste occorsa in Padova l'anno MDLXXVI* (Padua, 1576) 1v.

[85]   See Paolo Preto, *Peste e società*, 'Geografia del contagio', pp. 13–23.

[86]   See ASP, Sanità, b. 582, 7r (26 May 1438) and ASVer, SILT, 1457 (various dates). The *lazaretti* in Salò and Bergamo still survive. For Vicenza and Treviso see Gian Maria Varanini, 'Per la storia delle istituzioni ospedaliere nelle città della terraferma veneta nel Quattrocento' in Allen J. Grieco and Lucia Sandri (eds), *Ospedali e città: L'Italia del centro-nord XIII-XVI sec* (Florence, 1997), pp. 107–55. For Brescia, the 'first' *lazaretto* of San Bartolomeo was established in *c.*1438 outside the city walls in the area known as the Chiusure. Further temporary *lazaretti* were established in times of need throughout the fifteenth century according to Arnaldo d'Aversa, *Medici, epidemie e ospedali a Brescia* (Brescia, 1990), p. 26.

[87]   For Chioggia see Richard Goy, *Chioggia and the villages of the Venetian lagoon: studies in urban history* (Cambridge, 1985), p. 60 and ASV, Sanità reg. 12 47r (22 April 1527). For Corfu see Carlo Cipolla, 'Corfu: "chiave della cristianità" e la sua difesa contro la peste', in Carlo Cipolla (ed.), *Saggi di storia economica e sociale* (Bologna, 1988), p. 335.

[88]   For a good overview of the secondary literature for Italian responses see Grazia Benvenuto, *La peste nell'Italia.*

[89]   For example, Trieste, Mantua, Parma, Prato and Bologna.

[90]   The table constructed by Ann Carmichael is a useful guideline to the development of these institutions, although it should be handled carefully since it is based upon secondary sources and inaccurate in places. For example, the foundation of the *lazaretto vecchio* is not a reclassification of an old hospital and the decision regarding a permanent *lazaretto* in Florence was taken in 1464 not 1463; it can be found in Ann G. Carmichael, 'Plague legislation in the Italian Renaissance', *Bulletin for the history of medicine*, 57:4 (1983), p. 520. For the Milanese *lazaretto* see Luca Beltrami, 'Il lazzaretto di Milano', *Archivio storico Lombardo*, 9 (1882), pp. 403–41. The structure was completed by 1488. It is also described in A. Francesco La Cava, *La peste di S Carlo* which makes extensive use of the

a number of ports to protect trading centres against the importation of disease.[91] In Sardinia, the concern about the potential importation of infection led to the development of four *lazaretti*.[92] The use of multiple sites can be seen in Florence and Rome as well. In the latter city, the Ghetto was used to quarantine the Jews and the space was referred to as a *lazaretto*.[93] The scale of these structures increased through the sixteenth and seventeenth centuries.

Beyond the Italian peninsula, the institutions spread in France, where a *maison* or *hôpital pour pestiférés* was established in various cities from the mid-fifteenth century, with a particular flurry of foundations during the sixteenth century.[94] Examples were established in fifteenth- and sixteenth-century Spain, for example in Madrid in 1438.[95] *Pestspitale* were established as permanent institutions in the Swiss Confederation during the sixteenth century, in Bern in 1536 and Luzern

---

account by Fra Paolo Bellintano. The Florentine *lazaretto* was permanent from the 1490s. See John Henderson, *The Renaissance hospital*, pp. 91–6. In Naples, the *lazaretto* was founded in 1464 by Archbishop Carafa in an abandoned Benedictine convent with adjacent catacombs which were adopted as a cemetery. See Charlotte Nichols, 'Plague and politics in early modern Naples: the relics of San Gennaro' in Laurinda S. Dixon, *In sickness and in health: disease as metaphor in art and popular wisdom* (Newark NJ, 2004) p. 30.

[91]   For Trieste, Livorno, Ancona and Naples see Daniel Panzac, *Quarantaines et lazarets: l'Europe et la peste d'Oriente (XVIIe–XXe siècles)* (Aix-en-Provence, 1986). Panzac also considers the institution in Malta, which is also covered in Charles Savona-Ventura, *Knight hospitaller medicine in Malta 1530–1798* (Malta, 2004) p. 46. These ideas are also drawn out in Manlio Brusatin, *Il muro della peste: spazio della pietà e governo del lazaretto* (Venice, 1981).

[92]   Francesco Manconi, *Castigo de Dios: la grande peste barocca nella Sardegna di Filippo IV* (Rome, 1994), p. 224.

[93]   Cardinal Geronimo Gastaldi, *Tractatus de avertenda et profliganda peste politico = legalis. Eo lucubratus tempore, quo ipse Leomocomiorum primo, mox Sanitatis Commissarius Generalis fuit, peste urbem invadente Anno MDCLVI et LVII* (Bologna, 1684), p. 435. In Palermo, separate spaces were designated for the quarantine and treatment of criminals from prison. See Ingrassia, pp. 388–9.

[94]   Jean-Noël Biraben, *Les hommes e la peste en France et dans les pays européens et méditerranéens* (2 vols, Paris, 1975–76), volume two, pp. 171–5 describes institutions established in Bour en Bresse in 1472, Lyon in 1474 and Marseilles in 1476. His study makes a distinction between these institutions and the *lazaret* which developed as a quarantine centre in later centuries. The case of Toulouse, where a *lazaretto* was established in 1514, has been given separate attention by Robert A. Schneider, 'Crown and Capitoulat: municipal government in Toulouse 1500–1789' in Philip Benedict (ed.), *Cities and social change in early modern France* (London, 1989), pp. 195–220. See also the survey by Laurence Brockliss and Colin Jones, *The medical world of early modern France* (Oxford, 1997).

[95]   For the Hospital de San Antón founded in 1438 in Madrid see Teresa Huguet-Termes, 'Madrid hospitals and welfare in the context of the Habsburg empire' in Teresa Huguet-Termes, Jon Arrizabalaga and Harold J. Cook (eds), *Health and medicine in Habsburg Spain: agents, practices, representations* (London, 2009), p. 68. For the institutions in Seville see Kirsty Wilson Bowers, 'Balancing Individual and Communal Needs: Plague

in 1596.[96] England has had a reputation for being slow off the mark in terms of responses to the plague but this has been asserted on the basis of the late introduction of national instructions from London.[97] The work of Paul Slack has shown that temporary pesthouses were introduced in Shrewsbury, York, Windsor, Berwick, Durham, Nottingham and Newcastle during the sixteenth century.[98] A *lazaret* was introduced in Nuremberg in 1498 and in sixteenth-century Ulm.[99] Two were developed in Augsburg, in 1521 and during the 1570s but, according to Claudia Stein, these were used for people who could not afford to remain in household quarantine: travellers, soldiers and beggars.[100] As in France, various terms were used to refer to these German institutions including *Brechenhaus*, *Kranckenhaus*, *Lazaret* or simply *das Haus*.[101] In the Low Countries, cities established permanent institutions, such as Gorinchem in 1502 and Amsterdam, or temporary structures, like in Rotterdam and Haarlem.[102] Denmark did not construct a pest-house until 1619 but used policies of household quarantine from the 1580s.[103]

During the seventeenth century, plague hospitals were introduced in Europe which were architecturally distinct from earlier examples. The Low Countries are famous for the *pesthuis* which was built in Leiden in 1670, although the site was never used during an epidemic because the disease did not return to the city after

---

and Public Health in Early Modern Seville', *Bulletin of the History of Medicine* 81 (2007), pp. 335–58 and Linda Martz, *Poverty and welfare in Habsburg Spain* (Cambridge, 1983).

[96]   See Vera Waldis, 'Hospitalisation und Absonderung in Pestzeiten – die Schweiz im Vergleich zu Oberitalien', *Gesnerus*, 39 (1982), pp. 71–8.

[97]   Ole P. Grell has suggested that a small *lazaretto* was established for London in 1594 and that this introduction was preceded by self-imposed household isolation amongst the Dutch community of the city. See Ole P. Grell, 'Plague in Elizabethan and Stuart London: the Dutch response', *Medical history*, 34 (1990), pp. 424–39. Andrew Spicer kindly drew my attention to the fact that the Walloon community at Sandwich built a *lazaretto* in the 1570s. See his forthcoming article '"Pour avoir curez plusieurs de nostre eglise": Medical care and support for the poor in the French-Walloon communities at London and Sandwich, c. 1568–73'.

[98]   For introductions in England see Paul Slack, *The impact of plague in Tudor and Stuart England* (London, 1985), section two 'The social response', pp. 197–326.

[99]   Anne-Marie Kinzelbach, 'Hospitals, medicine and society: southern German imperial towns in the sixteenth century', *Renaissance studies*, 15:2 (2001), pp. 217–28. For Nuremberg see Roy Porter (ed.), *Cambridge illustrated history of medicine* (Cambridge, 1996), p. 210.

[100]   Claudia Stein, *Negotiating the French pox in early modern Germany* (Aldershot, 2008), p. 82.

[101]   Anne-Marie Kinzelbach, 'Hospitals, medicine and society', p. 221.

[102]   See Martinus A. van Andel, 'Plague regulations in the Netherlands', *Janus*, 21 (1916), p. 431.

[103]   Peter Christensen, '"In these perilous times": plague and plague policies in early modern Denmark', *Medical History,* 47:4 (2003), p. 437.

the completion of the building.[104] In earlier centuries, part of the St Caecilia's gasthuis had been used as a plague hospital, just as another part was used as an asylum.[105] The hospital of Leiden is typical of a seventeenth-century introduction: grand, visible and symbolic [Plate 1].[106] Like the *Hôpital St Louis* in Paris, built between 1607 and 1612, which has been described as 'the first monumental hospital in Europe for the exclusive treatment of the plague' and identified as a key part of the urban strategy of Henri IV for the city, these later introductions were impressive and often ceremonial in their design.[107]

Even where earlier institutions had existed, a number of Baroque redevelopments of *lazaretti* took place. On the Italian peninsula, these redevelopments were influenced by the policies of the Catholic Reformation. In Milan, Padua, Verona and Bergamo, for example, the existing large, rectangular structures of the sixteenth century had central, circular chapels added during the seventeenth century.[108] Often these chapels were made up of a number of open archways, so that the central altar (and the ceremony of Mass) would be as visible as possible from the surrounding hospital complex. This architectural addition reflected the intensification of the religious purpose of the *lazaretti* in many Italian cities during the early seventeenth century.[109] The Catholic Reformation redevelopment of the Italian *lazaretti* influenced later, purpose-built sites, such as the eighteenth-century *lazaretto* in Ancona.[110]

It was during the seventeenth century that some smaller localities recognised the need for a plague hospital, centuries after introducing policies of household quarantine. Plague hospitals had been established in some rural areas, such as in the countryside around Verona, in the previous century. In 1577, for example, a letter was sent by the Veronese authorities to Valleggio, a town in their territory, with instructions as to how to respond to the plague; the first of the five points concerned the development of a suitable and separate site on which to locate a *lazaretto* for those afflicted by the illness.[111] In addition to the hospital, the town

---

[104]   I am grateful to Jane Kromm for information on the institutions in the Netherlands.

[105]   See Jane Kromm, 'Domestic spatial economies and Dutch charitable institutions in the late sixteenth and early seventeenth centuries' in Sandra Cavallo and Silvia Evangelisti (eds), *Domestic Institutional Interiors in Early Modern Europe* (Aldershot, 2009), pp. 109–11.

[106]   For a discussion of the architecture of the Leiden plague hospital see Chapter 1, p. 76.

[107]   See Hilary Ballon, *The Paris of Henri IV: architecture and urbanism* (London, 1991), p. 166.

[108]   See ASP, Sanità b. 578 (13 October 1633) which makes reference to the new design.

[109]   See Chapter 1, pp. 40–42 and 73–7.

[110]   See Carlo Mezzetti, Giorgio Bucciarelli and Fausto Pugnaloni, *Il lazzaretto di Ancona: un'opera dimenticata* (Ancona, 1978).

[111]   ASVer Sanità reg. 33 124r (n.d. 1577).

was instructed to make use of *casotti* (huts) within the town to separate the sick from the healthy. References to public health in smaller, rural areas are few and far between and studies of rural responses to plague are lacking. Studies of the plague on the Venetian *terraferma* in 1630–31 have established that in Asiago (north west of Bassano del Grappa), for example, there was more than one *lazaretto*, with others in the surrounding villages of Gallio, Castelletto, Lusiano and Canova.[112] Such references are fleeting, however, and difficult to develop.[113]

Plague hospitals continued to be developed in later centuries, with examples founded in eighteenth-century Russia and nineteenth-century North America.[114] These later examples retained the name *lazaretto* but were sometimes developed in response to other contagious diseases. Many of the *lazaretti* sites were adopted for military purposes or as concentration camps during the twentieth century, leading to considerable structural alteration and damage. In Verona, for example, the *lazaretto* was in use until the eighteenth century and then was utilised as a storehouse for munitions and gunpowder. It was destroyed by two explosions there during the Second World War.[115] Nevertheless, some plague hospitals still survive; fine examples in Europe include those of Bergamo, Mahon and Salò.

Plague hospitals through the centuries varied in their nature and purpose. Many of the early modern examples were intended, as the Venetian versions were, to combine a charitable and medical purpose and are appropriately understood as a specific type of hospital. An important development in the historiography

---

[112] Elisabetta Girardi, 'La peste del 1630–1 nell'altopiano dei Sette Comuni', *Archivio Veneto*, 205 (2008), pp. 59–91.

[113] Paolo Ulvioni, *Il gran castigo di Dio: carestia ed epidemie a Venezia e nelle terraferma 1628-32* (Milan, 1989), for example, makes reference to some smaller *lazaretti* but provides no detail. Fragmentary information about Braunschweig Wolfenbüttel during the seventeenth century illustrates that sites including meeting houses, the poorhouse and the houses of private citizens were all proposed for the plague hospital. See Daniel E. Christensen, 'Politics and the plague: efforts to combat health epidemics in seventeenth-century Braunschweig-Wolfenbüttel, Germany' (unpublished PhD thesis, 2004, University of California Riverside). Rural plague hospitals and those of smaller settlements remain areas for future research.

[114] On later plague hospitals see John T. Alexander, *Bubonic plague in early modern Russia: public health and urban disaster* (London, 1980). This work takes the outbreak of 1770–72 as its focus but charts sixteenth-century outbreaks of the plague in 1506, 1508, 1552–53, 1563, 1566–68, 1570–71 and 1592. The plague hospitals are discussed on page 136 but the date of the original development of these institutions is unclear. For a North American example from Philadelphia, see Edward T. Morman, 'Guarding against alien impurities: the Philadelphia lazaretto, 1854–93', *The Pennsylvania magazine of history and biography*, 108:2 (1984), pp. 131–52.

[115] See Lia Camerlengo, 'Il lazzaretto a San Pancrazio e l'ospedale della Misericordia in Bra: Le forme dell'architettura' in Alessandro Pastore, Gian Maria Varanini, Paola Marini and Giorgio Marini (eds), *L'ospedale e la città: cinquecento anni d'arte a Verona* (Verona, 1996), p. 184.

of the hospital has been to consider the institution as rooted in its immediate environment: physical, social, political and economic. Like a number of other early modern hospitals, the *lazaretti* responded to the plague by combining medical and religious treatments; a genuine intention underpinning the establishment of these structures was the cure of the disease. Although their original purpose had been economic, the *lazaretti* undertook important charitable and social functions during the sixteenth century and should be aligned with these developing ideas about charity, poor relief and healthcare as specific hospitals for the plague-sick.[116] The *lazaretti* were shaped by these ideas as well as perceptions of the disease to which they were designed to respond.

The *Lazaretti* and the Plague

In its consideration of the plague, the path of this book does not lead through that well worn but rocky terrain of retrospective disease diagnosis. Too often, this route has been taken by historical travellers equipped with modern maps and guides, which tell them what to look for on arrival and how to interpret what they see. Such an approach to travel seems to me the most comfortable but least revealing when modern knowledge is used to limit rather than enhance historians' encounters with the past. The enduring questions of what plague was, why it advanced and why it retreated are important and intriguing. Their answers, however, remain, on the basis of our current knowledge and source material, a matter for informed speculation.[117] This work takes a different route. It prioritises what contemporaries thought about the plague and considers the ways in which these ideas shaped early modern responses to the disease.[118] This path does not dodge historical pitfalls. As difficult as it is to assess what the plague was in the past, it is equally troublesome

---

[116]   Giuliana Albini has developed a similar argument for fifteenth-century Milan. She claims that although the original function of the Milanese *lazaretto* was to provide isolation, it developed into a charitable institution providing care, with a decorative and symbolic function for the city in Giuliana Albini, *Città e ospedali*, p. 200.

[117]   Paul Slack drew to my attention two recent studies which have put forward forceful cases for the bacillus *Yersinia pestis* as the cause of early modern plague. As yet, these have not had sufficient response to know whether these will end the long-standing debate about the cause of the disease. Crucially, they do account for variations in the nature of the plague. See G. Morelli, Y. Song and C.J. Mazzoni et al, '*Yersinia pestis* sequencing identifies patterns of global phylogenetic diversity' *Nature Genetics* 42 (2010) 1140–43 and S. Haensch, R. Bianucci, M. Signoli et al, 'Distinct clones of *Yersinia pestis* caused the Black Death', *Public library of science, Pathogens* 7:6 (2010). The case against retrospective diagnosis of the plague was made forcefully in Samuel K. Cohn Jr, *The Black Death transformed: disease and culture in early Renaissance Europe* (London, 2003).

[118]   For the adoption of the approach for the pox see Claudia Stein, *Negotiating the pox* and Jon Arrizabalaga, John Henderson, and Roger French, *The Great Pox: the French disease in Renaissance Europe* (London, 1997).

to pin down its effects and explain contemporary responses. Epidemics have been described as watershed events – in particular, the dramatic episode of the Black Death of 1347–52, which swept through Europe with a mortality level estimated at between 40 and 60 per cent.[119] It is clear that death and devastation of this kind must have had effects: untangling the direct impact of epidemics remains a challenge for historians. This book contends that the episodes of plague during the fourteenth and fifteenth centuries stimulated governments to make institutional responses for public health on a new scale. These introductions were predicated on an idea which would prove to be influential throughout the early modern period and beyond: that the control of space and movement of the few could be enacted by increasingly powerful, centralised authorities and justified in terms of the common good. The reasons for this confinement and control need not be related to notions of individual sin or criminal behaviour. It is only when plague is viewed in context that the influence of early public health policies on later responses to social and religious groups can be seen.

The meaning of plague in context can be approached using the term itself. The language of the disease has entered our own vocabulary as well as that of most other modern European languages. The images and metaphors of disease feature in literary works across the centuries, including those by Shakespeare, Goldoni, Manzoni and Camus.[120] In English, contemporaries used the terms pest, pestilence and plague loosely and often interchangeably. Rather than precise meanings, the three terms could refer to some sort of strike or blow, a wound, a severe affliction brought on by God (akin to the biblical plagues of the Old Testament) or an outbreak of disease – for example the plague of leprosy. That the term was used in this way is an indication of the severity and social significance of outbreaks.

---

[119]   Valuable recent works on the Black Death, which indicate, amongst other things, the variety of source material now being used to say new things about plague include Samuel K. Cohn Jr, *The Black Death transformed*, Vivian Nutton (ed.), *Pestilential complexities: understanding medieval plague* (London, 2008), John Hatcher, *The Black Death: an intimate history* (London, 2008), Lars Bisgaard and Leif Sondergaard (eds), *Living with the Black Death* (Lancaster, 2009); Shona K. Wray, *Communities and crisis*. Rosemary Horrox's collection of primary sources remains valuable: *The Black Death* (Manchester, 1994). Samuel K. Cohn Jr, 'Plague and its consequences' in M. King (ed.), *Oxford Bibliographies Online: Renaissance and Reformation* (Oxford, 2010) provides an overview of the historiography, with particular reference to the Black Death.

[120]   On the language of disease see Margaret Healy, 'Discourses of the plague in early modern London' in Justin A.I. Champion, *Epidemic disease in London* (London, 1993), pp. 19–34 and *Fictions of disease in early modern England: bodies, plagues and politics* (Basingstoke, 2001) and Colin Jones, 'Languages of plague in early modern France' in Sally Sheard and Helen J. Power (eds), *Body and city: histories of urban public health* (Aldershot, 2000), pp. 41–9. Plague was often a metaphor for heresy: see Christine Boeckl, 'Plague imagery as a metaphor for heresy in Rubens's *The miracles of Saint Francis Xavier*', *Sixteenth century journal*, 27:4 (1996), pp. 979–95 and *Images of plague and pestilence: iconography and iconology* (Kirksville MO, 2000).

A similar malleability of meaning is true in other languages – in Italian the terms are *pestilenza* and *peste*.[121] Plague was a metaphor as well as a disease and its relevance was more than medical.

Plague epidemics were considered to be the most extreme form of illness. The plague could be sent by God as a punishment for sin or be a general consequence of the Fall of Man, which introduced corruption into a perfect, created world. In an early modern context, the divine and natural worlds were closely interlinked and the primary cause of disease – sin – was connected with secondary causes of miasmas and contagion in the environment. *Mal aria* (bad air) or miasmas (corrupt air) were sticky, rotten air particles caused by corruption. Once inhaled, this air introduced corruption into the body, causing various resulting symptoms. Conversely, corruption within the body could lead to the exhalation of miasmatic air, meaning that the diseases could be spread from person to person. Girolamo Fracastoro identified three principal forms of contagion in his famous work: direct, *ad fomites* (contaminated goods) and by distance.[122] In the second mode of transmission, adopting the contemporary metaphor put forward by Fracastoro of the seeds of disease, miasmatic air particles acted like burrs, fixing themselves to clothing and other materials that lacked a smooth surface.[123] It is no surprise, then, that early health legislation was particularly concerned about the importation of bedding, clothing and fabrics.[124] In place of the simplistic, nineteenth-century accounts of early modern medical thinking, historians have increasingly recognised the complexity of contemporary debates.[125] The ideas of miasmas and contagion were complementary rather than competing and both relied upon understandings of medicine and disease which were based on the writings of the Ancients. This framework for understanding disease causation remained fixed during the period of this study, despite innovation in treatment and public health responses.

The corpus of works by Hippocrates [*c*.450–*c*.370BC] and their summations by Galen [*c*.129–200AD] held the humoural theory at their centre, whereby the

---

[121]   Interesting examples are given in Samuel K. Cohn Jr, *Cultures of plague*, p. 24 of the terms being used to refer to heresy and the invasions of the Turks.

[122]   See the discussion in ibid., particularly pp. 9–10.

[123]   On the ideas of Fracastoro see Vivian Nutton, 'The seeds of disease: an explanation of contagion and infection from the Greeks to the Renaissance' in Vivian Nutton (ed.), *From Democedes to Harvey: studies in the history of medicine* (London, 1983), pp. 1–34.

[124]   See Zlata Blažina Tomić, *Kacamorti i kuga: utemeljenje i razvoj zdravstvene službe u Dubrovniku* (Dubrovnik, 2007), p. 89.

[125]   See, for example, Antonio dal Fiume, 'Medici, medicine e peste nel Veneto durante il sec XVI', *Archivio Veneto,* 116 (1981), pp. 33–59. For a reassessment of the distinction see John Henderson, 'Historians and plagues in pre-industrial Italy over the longue durée', *History and philosophy of the life sciences,* 25 (2003), pp. 482–4 and Anne-Marie Kinzelbach, 'Infection, contagion and public health in late medieval and early modern German Imperial towns', *Journal of the history of Medicine and Allied Sciences,* 61 (2006), pp. 369–89.

human body was made up of four humours (blood, phlegm, yellow bile and black bile) just as nature was made up of four elements (fire, water, earth and air).[126] Each individual person and season was characterised by a particular humoural or elemental balance, which determined the balance of the four contraries (hot, cold, wet and dry). There were nine possible mixtures or temperaments: an equal balance of each humour or a predominance of one or two. Sickness was an imbalance within these natural states. Age and sex affected the humoural balance of an individual. The temperament determined an individual's personality as well as their susceptibility to particular diseases. Similarly, the seasonality of diseases was explained with reference to the characteristics of the seasons.

Plague was characterised as hot and humid; those whose bodies were more naturally disposed towards these elements were seen to be most vulnerable.[127] An association with a fever and excess heat was common in descriptions of the sick. Various other symptoms were associated with the plague in medical treatises, including lethargy, weakness of breath, delirium, a lack of appetite, vomiting, a black tongue, a fast pulse, changes to urine or a headache.[128] These symptoms were echoed in accounts of people who served in plague hospitals. Paolo Bellintani, for example, provided his own ten signs for plague, based upon his experiences of serving in the plague hospitals of Brescia, Milan and Marseilles. He included fever, headaches, vomiting and extreme thirst, pain, swellings, nosebleeds, frenzy and a white tongue, although he says you cannot rely on this final sign because

---

[126]   Vivian Nutton, *Ancient Medicine* (New York, 2004) is a useful study of the process by which these ideas developed and were codified. See particularly chapter sixteen 'Galenic medicine', pp. 230–48. A helpful discussion of these ideas can also be found in Richard J. Palmer, 'Health, hygiene and longevity in medieval and Renaissance Europe' in Yosio Kawakita, Shizu Sakai and Yasuo Otsuka (eds), *History of Hygiene* (Toyko, 1987), pp. 75–98. This association was extended to link the humours to four principal organs within the body.

[127]   This axiom did not mean, however, that physicians agreed on which groups were more naturally disposed to these elements. Andrea Gratiolo, for example, lists infants, children, the young, women (most particularly virgins of about twenty years of age) amongst various other categories of those at particular risk, whereas Bernardino Tomitano identified men more than women, infants more than the young and the young more than the old. See Andrea Gratiolo, *Discorso di peste ... nel quale si contengono utilissime speculationi intorno alla natura, cagioni e curatione della peste, con un catalogo di tutte le pesti piu notabili de' tempi passati* (Venice, 1576) and Bernardino Tomitano, *De le cause et origine de la peste vinitiana* (Venice, 1556).

[128]   For descriptions of symptoms see, for example, Prospero Borgarucci, *Dove ciascuno potrà apprendere il vero modo di curar la peste et i carboni et di conservarsi sano in detto tempo* (Venice, 1565) 83r; Bernardino Tomitano, *De le cause et origine*, 14r, Andrea Gratiolo, *Discorso di peste* 32r and Nicolò Massa, *Ragionamento ... sopra le infermita che vengono dall'aere pestilentiale del presente anno MDLV* (Venice, 1556) 5v and 13r.

it can be very misleading.[129] Many of the same symptoms were identified beyond Italy too. Describing plague in England, William Bullein wrote that the sick,

> do swone and vomite yellow holour, swelled in the stomache with muche paine, breaking foorth with stinking sweate; the extreme partes very cold, but the internall partes boiling with heate and burning; no rest; blood distillyng from the nose ... corrupted mouthe, with blacknesse, quick pulse ... loss of memorie, cometyme with ragyng in strong people.[130]

The most noticeable signs (or swellings) included *carboni* (small pustules with black centres), *giandusse* (boils), tumours (red or brown), buboes behind the ear, under the arms and on the thigh and other *apostemi* (abscesses). Samuel Cohn has identified three different sorts of swellings in his work on plague in early modern Milan: buboes (swellings in the glandular areas), *carboni* (swellings elsewhere on the body) and *petecchie* (small, lentil sized spots or bumps which could be coloured).[131] The Paduan physicians who visited Venice in 1576 reported that these black marks on the skin (*petecchie*) were not only a symptom of the plague but also a sign of impending death from the disease.[132]

Despite these noticeable and nauseating symptoms, there was a notorious lack of consensus about diagnosis during plague outbreaks. The report presented to Venice by the Paduan physicians Hieronimo Capo di Vacca [d. 1589] and Gerolamo Mercuriale [1530–1606] in July 1575 is a well-known example of this. A Venetian notary wrote, in his account of the plague epidemic, that the two men were received like 'two Gods of medicine on earth' and were referred to as Sts Cosmas and Damian, the two patron saints of doctors, on their arrival in Venice.[133] The opening sentence of their report expressed their awareness of the varied and often contradictory advice which the Health Office officials had received and continued to receive regarding the nature of the disease and the best way to treat it. Just a few months earlier, the city's authorities had been given four reports from Venetian physicians, debating whether the disease was plague and whether it was contagious; the doctors were divided on both issues.[134] The variety of diagnoses

---

[129]   Paolo Bellintani, *Dialogo della peste*, Ermanno Paccagnini (ed.) (Milan, 2001), pp. 127–30.

[130]   Cited in Andrew Wear, *Knowledge and practice in English medicine, 1550–1680* (Cambridge, 2000), p. 301.

[131]   For a very useful discussion of swellings see Samuel K. Cohn Jr, *Cultures of plague*, pp. 48–54.

[132]   ASV, Secreta, MMN 55bis 1r (13 July 1576).

[133]   'restò la città tutta consolata, ammirandoli come duoi Dii in Terra della Medicina, e chiamavangli san Cosmo e Damiano, che fossero stati da Dio mandate à liberarla da tanti cruciati' in Rocco Benedetti, *Relatione d'alcuni casi*, p. 19.

[134]   The four doctors' reports are recorded in ASV, Secreta, MMN 95 127r–131v (11 February 1576).

widens further when printed physicians' treatises are added to the mix. The visiting Paduan physicians felt that the disease was not true plague but in fact a contagious, harmful and pestilential sickness.[135] They instructed the Republic to announce that there was no plague in Venice. Benedetti also recorded, however, that soon after their arrival in the city the situation worsened and they lost not only their admiration and fame but were also blamed for the increase in infection because people had been reassured by their assertion that the disease was not plague and had gone freely about the city, with little concern for public health. In 1675 the Venetian Protomedico Cecilio Fuoli reflected on his career of almost fifty years with the Health Office and referred to episodes in the city's history when many people had died because an insufficient number of doctors had diagnosed plague accurately, highlighting the outbreaks of 1575 and 1630 in particular.[136]

The problem of identifying the disease was exacerbated during outbreaks since diagnosis could be carried out by individuals who were not felt to have strong medical credentials, such as the female body searchers in England.[137] In the context of early modern Florence a contemporary wrote 'I have seen people who, having fallen from a horse, were wounded in the head and the arm. They were taken to the lazaret.'[138] Contemporaries were quite right when they observed that not everyone who was sent to the *lazaretti* was sick with the plague. The *lazaretti* were not intended as institutions for the sick alone – although, to be fair, neither were they intended for injured jockeys – since those suspected of the disease were also sent. The structure of two hospitals in Venice was designed to enable care to be given to those infected as well as those vulnerable to infection; nevertheless controversy regarding diagnosis endured.

Diagnoses were not only affected by medical views; they could be manipulated for a variety of reasons, often political or economic. Disease could be subjective. In her analysis of dirt, Mary Douglas wrote that 'there is no such thing as absolute dirt: it exists in the eye of the beholder'.[139] Douglas used dirt as a way of illustrating larger systems of conceptual thinking. The process by which disease was diagnosed and declared can also be used to open up considerations of the wider contexts of

---

[135] 'mali pernitiosi pestilentiali et contagiosi' in ASV, Secreta MMN b. 55 bis ('Scritta de Medici Capo di Vacca e Mercurial'). A pestilential fever was thought to be less virulent, less contagious and less deadly. On the distinction between the two see Vivian Nutton, 'The seeds of disease', p. 27.

[136] ASV, Sanità 743 96v (1676).

[137] See Richelle Munkhoff, 'Searchers of the dead: authority, marginality and the interpretation of plague in England (1574–1665)', *Gender and history*, 11 (1999), pp. 1–29 and Kevin Siena, 'Searchers of the dead in long eighteenth-century London' in Kim Kippen and Lori Woods (eds), *Worth and repute: valuing gender in late medieval and early modern Europe. Essays in honour of Barbara Todd* (Toronto, 2011), pp. 123–52.

[138] Cited in Giulia Calvi, *Histories of a plague year*, p. 180.

[139] Mary Douglas, *Purity and danger: an analysis of concepts of pollution and taboo* (London, 2002), p. 2.

societies, cities and states and the respective 'systems' at work. An epidemic, for example, is an event which is often discussed and accepted uncritically but it was a period which had to be declared at its beginning and end.[140] The level to which mortality had to rise or fall to be considered an outbreak was not quantitative but qualitative. In Turin, for example, this ambiguity was regulated through a policy of *quarantena compita*, a trial period at the end of an outbreak during which time the city was still cut off from the outside world but operated normally within the city.[141] The ideas which influenced decisions regarding public health were wider than simply medical and included political, economic and religious considerations. It was recognised that declaring an epidemic should only be done when absolutely necessary because of the effect on political reputations and economic profit. As a result, there was often more than a degree of reluctance in announcing the presence of the disease in cities.[142]

In place of great men and great discoveries, recent works in the history of medicine have made careful studies of the broad systems of care which were provided within early modern cities. This emphasis on the setting in which medicine was provided led to the development of the medical 'marketplace' idea; this is now, more convincingly, understood as a system of medical pluralism.[143] The variety of spaces within which medicine was provided, ranging from the home to the public *piazza* and the civic hospital, has been described. The key notion in these studies is that contemporaries would have made use of a number of the available treatments concurrently – an approach to health which resonates to the present day. In the face of illness, it appears that the human reaction is to consider any combination of change of diet or environment, the advice of doctors,

---

[140]   For an example of reluctance to declare an epidemic in nineteenth-century Venice, see Thomas Rütten, 'Cholera in Thomas Mann's Death in Venice', *Gesnerus* 66:2 (2009), pp. 256–87.

[141]   See Sandra Cavallo, *Charity and power*, p. 53.

[142]   See, for example, Anne-Marie Kinzelbach, 'Infection, contagion and public health', p. 383 on the fear of becoming 'ill-reputed' because of the plague. In Carlo Cipolla's seminal work, Prato's officials petition the Florentine government for permission to open the plague hospital but are denied for fear of inducing panic, *Cristofano and the plague*, p. 41. For the mention of a doctor imprisoned by the Spanish Viceroy for announcing plague in Naples before the authorities had decided to declare an epidemic see Charlotte Nichols, 'Plague and politics', p. 28.

[143]   The competitive nature of the marketplace has been replaced with a focus on the variety of medical spheres which were available in the early modern city and the ways in which these could coexist. The term 'medical marketplace' was coined by Harold Cook in *The Decline of the Old Medical Regime in Stuart London* (Ithaca NY, 1986). For medical pluralism see David Gentilcore, *Healers and healing in early modern Italy* (Manchester, 1998) and Margaret Pelling, *The common lot: sickness, medical occupations and the urban poor in early modern England* (London, 1998). For a discussion and revision of the concept of the medical marketplace see Mark S.R. Jenner and Patrick Wallis, *Medicine and the market in England and its colonies, c.1450–c.1850* (Basingstoke, 2007) .

the treatments of alternative medicines and the consolation and hope of religion. As yet, however, only some of these new approaches to the history of medicine have been applied to the plague.[144]

A number of distinctions must be made for the *lazaretti* in response to this ever-widening literature on early modern medicine. First, the boundaries of the institution were well defined – it was not a medical space which could be experienced concurrently with others, although this does not mean that the medicine offered within the *lazaretti* was isolated from that beyond its boundaries. Second, the medicine on offer was determined by the public health authorities not by individual patients, although there are hints that patients may have made use of a power of refusal regarding treatments within the hospitals. Finally, the emphasis on the commercialisation of medicine and the purchasing power of the sick applies only to the *lazaretti* when Venice was not infected with the plague. During epidemics, much of the care was provided free of charge and belongs, therefore, to the realm of charity. Beyond these distinctions, however, treatments in the *lazaretti* illustrate a number of similarities with those of other early modern hospitals and with responses to disease beyond epidemics. Medical, spiritual and practical care was provided through the combination of a number of different, early modern strategies for health.

The wide-ranging nature of early modern public health dictates the use of a diverse body of source material in this study, ranging from artistic and archaeological material to published accounts and archival records. The variety of sources is also, in part, bred by necessity: the sources for plague hospitals are fragmentary. Although there is no complete source for these hospitals, the hope is that each different type of source provides a further piece in the jigsaw. The majority of surviving contemporary descriptions of the *lazaretti* are reflective pieces, written by literate political or medical figures and published after an epidemic. An exception to this is the letterbook of the Health Office doctor Ludovico Cucino, who served in Venice during the plague of 1555–58 which is preserved in the Wellcome Library in London. This source, although a transcription of letters, does convey a sense of the progression of the plague as well as providing valuable information from a *lazaretto* doctor.[145] The other principal accounts of

---

[144] Recent studies which have used new approaches to study the plague include Gavin A. Bailey, Pamela M. Jones, Franco Mormando and Thomas W. Worcester (eds), *Hope and healing: painting in Italy in a time of plague, 1500–1800* (Worcester MA, 2005) using art, Samuel K. Cohn Jr, *Cultures of plague* using printed texts and Shona K. Wray, *Communities and crisis* using notarial records.

[145] The Cucino letterbook was purchased by the Wellcome library in 1903 at a sale of the books of Rev Walter Sneyd [1809–88]. Sneyd appears to have acquired the letterbook from a sale of items from the library of Matteo Luigi Canonici [1727–1806] who in turn had purchased the library of Giacomo Soranzo [1686–1761]. I am grateful to Helen Burton from the Special Collections and Archives at Keele University for providing me with a copy of the handlist of the Sneyd family papers.

lazaretti which claim eye witness status are contained within the description of
the plague outbreak of 1575–77 by the notary Rocco Benedetti, the description of
the *lazaretti* by Francesco Sansovino and, for Genoa, the fascinating account by
Father Antero Maria da San Bonaventura (Filippo Micone) [1620–86] who served
the *lazaretti* within the city during the devastating outbreak of 1656–57.[146] Father
Antero was an Augustinian monk, who remains one of the most famous preachers
of his day in Genoa and his service to the sick and poor is commemorated in a
monument within the city. His account of the plague hospital in Genoa, although
technically beyond the chronological boundaries of this study, is invaluable for
the rich description provided of conditions within the hospitals and also illustrates
ways in which the hospital structures changed over time in terms of their nature
and purpose; there is very little information available on the workings of the
lazaretti in Venice during the mid-seventeenth century because the city was not
affected by the outbreak of 1656–57. The description of Padua in 1575–77 by
Alessandro Canobbio includes detail on that city's plague hospitals. The account
by Fra Paolo Bellintani – who served in Milan, Brescia and Marseilles during the
plague – is rich, particularly with regard to religious healing within the plague
hospitals. These works are particularly vivid and wide ranging in their nature and,
as such, are used throughout the book.

This book also makes extensive use of archival material, principally from
the Venetian State Archive but including that of Padua, Verona and Treviso. The
nature of the Venetian Republic ensured the continued involvement of a number
of government bodies in the administration of the plague hospitals. The most
prominent bodies were the *Provveditori al Sal* (Salt Office), the *Procuratori di
San Marco* (Procurators of St Mark) *de citra,* the *Cinque Savi sopra la mercanzia*
(Board of Trade) and the *Provveditori alla Sanità* (Health Office). Archival material
relating to the *lazaretti* is split between the archives of these magistracies because
the government deliberately spread the responsibility for the administration of
these sites.

The Salt Office played a pivotal role in the establishment and development of
the Venetian *lazaretti*. The plague hospitals were established in Venice before the
foundation of the Health Office in 1486. In 1423, the Senate had instructed the Salt
Office to fund the construction of the *lazaretto vecchio* and to pay the salaries of
the workers.[147] The Salt Office also funded the building of the *lazaretto nuovo* in
1468 and paid rent to San Giorgio Maggiore for the use of the island.[148] During the
fifteenth century, the Salt Office appointed Priors to the *lazaretti* and administered
the hospitals. These areas of jurisdiction were largely handed over to the Health
Office during the sixteenth century but the Salt Office continued to pay the salaries

---

[146]   It should be noted that the account by Rocco Benedetti is available in a number of
different versions, including a manuscript at the Museo Correr, Venice. The page numbers
in the footnotes refer to the copy held at the Wellcome Library, London.

[147]   This is reprinted in *Venezia e la peste*, appendix seven, p. 365.

[148]   Reprinted in ibid., appendix nine, p. 366.

of workers, to assist with the high costs incurred by the Health Office during outbreaks and to fund occasional repairs to buildings. Surviving archival material predominantly concerns the significant sums of money which were paid for the hospitals by a body whose attention was fixed on preserving and improving the public appearance of the city. The Salt Office was an immensely rich branch of the Republic, which used its income from tax on salt as well as rents on warehouses and landing places to fund other public institutions and building projects, such as the rebuilding of the *Fondaco dei Tedeschi* (German Exchange House) and the rebuilding of the Rialto Bridge between 1588 and 1591.[149] The *lazaretti* had a particular function to fulfil in relation to the public face of the city. They were important institutions in terms of Venice's reputation in projecting a position of strength in the face of epidemic disease, as illustrated by the involvement of the Salt Office.

The interest of the Procurators of St Mark *de citra* in the *lazaretti* is attested to by the documentation surviving in their archive. The Procurators had been divided into three sections in 1319: the Procurators *de supra* were responsible for the Basilica of St Mark (the Doge's private chapel until 1807). The Procurators *de citra* and *de ultra* administered estates and private bequests, dividing the task according to the geography of the city.[150] In the archive of the Procurators *de citra* are copies of legislation, as well as copies of verdicts of cases involving the *lazaretti*, information regarding the elections of Priors, literary accounts of the development of the islands and a series of important account books relating to periods of building work. The Procurators were involved in the upkeep of the buildings in the *lazaretti* and commissioned carvings to decorate the hospitals.[151] The involvement of this branch of the Venetian Republic supports my emphasis on the charitable purpose of the hospitals.

Although underexplored, the role of the Board of Trade became increasingly prominent in the records of the *lazaretti*. Established in 1507, the purpose of this

---

[149]   Marin Sanudo records that rents were collected from small shops, cellars and warehouses at Rialto in Marin Sanudo, *De origine, situ et magistratibus urbis venetae ovvero la città di Venetia (1493–1530)* (Milan, 1980), p. 108. On the Salt Office see Jean-Claude Hocquet, *Il sale e la fortuna di Venezia* (Rome, 1990), chapter four 'L'organizzazione amministrativa del commercio del sale', pp. 97–130. The Salt Office referred to here is the Salinari Salis Maris, with responsibility for all salt coming into Venice except that of Chioggia, which had a separate magistracy (p. 100). In addition to payments to institutions such as the *Pietà* hospital the Salt Office also coordinated the funding of the construction of both the votive plague churches – the Redentore and the Salute. See ASV, Sal, b. 10 reg. 12 15v (16 April 1577) for the Redentore and Andrew Hopkins, *Santa Maria della Salute: architecture and ceremony in Baroque Venice* (Cambridge, 2000) for the Salute. These two churches are discussed in Chapter 6 pp. 230–31. For the *fondaco dei tedeschi* see Chapter 1, p. 59.

[150]   For information regarding the early role of the Procurators see R.C. Mueller, *The Procuratori di San Marco and the Venetian credit market* (New York, 1977).

[151]   These are discussed in Chapter 1, pp. 62–3.

branch of the Republic was to protect the 'prestige, profit and benefit which trade imparts' in the aftermath of the successful Portuguese voyage round the Cape of Good Hope.[152] For the purposes of this study, it is clear that the Board of Trade received copies of correspondence and, indeed, corresponded directly on the subject of public health and the *lazaretti* through the seventeenth century.[153] In 1609, for example, the Board of Trade made recommendations to the governors in Dalmatia and Albania regarding the site for a *lazaretto* and sent a model governing its form.[154] This is illustrative of the enduring importance of the hospitals for the structures of trade within the city. Further research into the role of this body in the administration of the *lazaretti* could be fascinating.

The Venetian *lazaretti* have always been considered in conjunction with the Health Office, created in 1456 and made permanent in 1486.[155] During the sixteenth century, this magistracy extended the spheres over which it held jurisdiction. It undertook a wide regulation of dangerous economic, social and spatial issues, such as meat markets, prostitution and the second-hand goods trade.[156] The archive of the Health Office is the most important from the point of view of the *lazaretti*, since it was this body which was responsible for the day-to-day running of the hospitals. This archival material, therefore, conveys the strongest sense of how these hospitals worked in practice and not simply in theory. The criminal archive of the Health Office, which would have provided fuller detail of transgressions against public health legislation, does not survive in Venice, although cases are sometimes referred to in brief in the records of the notary, the *notatorio*. This latter series, particularly the volumes relating to the sixteenth century, are full of references to the *lazaretti* and material from this archive underpins much of what follows in individual chapters.

This book is structured around the various stages in a patient's experience of the *lazaretti*. This is not intended to suggest a uniformity of experience amongst patients; indeed, illustrating the diversity of patient experiences is one of the most difficult challenges in working with early modern institutions. The intention underpinning the structure is to suggest that these hospitals should be considered from the point of view of contemporaries rather than later, often critical, observers. Part I of the book explores first impressions of the hospital from contemporary literary and artistic sources. These sources highlight metaphors

---

[152]   The founding statute of the Board of Trade is copied and translated in David S. Chambers and Brian Pullan (eds), *Venice: a documentary history 1450–1630*, pp. 168–9.

[153]   Engaging material can be found in ASV, Sanità reg. 16.

[154]   ASV, Sanità reg. 3 88v (6 October 1609).

[155]   For the development of the Health Office see Richard J. Palmer, 'The control of plague', pp. 51–86.

[156]   The best study is Patricia Allerston, 'The market in secondhand clothes and furnishings in Venice c.1500–c.1650' (unpublished PhD. thesis, European University Institute, 1996) and see also 'L'abito usato' in Carlo M. Belfanti and Fabio Giusberti, *Storia d'Italia vol 19: la Moda* (Turin, 2003), pp. 561–81.

which contemporaries use to describe the *lazaretti* and which connect the plague hospitals with other institutions in the early modern city, emphasising the often collective and connective nature of early modern isolation. The chapter considers the architectural structures of the Venetian hospitals and of plague hospitals across Europe. The Venetian hospitals did not serve as architectural models for *lazaretti* elsewhere – they were not purpose-built and lacked a clear overall design. Nevertheless the system of public health for the plague, firmly rooted in the social, environmental, economic and political structures of an individual city, proved to be influential across Europe and across the centuries.

In Part II, experiences of patients in quarantine are considered, including the process by which individuals were sent into quarantine and information on who was sent, engaging with the relationship between poverty and the plague. The staffing structure of the hospitals and the care provided by workers is then described – including the distribution of clothing and food and attempts to consider the emotional state of patients, regulating fear by allowing visits from friends and family, as part of the treatment of the 'non-naturals' of early modern medical thought.[157] The medical care provided to patients is also outlined, alongside the roles of medical practitioners within the hospitals and attention is drawn to a body of little-considered treatments marketed as secret cures for the plague.

In Part III, departures from the hospitals are explored, as a result of death as well as cure. Through a study of mortality statistics within the hospitals, the much debated issue of whether or not a stay in the Venetian plague hospitals was tantamount to a death sentence is considered. The hospital structures, which were designed to ensure that patients could die a 'good death', included facilities for burial and will-making and were intended to reintegrate the souls of the plague sick with the wider community through networks of charity. It is clear that a significant proportion of those sent to the Venetian *lazaretti* did die during plague epidemics but a number were thought to recover as a result of the care provided. The return to the city of those who survived the disease brings an important perspective to the study of groups within society, reminding us that people in the past were not always part of fixed, social categories. Perspectives of goods also altered according to circumstances: whether they had been owned by the rich or the poor and whether or not they had been disinfected by the Health Office or stolen and returned to the city illicitly all affected perceptions of danger and infection. Using influences from the material turn, the book ends by emphasising the significance of context for contemporary treatment of objects as well as people.[158]

---

[157] On fear as a response to plague epidemics over the longue durée, and on the fear of plague spreaders, see Paolo Preto, *Epidemia, paura e politica nell'Italia moderna* (Bari, 1987).

[158] It is nearly fifteen years since Lisa Jardine called for studies of the Renaissance that tackled culture, craftsmanship and commodities instead of individuals and ideas in *Wordly goods: a new history of the Renaissance* (London, 1996). A number of rich studies have been published in recent years. For Italy see in particular the work of Evelyn Welch, Tricia Allerston

Each of these chapters engages with the key ideas which underpin the analysis of this book: the nature of early modern public health and illness. In both cases, the book illustrates that these ideas were thought about differently in the past and their study reveals more about early modern social as well as medical history. The intention of the *lazaretti*, before 1650, was to separate the sick from the healthy and individuals from their goods but it was not to isolate individuals in the modern sense because of the way in which medical and religious ideas about care and cure were interwoven. Policies such as collective charity and prayer were considered to be as powerful (if not more so) as medical treatments prescribed by doctors in the fight against disease.[159]

Isolation in Venice meant the clustering and concentration of particular groups on sites encircled by water or enclosed by high walls. The visibility of these sites was important. Institutions were designed to acknowledge the presence of groups as well as to contain it; the sites also illustrated that governments were responding to problems on behalf of the populace. In the context of the plague hospitals, personal, economic and charitable links were maintained between these institutions and the wider city in order to gain the benefits of spiritual and physical healing, whilst keeping the threat of infection at arm's length. The rich resources of the city – economic, environmental and political – meant that the Venetian authorities were able to use early, permanent *lazaretti* to tackle the causes and effects of the plague. This was a daunting and undeniably difficult task but the *lazaretti* were used as genuine attempts at care and cure, even in the most difficult of circumstances.

---

and Marta Ajmar-Wollheim. See also, with a focus on early modern Germany, Ulinka Rublack, *Dressing up: cultural identity in Renaissance Europe* (Oxford, 2010).

[159]   Ingrassia, pp. 349, 352–3 discusses the tension between collective acts of penitence and notions of infection. On healing and religion see, for example, Andrew Cunningham and Ole P. Grell (eds), *Medicine in the Reformation* (London, 1993); *Health care and poor relief in Protestant Europe 1500–1700* (London, 1997); *Health care and poor relief in Counter Reformation Europe* (London, 1999); John R. Hinnells and Roy Porter (eds), *Religion, health and suffering* (London, 1999) and John Henderson, *The Renaissance hospital*. For work in a Venetian context see Paolo Preto, *Peste e società*, pp. 76–89 and see Richard J. Palmer, 'The control of plague' pp. 280–314 and Alexandra Bamji, 'Religion and Disease in Venice, *c.* 1620–1700' (unpublished PhD thesis, University of Cambridge, 2007).

Chapter 1
'From a distance it looks like a castle': First Impressions and Architectural Design

The striking environment of the Venetian lagoon, with its marshes and sandbanks, presents an ever-changing picture of land interweaving with water. The lagoon breaks the landmass into separate islands of varying sizes. The largest of these islands have supported significant populations during their histories. In the medieval and early modern periods, some of these larger islands were administered in the same way as the principal cities of the *terraferma*, illustrating a degree of political independence from Venice. The smaller lagoon islands were often used by the religious orders, although a number of these sites were abandoned during the medieval period, because of the poor quality of the air and issues of indiscipline within the communities.[1] Two of these smaller islands were adapted for use as Venice's plague hospitals during the fifteenth century. The site of the *lazaretto vecchio* lies just off the Lido, one of the protective islands which shelters Venice from the sea, approximately three kilometres from the city. The second island, which housed the *lazaretto nuovo*, lies three kilometres northeast of Venice, separated by a small channel of water from Sant'Erasmo, the island known as the garden of Venice. In this chapter, we will consider the views of these *lazaretti* islands, from city and beyond. First, the view of the *lazaretti* as important religious and civic institutions will be described. Second, the impression made on visitors, as recorded by contemporaries in literary and visual sources will be illustrated, including the notable views of the sites as Hell and Purgatory, and, as extensions of Venice in times of health, as Paradise.[2] Third, the protective nature of the architecture at the *lazaretti* will be explored using the contemporary metaphor of the castle. In the final sections, the architecture of the hospitals will be described in more detail, including both the structure and decoration of plague hospitals within and beyond Venice. Each of these sections illustrates that the Venetian *lazaretti*

---

[1] Mary Laven, *Virgins of Venice: broken vows and cloistered lives in the Renaissance convent* (Harmondsworth, 2003), p. xxiv.

[2] These metaphors in literature are likely to have been influenced by Dante's *Divine Comedy*. I am grateful to Mary Laven for pointing out to me that Arcangela Tarabotti adopted the same device: *L'inferno monacale* was followed by the less famous sequel *Paradiso monacale*. For these images applied to prisons, in a poem by a Venetian as well as other contexts, see Guy Geltner, *The medieval prison: a social history* (Princeton NJ, 2008), pp. 118–19.

can fruitfully be compared with other contemporary institutions in terms of the use of space within the city and the nature of the isolation employed within the sites.

Religious associations, ideas and language infuse contemporary accounts of the *lazaretti*, from the earliest examples. Discussions of Venice's first plague hospital, the *lazaretto vecchio*, refer to the role of St Bernardino of Siena in determining the location and foundation of the site. St Bernardino, visiting Venice in 1422, preached for a year and it is said that he had such success that the Doge of the city promised him two wishes. Having served in the plague hospital in Siena during the epidemic of 1400, St Bernardino wished that the Venetian authorities should establish a plague hospital on an island of the Venetian lagoon and he stressed the need for a spacious and remote location.[3] In a wider Italian context, it is not unusual to see the involvement of a prominent religious figure with the *lazaretti*, although the Venetian *lazaretti* were in the hands of the political authorities and were never staffed by religious orders. In Milan, St Carlo Borromeo worked within the *lazaretto* during the terrible outbreak of plague of 1575–77 – sometimes known as the plague of St Carlo.[4] Various contemporary writings described Borromeo's work as that of the model for a perfect pastor during outbreaks of epidemic disease and in this, service within the *lazaretti* was prominent.[5] His worked bridged spiritual and physical care. He was renowned for distributing clothing and food. In the image of his ministry [Plate 2], we see the connections between piety and medicine: even the *putti*, in the top left, are put to work perfuming and purifying the air.

In some places during the late sixteenth and seventeenth centuries, the context of plague was talked of in the light of the Catholic Reformation and epidemics were said to provide an opportunity for the humble giving and receiving of charity, for developing an attitude of compassion and, where necessary, for acts of submission and conversion to Christianity. Plague, for example as Thomas Worcester has shown, was described by the Jesuit Etienne Binet [1569–1639] as a time when many were saved because it was 'blessed by God'. This meant it was not only an opportunity for the conversion of souls but a time ripe for the making of saints and martyrs, although the latter was the cause of some debate.[6]

---

[3]   This is discussed in Iris Origo, *The world of San Bernardino* (London, 1963).

[4]   Luca Beltrami, 'Il lazzaretto di Milano', *Archivio storico lombardo*, 9 (1882), p. 429.

[5]   See, for example, Paolo Bisciola, *Relatione verissima del progresso della peste di Milano ... dove si raccontano tutte le provisioni fatte da Monsignor Illustrissimo Cardinal Borromeo ... dove si può imparare, il vero modo d'un perfetto Pastore amator del suo gregge e come in Principe deve governar una città nel tempo di peste* (Bologna, 1630) and Paolo Bellintani, *Dialogo della peste*, Ermanno Paccagnini (ed.) (Milan, 2001). For other sources on San Carlo's plague experience see Samuel K. Cohn Jr, *Cultures of plague: medical thought at the end of the Renaissance* (Oxford, 2010).

[6]   Thomas Worcester 'Plague as spiritual medicine and medicine as spiritual metaphor: three treatises by Etienne Binet S.J. (1569–1639)' in F. Mormando and T. Worcester (eds), *Piety and Plague: from Byzantium to the Baroque* (Kirksville MI, 2007) p. 230.

Binet highlighted that illness and the necessary medical response created opportunities for effective spiritual care. He particularly praised the example set by Carlo Borromeo in the care of the sick in Milan between 1575 and 1577.[7] Binet begins his treatise by asking whether the plague brings more ill than good and concludes that, without the plague, there would be less devotion and fewer saints.[8]

The *lazaretto* in Genoa was thought to have a clear charitable and religious purpose, tailor-made for the purposes of the Catholic Reformation in the written description by Father Antero Maria da San Bonaventura, the Rector at the hospital for the outbreak of 1656.[9] Father Antero recorded the 'scandalous' behaviour of some patients within the *lazaretto,* who ate meat on a Friday and Saturday and did not go to Mass or act with any reverence towards the Mass. One example of such patients was four Dutch sailors.[10] All of these sailors were said to have converted in the *lazaretto* and become very devout. Father Antero wrote that they converted during their period of sickness and praised God that they were healed. Here, religious and physical healing went hand-in-hand. The healing of these sailors was said to have been particularly extraordinary (and all the more obviously miraculous) because it happened at the beginning of July, when few in the plague hospital survived. Father Antero described his own reaction to their conversion as one of recognition that he had witnessed 'a great miracle, similar to that which I read about in the report from Japan by PP Giesuiti, of five blind persons, who were baptised and all had their vision restored'. Here, the concurrent healing of soul and body is emphasised by the restoration of sight in both the religious and physical sense, making use of a common metaphor for conversion. Elsewhere in his text, Father Antero also employed the metaphors of slavery and freedom and disease and cure. The Italian *lazaretti* were seen to fulfil both a general religious and specific Catholic-Reformation function, making the involvement of religious figures appropriate.

Conversion was also a feature of *lazaretti* elsewhere in Europe. In Malaga, Mary Elizabeth Perry has recorded the case of a slave girl, Fatima, who is said to have converted to Christianity in the plague hospital.[11] Fatima was said to have been given the baptismal name Ana, recovered from her illness and left the hospital. She was then said to return to her Muslim faith and deny that her baptism had taken place. When pressed during an investigation by the Inquisition, Fatima eventually

[7]   Ibid., p. 234.

[8]   Ibid., p. 229.

[9]   Discussed in more detail in Jane L. Stevens Crawshaw, 'Charity, compassion and conversion in Counter-Reformation plague hospitals' in the forthcoming edited volume of conference proceedings, Teresa Huguet Termes (ed.), *City and hospital in the European West (13th–17th centuries).*

[10]   Father Antero Maria da San Bonaventura, *Li lazaretti della città*, p. 22.

[11]   Mary Elizabeth Perry, 'Finding Fatima, a slave woman of early modern Spain', *Journal of Women's History*, 20:1 (2008), pp. 151–67.

acknowledged the baptism but explained it by saying that she had been 'crazy and without sanity and without judgement'. This is a shrewd defence by someone who had recovered from the plague, since madness was widely acknowledged to be a common characteristic of the plague sick. The cleric who had carried out the baptism also spoke directly to this aspect of conversions amongst the plague sick, saying, 'that since the said Moor [Fatima] continued to ask for baptism and since she was not frenetic but in her sound mind and it was for her remedy and salvation, he had baptized her'. One of the specific features of plague hospitals was their locations on the outskirts of cities – whether beyond city walls on the mainland or on islands close to ports. This allowed them to be used by city authorities to protect populations from perceived threats – whether that was the Protestants for the Atlantic-facing Genoese or the Muslim slaves of Malaga. The sites offered the opportunity to prevent the importation of heresy and immorality as well as epidemic disease.

The religious function and potential of plague hospitals enhanced their importance for cities. The civic purposes of hospitals were explored in John Henderson's 2006 monograph, in which he established Florence as the home of 'The Renaissance Hospital'. Henderson's work has described the aim of medieval and early modern hospitals as that of 'healing the body and healing the soul' in equal measure.[12] He cites a contemporary who describes Florence's hospitals as, 'beautiful and capacious ... adapted and organised to receive any sick or healthy person who is wretched and needs to be received for whatever reason'. Florence, however, cannot claim the invention of the Renaissance plague hospital: the same contemporary goes on to say 'except those who are sick from plague'. At the point of writing, early Renaissance Florence lacked a *lazaretto* and instead made a 'third class' response to plague, using temporary sites during periods of emergency. Henderson writes that the use of these temporary sites 'should not be confused with the general tenor of attitudes that underlay society's mechanisms to deal with the poor'. The consensus of historians has been that temporary *lazaretti* cannot be aligned with the broader context of developing ideas on poor relief, which is why so much attention has been paid to the introduction of permanent Health Boards, particularly in Italy.[13] Where permanent *lazaretti* were established, however, the

---

[12]   See John Henderson, 'Healing the body and saving the soul: hospitals in Renaissance Florence', *Renaissance Studies,* 15:2 (2001), pp. 188–216 and *The Renaissance hospital: healing the body and healing the soul* (London, 2006).

[13]   For Venice and its territory useful sources are Richard J. Palmer, 'The control of plague in Venice and Northern Italy 1348–1600' (unpublished PhD. thesis, University of Kent, 1978). Michelle A. Laughran, 'The body, public health and social control in sixteenth-century Venice' (unpublished PhD. thesis, University of Connecticut, 1998). Salvatore Carbone, *Provveditori e sopraprovveditori alla sanità della repubblica di Venezia: carteggio con i rappresentanti diplomatici e consolari veneti all'estero e con uffici di sanità esteri corrispondenti inventario* (Rome, 1962). Ciro Ferrari, 'L'ufficio di sanità di Padova nella prima metà del sec. XVII', *Miscellanea di storia veneta*, 3:1(1910), pp. 1–267. Katerina

decision was informed by ideas about charity and welfare. Indeed, Henderson's work reflects this: in 1479, when the decision was taken to set up a permanent plague hospital, it was said to be 'couched in terms of Christian charity to show the world that the city's door of charity was as open as in other parts of the world' and justified on the grounds that 'the greater the danger to those who look after the sick and the more these people are abandoned by everybody, the greater the merit in the eyes of God to whomever receives them and provides for their needs'.[14]

In discussions of the origins of the Venetian *lazaretti*, there is dispute as to where the original charitable impulse lay. The role of St Bernardino of Siena has already been discussed. In his study of Doge Francesco Foscari [1373–1457], Denis Romano gives the responsibility for the hospital's proposal to Foscari himself and uses it as an illustration of the Doge's paternal care for the community. In a way that is characteristic of Venetian history, the credit for the foundation of the *lazaretto* is given to the figure who represented the Republic. Regardless of the point of origin, Venetian authors came to associate the *lazaretti* with particularly Venetian virtues: piety, longevity, stability and prosperity. The hospitals were written into the long tradition of panegyric writing, in which Venice was described as an earthly Paradise. During the Renaissance, the mould was created for the genre of 'praise of city' writing, which shaped the amorphous myth of Venice.[15] Once formed, the myth was brought out for use on special occasions through the early modern period. According to the myth, the beauty and calm of the natural environment permeated the social and political structures of the city. This close connection between the nature of the environment and the nature of the place, however, became problematic in times of plague because explanations of disease causation were so closely linked to physical environment.[16] For contemporaries, it could be difficult to explain how the source of the disease could lie in Venice's physical environment; a number of the accounts in the section which follows aimed to diffuse this tension.[17]

Early modern accounts of the plague engaged with broader ideas about cities and their moral and physical fabrics. Many of these accounts used religious language. Sometimes, however, the vocabulary was of a surprising kind: the *lazaretti* in Venice were said to resemble gardens and Paradise as well as Purgatory

---

Konstantinidou, 'Gli Uffici di Sanità delle isole ionie durante il seicento e il settecento', *Studi veneziani*, 49 (2005), pp. 379–91. Alessandro Pastore, 'L'organizzazione sanitaria nella Repubblica di Venezia al tempo di William Harvey' in Giuseppe Ongaro, Maurizio Rippa Bonati and Gaetano Thiene (eds), *Harvey e Padova* (Padua, 2006), pp. 201–17. See also the classic works by Carlo Cipolla on the Health Boards of Tuscany, cited on p. 4 note 10.

[14]   John Henderson, *The Renaissance hospital*, p. 94.

[15]   For the myth of Venice see the Introduction, p. 2 note 7.

[16]   For a discussion of Palermo's environment and the effects of tuna fishing in causing the plague there see Ingrassia, pp. 134–7.

[17]   See Jane L. Stevens Crawshaw 'Bodies politic: the environment, public health and the state in early modern Venice', in the forthcoming special issue of *Renaissance Studies*.

and Hell. Some of these comparisons are also expressed visually in artistic depictions of the Venetian *lazaretti*. The imagery applied to the *lazaretti* can tell us more about these hospitals and highlight connections between the plague hospitals and other early modern institutions. The echoing of imagery around the city allows us to explore the relationship between the *lazaretti* and other sites of trade and welfare which made use of defensive and protective architecture. Contemporary descriptions, then, are considered in three sections which follow based around descriptions of the *lazaretti* as Paradise, as Hell and as castles. The third of these sections, which highlights the connections with other Venetian institutions, is not intended to suggest that any of the institutions under consideration were unique to Venice; rather contemporaries described institutions and policies using a general language of public health and care for the poor, which was spoken in Venetian dialect, in order to tie these institutions into general histories of the city. The final section of the chapter considers the architectural design of plague hospitals in Venice and beyond in order to highlight the organisation of space within early modern social policies.

Contemporary Descriptions

Few contemporary accounts survive which describe experiences of early modern quarantine, not least because of the moderate literacy levels of society at the time. A French visitor to Venice wrote an account of the hospitals of the city in *c*.1500. In this, he noted the provisions made within the structures at the *lazaretto vecchio* to care 'for the bodies and souls of these sick persons, both in death and in life'. His description of the *lazaretto nuovo* referred to it as 'large and beautiful and in a pleasant spot' before outlining its purpose in providing quarantine outside the city.[18] The brief nature of this account is by no means uncommon, neither is the superficial nature of the description. Lengthy accounts of the hospitals are unusual. Two exceptional descriptions of the Venetian *lazaretti* are used in this chapter to explore contemporary perceptions – both are packed full of vivid detail. Each was written by a Venetian – one a nobleman and the other a notary – and both describe the *lazaretti* during the outbreak of 1575–77.[19] The first, from 1580, was recorded by Francesco Sansovino [1521–86] as part of his guidebook to the

---

[18]   This anonymous account has been widely reprinted and is available in an Italian translation from the French in *Venezia e la peste 1348–1797* (Venice, 1980), p. 91 and in an English translation in David S. Chambers and Brian Pullan (eds) with Jennifer Fletcher, *Venice: a documentary history, 1450-1630* (Oxford, 1992), pp. 302–3.

[19]   Benedetti was a Venetian notary, active between 1556 and 1582 according to the index in the Venetian *Archivio di Stato*. On literature in response to plague see Samuel K. Cohn Jr, *Cultures of plague*. An engaging case is provided in Ann G. Carmichael, 'The last past plague: the uses of memory in Renaisance epidemics', *Journal of the history of medicine*, 53 (1998), pp. 132–60.

city, *Venetia città nobilissima et singolare*.[20] The second, by Rocco Benedetti, was published in Urbino in 1577 and then Bologna in 1630 as the second part of a short volume containing an account of the plague in Milan in 1576–77, detailing the works of Carlo Borromeo.[21] Both authors published other works in addition to these descriptions. Those of Sansovino are well-known to those interested in the history of Venice.[22] Sansovino's account of the *lazaretti* forms part of a larger work, one of the official histories of the Venetian Republic. Like Gasparo Contarini's [1483–1542] *Della republica et magistrati di Venetia* and Marc'Antonio Sabellico's [?1436–1506] *Le historie vinitiane,* Sansovino's text is part of the 'praise of the city' tradition within Venetian historiography.[23] Rocco Benedetti wrote a trio of publications which reflected upon key events of the 1570s for Venice: the other two being the naval victory at Lepanto in 1571 and the entry of Henri III of France to Venice in 1574.[24] The two authors offer opposing views of the Venetian institutions: Sansovino portrayed the *lazaretti* as Paradise and Benedetto used the imagery of Purgatory and Hell.[25]

The Lazaretti *as Paradise*

Francesco Sansovino provided a lengthy and fascinating account, which focused upon the Venetian *lazaretto nuovo*. It contained hints about the operation of the hospital, about the way in which the Republic viewed these institutions and how the authorities wished them to be perceived from abroad. Sansovino's text was written 'as an everlasting testimony to the glory of this Christian and pious city'

---

[20] Francesco Sansovino, *Venetia città nobilissima et singolare: descritta in XIII libri* (Venice, 1663), book five, p. 232.

[21] Rocco Benedetti, *Relatione d'alcuni casi occorsi in Venetia al tempo della peste l'anno 1576 e 1577 con le provisioni, rimedii et orationi fatte à Dio Benedetti per la sua liberatione* (Bologna, 1630). This work was also published in Urbino in 1577. It is the later edition to which page numbers cited in the following footnotes refer. A section of this account, that relating to the *lazaretti*, is reprinted in translation in David S. Chambers and Brian Pullan (eds) with Jennifer Fletcher, *Venice: a documentary history*, pp. 117–20.

[22] For a discussion of these works see Paul F. Grendler, 'Francesco Sansovino and Italian popular history 1560–1600', *Studies in the Renaissance*, 16 (1969), pp. 139–80.

[23] For a discussion of the 'praise of city' writings see Edward Muir, 'The myth of Venice' in *Civic ritual*, pp. 1–64.

[24] In addition to the work on the plague cited in note 21, Benedetti published the *Ragguaglio delle Allegrezze, Solennità, e feste, fatte in Venetia per la felice Vittoria* (Venice, 1571) and *Le feste et trionfi fatti dalla serenisima signoria di Venetia nella felice venuta di Henrico III. Christianissimo re di Francia et di Polonia* (Venice, 1574). According to the online resource Edit 16, Benedetti published thirteen works, including those mentioned above, a number of which were dedicated to prominent political and religious figures.

[25] On the *lazaretti* elsewhere as Hell, see Carlo Cipolla, *Cristofano and the plague: a study in the history of public health in the age of Galileo* (London, 1973), p. 27. For a point of comparison with the same image applied to prisons see Guy Geltner, *The medieval prison.*

and 'as an example to foreign princes' so that they could appreciate 'the charity of the fathers and governors to the populace in times of urgent need'. Throughout the account he was keen to articulate the ideal of the godly Republic. Sansovino's account emphasised the important role which the *lazaretti* played in making Venice's responses to disease visible to trading partners. It also highlighted the charitable and pious aspect of the institutions.

Sansovino's description of the *lazaretti* was partly indebted to earlier 'praise of city' accounts, works which describe the city of Venice, as well as its constituent parts, as idyllic. Marc'Antonio Sabellico described the *lazaretti* as 'magnificent buildings' which 'from afar were reminiscent of well-guarded castles', as well as stating that the function of the *lazaretto vecchio* was to provide care for the sick and help the poor.[26] Gasparo Contarini's work was more concerned with the responsibilities of the Health Office than with details of the *lazaretti* but he described the hospitals in brief, as 'ample houses built in the lagoon three miles off from the city' near to 'gardens of great beauty'.[27] Sansovino's text drew on these earlier works. He dedicated a short space to the description of the *lazaretto vecchio*, mentioning the 'various comfortable and spacious rooms' and referring specifically to Sabellico's description of its function. In his developed description of the *lazaretto nuovo*, Sansovino relied on Sabellico's text for his introductory statements. He described it as having 'one hundred rooms and an enclosed vineyard: it is so big that from afar it resembles a castle'. After this initial reference to earlier texts, however, Sansovino claimed to develop his own knowledge of the institution in which he said he had stayed following the death of his eleven-year old daughter and the sickness of his wife.[28]

Sansovino praised the institution of the *lazaretto nuovo*, emphasising the tranquil nature of the setting. Developing Contarini's description of a spacious and pleasurable site, Sansovino described the *lazaretto nuovo* as a 'land of plenty' [*Cucagna*], in which supplies were bountiful, being delivered daily in ample quantity. The image of '*Cucagna*' was applied to *lazaretti* elsewhere. This may

---

[26] 'opera nova et apparecchiata magnificamente per tale effetto. La quale a chi la vede di lontano ha forma d'un Castello, molto ben guernito'. Marc' Antonio Sabellico, *Le historie vinitiane* (Venice, 1543), book six, p. 225. For the language of invasion and defence in the context of plague see Samuel K. Cohn Jr, *Cultures of plague*, p. 299 note 18. The image of the castle was a common one, applied to a number of early modern institutions. It also links with the widely held notion that armies and warfare were instrumental in the spread of epidemic disease – although this remains an area which warrants further study from historians. See John L. Flood, '"Safer on the battlefield than in the city": England, the "sweating sickness" and the continent', *Renaissance studies*, 17:2 (2003), pp. 147–77.

[27] 'edificate nelle lagune certe case ampissime, lontane tre miglia dalla città, vicino lequali sono certi horti con molta leggiadria', Gasparo Contarini, *Della republica et magistrati di Venetia* (Venice, 1591), book four, p. 85. Contarini's text was first published in Italian in 1544.

[28] For Sansovino's claim and the issue of the nobility in the plague houses see Chapter 2, pp. 93–6.

seem to be an odd description of an early modern plague hospital but in his account of the hospitals in Sardinia, Manconi points out that conditions in the *lazaretti*, even during outbreaks of plague, were probably no worse than within the city.[29] In Genoa, Father Antero Maria da San Bonaventura recorded that problems of supply at the *lazaretto* came about because of the same problems within the city.[30] It may even have been that there was some advantage in terms of provision to being in the plague hospitals during epidemics. In Florence in 1633, the *lazaretto* was closed temporarily because of its unpopularity. The site was, however, soon reopened because of the cost of supplying the sick within a decentralised system of household quarantine. In Venice, Sansovino suggested that on the *lazaretti* there was unceasing provision, saying, 'It was a wonderful thing to see the large number of boats visiting these groups of people with various types of refreshments.' Food was said to have been distributed with 'order and calm' because everyone knew that they were well provided for.

Sansovino describes the experience of patients from the moment of their arrival at the *lazaretto*. Those arriving to carry out a period of quarantine were welcomed with joyous applause and widespread cheer. Those on the island declared to the new arrivals that they should be glad, because there was no need to work. Sansovino's account played on the original monastic function of the islands. In place of worldly occupations, the *lazaretto nuovo* offered an uninterrupted opportunity for piety, humility and goodness. Patients, he wrote, spent their time in worship and prayer with 'the harmony of voices praising God; some singing litanies, others psalms'. Such an approach to quarantine was encouraged explicitly by Carlo Borromeo, for example, in sixteenth-century Milan, who advised that,

> Each person should prepare themselves to use this time well, and treat every day of this quarantine as being like the holy time of Lent: and just as Our Lord fasted for forty days in the desert – away from conversation with other men, interacting only with God through prayer: so should each father of a family ensure that within his household, in this public time of sadness and solitude, not only do members of his family retreat from conversation with those outside their house; but even more that they retreat inside themselves in prayer, in holy meditation, in the examination of their consciences, in the consideration of universal and individual judgement, the sufferings of hell, the glory of Paradise and other

---

[29] Francesco Manconi, *Castigo de Dios: la grande peste barocca nella Sardegna di Filippo IV* (Rome, 1994) p. 177.

[30] Father Antero Maria da San Bonaventura, *Li lazaretti della città e riviere di Genova del MDCLVII ne quali oltre à successi particolari del contagio si narrano l'opere virtuose di quelli che sacrificorno se stessi alla salute del prossimo e si danno le regole di ben governare un popolo flagellato dalla peste* (Genoa, 1658), p. 13.

similar things, listening with devotion to those things which God speaks to their hearts and deciding to act on these things without exception.[31]

Borromeo's text illustrates a contemporary perspective on idealised quarantine, as well as emphasising the significance of the unit of the family for regulating morality.

Jacopo Strazzolini recorded that during the plague outbreak of 1598–99 in Cividale del Friuli, church services were stopped but each time the bells of the main church rang, all of those in the *lazaretti* and in household quarantine, those serving and working, fell to their knees and prayed until the end of the Mass, which was marked again by the ringing of the bells. In seventeenth-century Rome, the ministers of the *lazaretto* were encouraged to ensure that those within the hospital lived 'quietly, without complaint and without gaiety, without obscene language and instead with the cheerfulness and tranquillity becoming to good Christians, and indeed, more akin to religious orders than to simple Christians'.[32] Sansovino developed similar ideas but connected the behaviour of patients to the actions of the Venetian government. At night time the island was said to be silent, as if totally uninhabited. Rather than being 'overwhelmed and occupied by compassion and grief' in the midst of such a horrendous outbreak of disease, the patients in the *lazaretti* were, instead, overwhelmed by 'applause and joy' at the goodness of the Republic. The islands were portrayed as offering respite from an infected world.

The idea of idealised provision and shelter provided by the Republic was extended to Sansovino's observations of other islands. Sansovino described the marvellous sight of the wooden huts constructed on the Lido which, he said, had the form of a new city, the sight of which moreover had a pleasant and jolly aspect

---

[31] 'Ciascuno per meglio disporsi a passar bene questo tempo, per ottenar il fine che si pretende, ogni giorno faccia conto, che questa quarantena sia a punto come un'altro sacro tempo della quadragesima: e come già Nostro Signore digiunò quaranta giorni nel deserto, lontano da ogni conversatione de gli huomini, trattando con Dio solo per mezo dell'oratione: cosi procurate voi padre di famiglia ciascuno nelle vostre case, che in questo tempo di publica mestitia, e solitudine, non solo vi sia ritiramento dalle conversationi esteriori di fuori di casa; mà molto più si ritiri ciascuno interiormente all'oratione, alle sante meditationi, alli essamini della conscienza, alla consideratione de gli giudicio universale e particolare, delle pene dell'inferno, della gloria del Paradiso et altre simili, ascoltando con divotione quello, che in cosi fatte consideratione vi parlerà Dio al cuore, e determinando con fermo proposito di metterlo in essecutione senza alcu' fallo.' in the volumes of the Constitutiones of the 6 Provincial Councils held in 1565–82 and Acta of the 11 Diocesan Synods held in 1564–84 in the *Acta Ecclesiae Mediolanensis* (Milan, 1682), volume two, p. 976. This forms part of the section on indulgences and instructions to the clergy in times of plague which runs from pp. 966–79.

[32] Cardinal Geronimo Gastaldi, *Tractatus de avertenda et profliganda peste politico = legalis. Eo lucubratus tempore, quo ipse Leomocomiorum primo, mox Sanitatis Commissarius Generalis fuit, peste urbem invadente Anno MDCLVI et LVII* (Bologna, 1684), pp. 581–4.

(*per altro di grato, et giocondo aspetto*), souls which could have been terrified at the sight of so much sickness, did not feel oppressed or occupied by extreme pity and pain. This image diffused some of the tension created when the most Serene Republic was infected with the plague because, crucially, for Sansovino, the lagoon provided the source as well as the solution to Venice's public health problems.

In Venice the lagoon islands had traditionally provided relief from the city. They were spaces to escape to; many patricians owned property on the islands where they took advantage of the verdant, spacious environment for entertainment and enjoyment.[33] Murano, in particular, was thought of as refreshing.[34] The island contained botanical gardens and was seen to have good air as a result of the furnaces which served the glass industry. In Tommaso Porcacchi's [*c.*1530–85] description of Murano, he explains that many Venetian nobles lived on Murano during the summer and he describes the island as Venice in miniature (*é una picciola Venetia*) because it too was divided down the middle by a large canal. In 1530, Doge Andrea Gritti [1455–1538] went to Murano to relieve his symptoms of gout and, during an outbreak of plague, he went to Ca' Vendramin for its fresh air (*andato per mutar aiere*).[35] Doge Francesco Venier [1490–1556] went there in the year of his death to try to improve his general state of health.[36] In addition to travelling to the mainland to escape disease, Venetians made use of the lagoon islands to benefit their health.

The association between the lagoon islands and gardens is significant from the point of view of early modern medicine. Gardens were thought to improve both the physical and spiritual health of the viewer and visitor. Many religious communities maintained gardens which offered spaces for repose, comfort and spiritual reflection in addition to supplying herbs and foodstuffs.[37] Monastic houses in England had maintained closed gardens, supposed to represent Eden and to act as a focus for contemplation – known as 'paradyse'.[38] Gardens were thought to soothe the observer and Renaissance gardens often contained inscriptions which

---

[33] Patrick Monahan, 'Sanudo and the Venetian villa surburbana', *Annali di architettura*, 21 (2009), pp. 151–67 although concerned with the architecture of patrician homes does consider the function of these spaces.

[34] Pompeo Molmenti, *La storia di Venezia*, volume II 'Lo splendore', chapter eleven, pp. 386–9 and 380–81 for his praise for the gardens of Murano, the Giudecca and Vignole.

[35] *I Diarii di Marino Sanuto*, Rinaldo Fulin (ed.) (58 vols, Venice, 1879–1903), vol. 53, p. 342.

[36] Andrew Hopkins, 'Architecture and "infirmitas": Doge Andrea Gritti and the chancel of San Marco', *Journal of the society of architectural historians*, 57 (1998), p. 187. Cini, Mantova b. 1489 bb. 62 (16 April 1556 and 12 May 1556).

[37] For the cloister garden of the Dubrovnik Franciscan monastery see Mladen Obad Šćitaroci, 'The Renaissance gardens of the Dubrovnik area, Croatia', *Garden History* 24:3 (1996), p. 186.

[38] Carole Rawcliffe, 'Delectable sightes and fragrant smelles: gardens and health in late medieval and early modern England', *Garden History*, 36:1 (2008), pp. 3–22.

reflected upon the intended beauty and calm of the spaces.[39] The predominant colour of green was one which was thought to be the perfect medium between white and black which, therefore, would refresh and nourish the eye. Francis Bacon wrote of the sweet odours and varied colours, appropriate to the season, which could come from a well-planned garden, which emulated the first garden, which had been of divine creation.[40]

Although connections with ideas on health are not developed, gardens feature in Renaissance architectural treatises on the ideal cities. Andrea Palladio [1508– 80] described tree-lined streets as having the potential, with their beauty and verdure to enliven and please the soul and to provide shade and certain comfort; fresh air was also said to sharpen the wits. In treatises on the ideal city, hospital architecture is often considered. In these works, however, the emphasis tends to be placed on constructing subdivided structures which enable the separation of the sick. Gardens feature in some architectural plans for the ideal hospital, such as those by Giorgio Vasari the Younger. Vasari the Younger also included a prominent garden in a plan of a site in which slaves could be held during their time in ports.[41] There was some overlap between these institutions and plague hospitals – indeed, *lazaretti* were sometimes used to accommodate slaves.[42]

Archival sources show that gardens featured in *lazaretto* structures. In Verona, for example, after the outbreak of 1575–77, the hospital structure was said to be overgrown. A custodian was elected and was given a series of responsibilities, foremost amongst which was to keep the rooms and the portico clean. He was also to oversee the development of the courtyards. Hedges were to be planted. A large ditch was to be dug around the structure and hedges of a species of hawthorn were to be planted for the security and beauty of the structure.[43] In Venice, the issue of gardens within the *lazaretti* was a source of much debate. Repeatedly during the sixteenth and seventeenth centuries, the Health Office officials determined that the grassed area and vineyards should be stripped back to open land and used for the disinfection of goods because of the pressure on space. In 1549 an instruction was issued to reduce the vineyard in the *lazaretto nuovo* to open grass land (*prado*). The vineyard was considered to be less important than space for the disinfection of goods. In 1560, though, it was noted that the cleared land was running the risk of becoming waterlogged and swampy, with obvious implications for the health of the sites. The Priors were given the right to grow herbs or plants on the land. It was stipulated that if the space was needed for the disinfection of goods, they

---

[39]   See, for example, Mladen O. Šćitaroci, 'The Renaissance gardens', p. 189.

[40]   See Francis Bacon, 'Of gardens' in his *Essays* (London, 1992), pp. 137–43.

[41]   Gianni Carlo Sciolla (ed.), *La città ideale nel Rinascimento* (Turin, 1995), pp. 146–7.

[42]   See the account of a slave and a conversion narrative in Mary Elizabeth Perry, 'Finding Fatima, a slave woman of early modern Spain', *Journal of Women's History*, 20:1 (2008), pp. 151–67.

[43]   ASVer, SILT 28 42v (23 January 1591).

would not be compensated for the lost plants.[44] Two years later, space was needed to expose wool and animal skins to the air and the Priors were ordered to clear all of the empty land on the islands. The Priors repeatedly tried to cultivate the land but open space was in short supply. In the end, the disinfection of goods was felt to be of greater benefit to health than the tranquil space of the garden.

Although the gardens were stripped back within the Venetian *lazaretti*, these elements of the structures were emphasised in some of the artistic depictions of the hospitals. For the most part these survive within maps of Venice although some plans of the institution are extant in the Venetian *Archivio di Stato*.[45] A genre of books containing illustrations of the islands is that of the *Isolario*, or book of islands. These illustrated a number of countries – on the pretext that all continents were islands – but very few cities. Tenochtitlan (the site of present-day Mexico City) and Venice were the most commonly illustrated. In Tommaso Porcacchi's *L'isole piu famose del mondo* (1572) Venice is the starting point. Porcacchi includes a surprisingly distinct impression of the city [Plate 3]; most early modern maps were variations on a theme. Porcacchi emphasises the fragmented nature of Venice and illustrates a number of zones as being particularly isolated. He shows some of the 400 public and private bridges of the city. In his map, the two *lazaretti* are shown in the same style as the other islands of the lagoon [Plates 4 and 5].[46] The churches, cloisters and gardens are illustrated. When the islands were converted to public health use, they retained many of the architectural features of the earlier monastic structures, particularly the prominent chapels. The emphasis upon the religious features of the islands was part of the architectural reality as well as the symbolic significance of the hospitals.

Prominent gardens were emphasised by Sansovino and others in order to associate the islands with qualities of peace and an opportunity for religious reflection. For contemporaries keen to praise the Republic of Venice, a focus on this description was a clever way of describing the strain of plague epidemics without tainting the reputation of the city. The depiction of the *lazaretti* as places of pleasure and provision, where the sick could rest without fear, also emphasised important elements of early modern public health, which tackled the body, soul and emotions of patients.

Although the same space of the garden featured in a second account of the Venetian *lazaretti*, by Rocco Benedetti, it was used to different effect. This time, it was the cruelty of the natural world, not its potential for healing, which was emphasised. The early modern world had a close relationship with the environment.

---

[44]   ASV, Sanità 730 295r (20 December 1560).

[45]   The best study remains that of Jürgen Schulz for its breadth of coverage and detail of analysis: 'The printed plans and panoramic views of Venice (1486–1797)', *Saggi e memorie di storia dell'arte*, vol. 7 (Florence, 1970). These sources are also well discussed in Bronwen Wilson, *The world in Venice: print, the city and early modern identity* (Toronto, 2005).

[46]   This style is used in the maps of Venice by Guillaume Gueroult (1553), Matteo Pagan (1559) and Paolo Furlani (1565), amongst others.

Contemporaries were familiar with the idea that nature was a force to be fought as well as harnessed. The gardens of the *lazaretti*, in Benedetti's description provided the location in which blood-coated bodies were found, entangled and damaged by the sharp spines of nature, red in tooth and claw. Benedetti's sense of the hospitals was of strained institutions in which individuals suffered instead of being healed. Benedetti focused upon the *lazaretto vecchio*. His publication was said to be based upon his own experiences of the city in 1576–77 (although the epidemic began in 1575). In the course of the plague epidemic he described undergoing household quarantine for forty days following the deaths of his mother, brother and nephew. Unlike Sansovino, he described the horror of the plague epidemic and the transformative touch of the disease on the city before considering the two *lazaretti*.

The Lazaretti *as Hell*

Benedetti's first mention of the *lazaretto vecchio* utilised religious language of a very different nature to that of Sansovino, this time from the Book of Leviticus when God ordered Moses to expel the lepers (and, Benedetti added, anyone infected with contagious diseases) from the camp.[47] In Benedetti's description of the expulsion of the sick, there was more a sense of abandonment than of care. The pure and holy were separated from the contaminated; Christian charity and provision were absent. In the section of his account which dealt with the *lazaretti*, Benedetti gave them no introduction; his first comment launched into a description of the *lazaretto vecchio* as 'Hell itself'. Instead of Sansovino's prayers and quiet, Benedetti described 'groans and sighs ... without ceasing'. Instead of plentiful supplies, Benedetti spoke of plentiful and suffocating 'foul odours [and] clouds of smoke from the burning of corpses'. Instead of patients occupied in prayer and thanksgiving, Benedetti told of those 'driven to frenzy by the disease, especially at night, [when they] leapt from their beds and, shouting with the fearful voices of damned souls, went here and there, colliding with one another and suddenly falling to the ground dead'. This cuts dramatically across the characterisation of the islands as ordered, harmonious structures of salvation, setting them up instead as sites of filth, chaos and madness.

For Benedetti, it was the *lazaretto vecchio* which represented a true horror, with the *lazaretto nuovo* seeming 'a mere Purgatory' in comparison. It is important to remember that Purgatory was a place of trial – often by ice and fire and that the association with the latter meant that medieval thinkers sought the mouth of Purgatory in volcanoes.[48] This was a state in which suffering was cleansing. In Benedetti's Purgatory, the problems included the impossibility of maintaining adequate supplies and the depressed, reflective state of the individuals who remained and 'suffered and

---

[47]   Rocco Benedetti, *Relatione d'alcuni casi*, p. 17. The passage in question is OT, Leviticus 13:46.

[48]   Jacques Le Goff, *The birth of Purgatory* (trans.) Arthur Goldhammer (Aldershot, 1990).

lamented the death of relatives, their own wretched plight and the break-up of their homes'. He also emphasised the issue of overcrowding by providing estimates of the number of people contained within both institutions at the height of the epidemic. He described 7,000–8,000 people within the *lazaretto vecchio* and 'a good 10,000 persons' both within, and on boats surrounding, the *lazaretto nuovo*.

The use of boats to augment quarantine hospitals was recognised to be a successful Venetian initiative.[49] Benedetti's work is detailed and serves as a partial corrective to Sansovino's idealised account. He illustrated, for example, that the *lazaretti* were not sufficient to meet the needs of the city during periods of infection and recorded that other islands were used as overflow hospitals and a variety of temporary constructions were utilised. Nevertheless Benedetti's application of the description of Hell to the hospitals was not original and tapped into a broader genre of writings, just as Sansovino's image did. Descriptions of the plague hospitals and household quarantine as hellish were used across Europe. One contemporary wrote of the 'horror of heart' inspired by these sites, which caused the soul to sink.[50]

For Benedetti, the hellish conditions created by plague had originated as a form of punishment: he saw the Venetian naval victory of 1571, the civic celebrations marking the entry of Henri III in 1574 and the sickening suffering of 1576–77 as intertwined.[51] Benedetti was conscious of the notion that the extravagance of past celebrations may have invoked the wrath of God upon the city. He acknowledged that a fortune had been spent on all three occasions described in his publications but was highly critical of this in the case of the public health for the plague. Benedetti carried imagery and language through the three accounts. In the case of 1571 and 1576, Benedetti described the spoils (*spoglie*) returned to the city after the famous Venetian victory over the Turks at Lepanto in 1571 as well as the spoils of the plague, which were misery. In 1571, Benedetti wrote, prisons were opened whereas in 1576 many individuals were imprisoned in the plague. In 1571, the music played in the city was said to be exceptional, making the city feel like Paradise. By 1576, as has been seen, Venice and the islands surrounding it had become hellish in Benedetti's eyes.

Benedetti also used similar language in his tracts on 1574 and 1576. His emotive and forceful language described the 'sad and sorrowful triumph of death' hanging over the city during the plague – particularly cruel since it appeared 'as the other side of the coin to the splendid and sumptuous celebrations held previously … to welcome the Most Christian King of France'. In 1574, the lagoon islands were sites to which the King of France was accompanied before entering the city. By 1576, many of the islands were becoming plague hospitals. The imagery of an armada was also used to describe the celebrations of 1574, when the French

---

[49]   Ingrassia, p. 377.

[50]   Cited in Andrew Wear, 'Fear, anxiety and the plague in early modern England' in John R. Hinnells and Roy Porter (eds), *Religion, health and suffering* (London, 1999), p. 357.

[51]   See the works referenced in note 24.

King was transported on the ceremonial boat of the Bucintoro encircled by many galleys – large and small – with brigs and *palaschermi*, each differently adorned. There were an infinite number of flags of every colour and of gondolas and boats of every type. In truth, Benedetti wrote, the scene resembled an enormous armada (*armata*) with a great stream of flags in the middle of the water. This same image of an armada is used to describe the quantity of boats surrounding the *lazaretto nuovo* during the plague epidemic. Benedetti, like Sansovino, linked the plague with the city's history but portrayed the epidemic as an extraordinary episode of difficulty and strain, a harrowing reminder of the city in happier, healthier times.

The written accounts and visual images of the *lazaretti* were carefully constructed, with developed imagery. They can be grouped around images of Paradise and Hell: one extols what has come to be known as the 'Myth of Venice' and the other includes elements of the 'Antimyth'. For our purposes, both are telling with regard to the perceptions of the hospitals, which appear to have varied considerably depending on the context in which accounts were written. Sansovino put pen to paper when the city was making a surprising recovery from the devastation of the plague. Economically and demographically Venice seemed to be bouncing back from recent strains, and confidence in the longevity of the Republic was high – as was the government's determination to develop the confidence of outsiders, particularly those with a potential economic interest in the city. In contrast, Benedetti's account was first published during 1577 and then reprinted in 1630, during the two most devastating outbreaks of the early modern period, when mortality rates were high and the city may have seemed hellish indeed. Crucially, the two accounts also consider two different *lazaretti* and the polarised accounts warn against oversimplifying the history of these two institutions. In both cases, the accounts of the *lazaretti* portray them as fully contextualised, rooted in Venetian history and culture. Further support for the deliberate depiction of the *lazaretti* as Venetian institutions can be seen in the parallels between the imagery used to describe the *lazaretti* and that used to describe other institutions within the city, considered in the next section around the image of the castle.

The Lazaretti *as Castles*

The description of the *lazaretti* by Sabellico, adopted by later authors, portrayed the hospitals as well-guarded castles. This was a metaphor used by contemporaries to describe other sites in the city as well. Although one of the six *sestieri* into which Venice has been divided since 1171 was known as Castello, this was after a fortress which had originally stood on the site of San Pietro di Castello rather than being a symbolic statement on the social make-up or topography of the area. The small island was originally called Castello Olivolo and then shortened to Castello.[52] In other contexts, though, the term was used less literally. The blocks

---

[52]   Francesco Sansovino, *Venetia città nobilissima et singolare, descritta in XIII libri* (Venice, 1663), p. 5.

of houses in which prostitutes were supposed to live were termed *castelletti* (little castles) because they were only accessible through one bridge and could therefore be closely monitored.[53] The Ghetto was referred to as a *castello* and had been placed on a self-contained island within the city.[54] It was founded in 1516 on the island on which the waste products from an iron foundry had been thrown (the 'geto'). In his description of the site, Marin Sanudo emphasised that it had only one entrance which could be closed up and guarded.[55] The site was encircled by water, allowing a clear separation between Jews and Christians.[56]

Purification using protective spaces, as in a castle, could apply to individuals on both sides of the walls. Isolated sites facilitated some degree of interaction while limiting the perceived dangers of a permanent presence of particular groups. For the Jews, as for other national communities and institutions, there could be a sense of reciprocal advantage in the development of these spaces. These groups could develop and maintain their own identities whilst still living under Venetian law and according to Venetian rules. The separation could be seen by the Jews as a form of protection. In Leon Modena's account of the outbreak of epidemic disease in 1630–31, for example, he describes how far fewer Jews died than Christians during the plague and that, for a period, the wondrous division between the camp of Israel and the city meant that no one died or became ill in the two Ghettos.[57] This manipulation of urban space as a form of protection is important for understanding public health policies of the period and the use of closed sites.

Closed sites were also used to care for the poor. During the sixteenth century, a number of smaller medieval hospitals (often accommodating up to ten people at a time) were absorbed into larger, often specialised hospitals.[58] Some hospitals had wings for specific ailments. These larger, specialised hospitals fell under the administration of religious groups, although they increasingly stood on the boundaries between secular and religious and public and private institutions. In Venice, the city's authorities developed four *Ospedali grandi* – the *Pietà* which

---

[53] For the *castelletti* see Michelle A. Laughran, 'The body, public health and social control in sixteenth-century Venice' (unpublished PhD. thesis, University of Connecticut, 1998), p. 57.

[54] Sanudo described the Ghetto as 'come un castello' in *I Diarii di Marino Sanuto*, Rinaldo Fulin (ed.) (58 vols, Venice, 1879–1903), volume 22 cols 72–3. For the development of Ghettos see Donatella Calabi and Paola Lanaro, *La città italiana e i luoghi degli stranieri XI –XVIII sec* (Rome-Bari, 1998), p. 152 and, for Venice, references in the Introduction note 45.

[55] Marin Sanudo cited in Ennio Concina, Ugo Camerino and Donatella Calabi, *La città degli Ebrei*, p. 27.

[56] Concina has compared this to the waters around the Arsenal and around the *lazaretto nuovo*, illustrating a protective and purifying function in ibid., p. 31.

[57] Mark R. Cohen, *The autobiography of a seventeenth-century Venetian rabbi: Leon of Modena's Life of Judah* (Princeton NJ, 1988), p. 135.

[58] For a history of hospital development see the Introduction, pp. 17–18.

was a foundling hospital, the *Incurabili* for the incurable sick, the *Mendicanti* for beggars and the *Derelitti* for the destitute.[59] Brian Pullan has drawn attention to the religious, social and political contexts of this development and Bernard Aikema has illustrated the architectural similarities in design of the new institutions.[60] The *lazaretti* can be usefully juxtaposed with the institutions explored in these works.

Military imagery of castles and armadas, used to describe the *lazaretti*, highlighted ideas of confinement. The imagery illustrated the location of the *lazaretti* on the outskirts of the city, acting as fortifications. The impression of institutions closed off from the city is given in artistic depictions of the islands in the maps of Erhard Reeuwich, in designs from surviving maps in the Venetian *Archivio di Stato* and in the depiction by Benedetto Bordone [Plate 6].[61] In Bordone's map, for example, the *lazaretti* are depicted as being distinct from the other islands in the lagoon [Plates 7 and 8]. It is worth noting that Bordone places the *lazaretti* equidistant from other islands. The two *lazaretti* were three kilometres from Venice but were much closer to other islands. The *lazaretto nuovo* is sufficiently close to Sant'Erasmo that, once turned over to military use, a bridge was built to link the two islands so that the warehouses of the *lazaretto nuovo* could be used to store military equipment for Sant'Erasmo. The buildings of the *lazaretti* are shown, in Bordone's map, to be entirely enclosed, expressing security and protection. In Bordone's image, only the landing station and the distinctive Venetian chimneys are visible. The rest of the structure is hidden from view. The early structures of the *lazaretti*, however, with their original monastic walls did not use the whole of the islands. Records refer to the use of space outside the walls.[62] The sense of the entire structure being enclosed is a reflection of desire and image rather than the reality of the islands.

Confinement was used for institutions designed to hold valuable commodities, dangerous but potentially lucrative social groups and those in need of charity and welfare. The policy could be used to protect those within or beyond the walls of

---

[59]   For the *Pietà*, including European comparative material, see Brian Pullan, 'Orphans and foundlings in early modern Europe', *Poverty and charity: Europe, Italy, Venice, 1400–1700* (Aldershot, 1994) III, pp. 5–18. For a comparative study of the *Pietà* hospitals in Bologna and Florence see Nicholas Terpstra, *Abandoned children of the Italian Renaissance: orphan care in Florence and Bologna* (London, 2005). For comparative material on the *Incurabili* see Jon Arrizabalaga, John Henderson and Roger French (eds), *The Great Pox: the French Disease in Renaissance Europe* (London, 1997), chapters six and seven.

[60]   See the works cited on p. 14 note 47.

[61]   A depiction from 1552 of the *lazaretto nuovo* again shows it enclosed by a perimeter wall. The hospital is portrayed as a square structure with a chapel in one corner, arched porticoes surrounding the rooms and the cemetery in close proximity to the chapel. A similar, less elegant view, dating to the early sixteenth century, survives in the *Archivio di Stato*. A number of these are reprinted in Gerolamo Fazzini (ed.), *Venezia: isola del lazzaretto nuovo* (Venice, 2004).

[62]   Cucino 93v (2 June 1557).

these institutions. A number of sites, like the *lazaretti,* straddled this divide and are explored in this section. A number of examples could be given from the early modern city: here, the *fondaci* (institutions which were used to house valuable goods as well as foreign traders), the Venetian Ghetto (for the city's Jews), hospitals and convents will be considered as representative of the different types of confinement employed.

Architecture was often designed to convey a sense of safe space between institutions and the city. In Venice, there was an emphasis upon safe space in the context of the city's *fondaci*.[63] These developed as part of the structures in place for visiting merchants across the trading cities of the early modern world.[64] In Venice, *fondaci* were established for valuable commodities for the city and for foreign merchants.[65] These institutions were separate spaces, containing things of worth and wealth. The German author Felix Faber [*c.*1441 –1502], who left accounts of his travels in Europe and beyond, described the *fondaco* as a 'building from which goods flow towards other districts like water from a fountain', giving the sense of provision to the point of overflowing.[66] This is an appropriate simile, given the association between trade and lagoon water and the quantity of goods coming in to the city. It is also an interesting image given the problems of water supply within Venice. Although a number of fountains were decorated in other European cities as signs of the state's benevolence in providing for its citizens' needs, Venice's most famous early modern fountain was of wine rather than of water.[67]

An example of a closed *fondaco* for a commodity which required protection is the *fondaco della farina*. This institution was developed to deal with the problem of famine, which affected Venice on a number of occasions during the sixteenth century. Alongside land reclamation to boost harvest yields and the regulation of prices, attempts were made to keep grain reserves for the city. According to Brian Pullan, a number of cities in the Venetian state – Venice included – took measures to accumulate grain stores between 1540 and 1560. Two-thirds of the wheat which was brought to Venice was placed into the two *fondaci* at Rialto

---

[63] The Italian term developed from the same root as the Arab term *funduq*. These institutions were common features of the medieval Byzantine and Islamic worlds. See Deborah Howard, *Venice and the East: the impact of the Islamic world on Venetian architecture 1100–1500* (London, 2000) ,'The *fondaco*', pp. 120–26 and 'The *Venetian fondaco*', pp. 126–31.

[64] See Olivia R. Constable, *Housing the stranger in the Mediterranean world: lodging, trade and travel in late Antiquity and the Middle Ages* (Cambridge, 2003).

[65] A decision was made to establish a *fondaco* for Turkish merchants in 1573 but a site was not chosen until 1621. See Deborah Howard, *The architectural history of Venice* (London, 2002), pp. 33–4.

[66] 'una casa della quale le merci profluiscono verso altre contrade come l'acque della fonte' cited in Ennio Concina, *Fondaci: architettura, arte e mercatura tra Levante, Venezia e Alemagna* (Venice, 1997), p. 9.

[67] Robert C. Davis, 'Venetian shipbuilders and the fountain of wine', *Past and Present*, 156 (1997), pp. 55–87.

and St Mark's Square.[68] These were institutions of protection both for the city and for the commodities they contained. Closed architecture was employed in other contexts where protection was needed for valuable contents. The Venetian *Zecca* (Mint) was described in 1561 as a 'worthy prison for precious gold'.[69] In architectural treatises, the institution of the Mint was paralleled with prisons. Palladio, for example, said that both should be located in the securest of locations and surrounded by tall walls and guarded with force. In both cases, the architecture of the institutions would have made the sites deliberately visible.[70] The Venetian *Zecca* was built in a similar architectural style to the salt warehouses at the Dogana and west on Giudecca.[71] These structures were large, with twenty-two warehouses placed side-by-side. The warehouses adopted the names of the original, religious structures which had stood on the site – San Gregorio, Trinità, Gesuiti, Spirito Santo and Umiltà. Each of these buildings was a closed, high roofed and spacious structure, designed to withstand the enormous pressure of the tons of salt placed inside as well as a high risk of internal erosion. The commodity which they contained was valuable and they were well-protected. These imposing structures also acted as a show of wealth for the city.

The architecture of the Venetian Arsenal also exemplified the preference for closed, bastion-like structures that expressed the city's wealth and commitment to trade. In Tommaso Porcacchi's map of the city, the separate nature of the Arsenal (and its size) are clear to see in the top right of the image [Plate 3]. The Arsenal's scale, purpose and structure focused on the production of high quality ships and its skill and production time were the inspiration for urban myths.[72] The Arsenal was surrounded by high walls. Its warehouses were the largest buildings in the city and show various parallels with those of the *lazaretti*. As a complex, it was hidden from view. It was also an island. The closed architecture was thought to be appropriate for protection and to deter thieves – two ideas which are also relevant to the design of the *lazaretti*. The Arsenal, on its island location, fostered a strong sense of identity amongst those who worked there. The site was so closely connected with the place where workers lived that they called it the *casa* or house.[73] It was a practical, working structure but still contained loaded architectural elements. It

---

[68]   See Brian Pullan, *Rich and poor in Renaissance Venice: the social institutions of a Catholic state, to 1620* (Oxford, 1971), pp. 287–96 for the problem of famine and the state response.

[69]   Cited in Ennio Concina, *Fondaci*, p. 171.

[70]   On the visibility of prisons, see Guy Geltner, *The medieval prison*, p. 4 and p. 71.

[71]   Manuel Cattani and Nicola Berlucchi (eds), *I magazzini del sale a Venezia: indagini storiche e diagnostiche per un intervento di restauro conservativo* (Venice, 2006), p. 20.

[72]   For example, contemporary observers often retold the story of an entire galley ship built and launched in 1574 for the entertainment of the French King Henri III in the time it took him to eat dinner. See Robert C. Davis, *Shipbuilders of the Venetian Arsenal: workers and workplace in the pre-industrial city* (Baltimore MD, 1991), p. 4.

[73]   See ibid. for the importance of the site in terms of identity.

included images of saints on the buildings, including St Giustina and had its own church, Santa Maria delle Vergini. The Arsenal is a classic example of the way in which enclosed space could strengthen the identity of those within it.

Identity, protection, wealth and provision for the city were at the heart of the establishment of *fondaci* for foreign merchants as well. In the case of the *fondaci* for merchants, the institutions were designed to keep a demarcated distance between the foreigners and the wider city whilst facilitating contact between them for trade. The German *fondaco* had an entrance which was locked up at night, like the *lazaretti*. Milesio described the *fondaco* as completely cut off ('tutto in isola'), highlighting an obvious parallel with the Ghetto as well as other public health sites.[74] The *fondaco* was designed to protect Venetians, particularly in the aftermath of the Reformation and the German threat of heresy, and allow the Germans safety within the structure. Sansovino described it as 'a small city within the body of Venice, in other words a city within a city'.[75] One contemporary compared the German *fondaco* to a college, writing that the merchants, artisans and servants, 'live as in a college, having everything in common, and they eat in the same place at a set hour, which proves very convenient for their business'.[76] Contemporaries recognised that the separation made between Germans and the wider city, designed as a form of protection, could pose its own dangers in allowing unsupervised behaviour. The Germans had their own tavern. The Papal Nuncio who made this observation went on to record the disreputable behaviour of the Germans and wrote that the freedom given to the foreigners within the city was akin to 'nurturing a viper in their own bosom'. Nevertheless, the site was prominent within the city and it too operated as a show of wealth. The German *fondaco* was famously rebuilt following a fire in 1505. The rebuilding was funded by the Salt Office and it was decorated with external frescoes facing the Grand Canal by Giorgione and by Titian.[77]

The location of the *lazaretti* on islands of the Venetian lagoon or outside the walls of *terraferma* cities is also comparable to the sites chosen for religious communities, which were some of the most important closed institutions of the early modern period. These institutions required space for living quarters, chapels, gardens and vineyards but were also intended to be kept at a safe distance from potentially

---

[74] Giovanni B. Milesio, *Beschreibung des deutschen Hauses in Venedig* (Munich, 1881), p. 29. On similarities between the Ghetto and the *fondaco* see Ennio Concina, Ugo Camerino and Donatella Calabi, *La città degli Ebrei*, pp. 211–16.

[75] 'una piccola città nel corpo di Venezia che val a dire una città entro l'altra' cited in Ennio Concina, *Fondaci*, p. 159.

[76] Alberto Bolognetti (papal nuncio in Venice 1578–81) in David S. Chambers and Brian Pullan (eds) with Jennifer Fletcher, *Venice: a documentary history*, p. 330. Bolognetti's reference to a college is likely to be religious.

[77] See Simon P. Oakes, 'The presence, patronage and artistic importance of the German community in early Cinquecento Venice' (unpublished PhD. thesis, University of Cambridge, 2006) particularly chapter one 'The typology of the *fondaco dei tedeschi*'.

polluting elements. Mary Laven writes of enclosed early modern convents, the 'blind windows, concealed corridors, forbidding walls ... [were] the concrete mechanisms by which nuns were once kept secluded and isolated from contact with the rest of society, and their function was symbolic as well as practical'.[78] Helen Hills has written that the closed architecture of the convent revealed what it hid in its symbolism of inaccessibility and protection for female bodies.[79] In some cases, convents were used as prisons to house female criminals.[80] A similar sense of inaccessibility and protection was intended for the *Convertite*, a convent for repentant prostitutes, which, Laura McGough has written, was used to 'quarantine beauty'.[81] The *Convertite* was located on the island of the Giudecca, McGough writes, for the protection of the women and the benefit of the wider city. The island had also been used for Jews, exiled Venetians and Eastern Orthodox communities during its history.[82] Even for the convents within the city itself, a careful balance was sought regarding the location. The convents required the services of male clergy, the delivery of goods and some supplies and also accepted the visits of authorities keen to discover whether enclosure was being maintained. The maintenance of their enclosed communities relied upon some degree of interaction and access. Too large a distance between the convents and the city placed them at risk of a lack of supervision and, therefore, indiscipline. At the same time, their separation was a form of protection, enabling their purifying function to be maintained. These were institutions which the authorities struggled to keep closed and the boundaries of which individuals often transgressed.

The institutions that have been considered here for their architecturally-closed building structures were associated with the financial and spiritual wealth of the city. They had an economic function and also contributed to the reputation of Venice as a pious Republic and, perhaps counter-intuitively, a city that was open to foreigners. The *lazaretti* were important parts of defences against the importation of disease and, therefore, of the mercantile structures of the city. They were sites for the disinfection of large quantities of goods. They facilitated trade by ensuring that goods entered the city safely, thereby contributing to the wealth of the city. The *lazaretti* also fulfilled an important social and charitable function in providing care of the sick on behalf of the city. Such structures were considered to be important and pleasing to God. Both the idea of protection and of piety shaped the images used to describe the Venetian *lazaretti* as well as the

---

[78]   Mary Laven, *Virgins of Venice*, p. xx.

[79]   Helen Hills, *Invisible city: the architecture of devotion in seventeenth-century Neapolitan convents* (Oxford, 2004).

[80]   Guy Geltner, *The medieval prison*, p. 23.

[81]   Laura McGough, 'Quarantining beauty: the French disease in early modern Venice', in Kevin Siena (ed.), *Sins of the flesh: responding to the French disease in early modern Europe* (Toronto, 2005), pp. 212–37.

[82]   Ibid., pp. 231–2.

development of particular architectural features. The rest of this chapter explores these architectural elements, initially in Venice and then in Europe more generally.

The Design of the Venetian *Lazaretti*

In Venice, it is difficult to use surviving buildings as a guide to the early modern *lazaretti*. As noted in the Introduction, the use of the two *lazaretto* islands as military sites from the late eighteenth century led to significant alterations being made to the physical structures on both islands. These make reconstruction difficult. Some indication of the sixteenth-century structure can be gleaned from a series of account books for sixteenth-century building work and descriptions and seventeenth-century plans and notes within the Venetian *Archivio di Stato*.[83] Descriptions of the physical structures of the Venetian *lazaretti* also date from the eighteenth and nineteenth centuries. In addition, the structure of the *lazaretto nuovo* can be considered through the available archaeological evidence collated by the *Archeoclub d'Italia*. These sources illustrate that there were a number of parallels in the design of the two *lazaretti*. The two islands were approximately 2.5 hectares in size.[84] The hospitals were surrounded by tall perimeter walls, about twelve feet high.[85] Both hospitals had landing stations, for obvious reasons. In theory, the chapels stood at the centre of both *lazaretti*, although the gradual development of the buildings meant that, architecturally at least, the chapels did not take centre stage. Beyond these similarities, the structures of the two *lazaretti* developed differently, in line with the different functions of the islands.

The physical structure of the *lazaretto vecchio* during the sixteenth century included many of the original monastic buildings on the island. These were supplemented with structures relevant to the new function of the island. New additions and monastic features are visible in the plan from 1813, said to be based on an earlier plan of 1597 which had been updated with necessary adjustments [Plate 9]. Part of the hospital incorporated the cloisters of the old monastery,

---

[83] The account books, held by the *Procuratia di San Marco di citra* (Procurators), cover the years 1439, 1466–1540, 1542–50, 1547–49, 1548–49, 1549–51, 1561–62 and finally 1586–88. Of this series, the first two are in a poor state of conservation. Some of the later books are only a quarter full and often include entries for unspecified tasks, or simply name the individual to whom a sum of money was to be given, without listing the activity which had been carried out. Nevertheless they provide a useful source for a partial reconstruction of the Venetian structures.

[84] According to Richard Goy, the environment of the Venetian lagoon has remained remarkably constant since the early modern period, with the exception of the island of Cavallino and the islands that have been lost near Torcello. See Richard Goy, *Venetian vernacular architecture: traditional housing in the Venetian lagoon* (Cambridge, 1989), pp. 12–13.

[85] ASV, Sanità 753 222r (7 January 1742).

which formed three sides of the square courtyard around a well and adjacent to the church.[86] The area of the chapel is visible on the left-hand side of the plan. A small cemetery can also be seen, which would have belonged to the earlier monastery. An eighteenth-century description by Vicenzo Coronelli describes a sizeable church, with three altars, a sacristy and a bell tower. Flaminio Corner recorded that in 1716 there was only one, wooden altar in the church but that a marble altar was added dedicated to Mary, mother of health, like *Santa Maria della Salute,* the votive church built after the outbreak of plague in 1630–31. During the eighteenth century, two marble altarpieces were added to the church – dedicated to the plague saints Roch and Sebastian and an image of St Bernardino of Siena was added to the altar of St Sebastian in recognition of his role in the foundation of the hospital.[87] Fifteen inscriptions are recorded by Emmanuele Cicogna [1789–1868] from within the church, thirteen date from the eighteenth century and two from the nineteenth. Only one is from the sixteenth century.[88] There is nothing to suggest, however, that this is because the church was extended after the sixteenth century. Later developments are in the internal decoration of the church rather than the structure. Eighteenth and nineteenth-century accounts describe the church as having deteriorated into a poor state of repair. The main altarpiece was said to be faded and damaged with two other altars without decoration at all – indications that these structures had stood the test of time, albeit unsuccessfully.

Very little information survives about decorative elements within the chapel. Occasionally the donation of items is recorded in archive documentation. In 1590, for example, the main altar at the *lazaretto vecchio* was embellished on Christmas Eve with a screen (*palio*) with a gold heart (*de cuorre d'oro*), a hanging lamp (*cesendelo)* to be placed in front of the altar displaying the figure of Christ and vestments for saying the Mass, made of crimson damask complete with adornments.[89] Such mentions, however, are fragments. A relief survives from 1525 [Plate 10] which was commissioned for the *lazaretto vecchio* by the Procurators of St Mark *de citra* and which is now held as part of the collection at the Museo Correr. In the carving, St Mark, the patron saint of Venice since *c.*828 when his relics were said to have been brought from Alexandria by Venetian merchants, is flanked by St Roch and St Sebastian. In the carving, the two plague saints are dwarfed by the mighty St Mark. This was a loaded image, designed as a reminder of the pre-eminence of the city. The sizing of the figures was significant since the image was placed over the doorway of the chapel on the island.[90]

---

[86]   This is repaired in ASV, PSMc b. 360 book 5 *poliza* 110 (28 marzo 1587).

[87]   Flaminio Corner, *Notizie storiche delle chiese e monasteri di Venezia e di Torcello* (Venice, 1990), pp. 554–6.

[88]   This inscription is discussed in Chapter 3, p 120.

[89]   ASV, Sanità 736 40r (24 December 1590).

[90]   The commission for the relief is reprinted in *Venezia e la peste*, p. 88. It is described in ASV, PSMc, b. 361, D6, 15r (undated) which mentions 'la chiesa [d]ove sopra la porta stessa vegonsi le imagini di Ssti Marco, Rocco e Sebastiano'.

St Roch is depicted on St Mark's right, bearing his customary staff and with his upper thigh and bubo exposed. He was himself said to have contracted the plague on returning from a pilgrimage to Rome but survived thanks to the services of an angel and a small dog that brought him food. St Sebastian was a popular intercessor because of the suffering he endured in life. As a soldier who had converted to Christianity, he was condemned to death, tied to a column and shot with arrows but did not die; he was then seized and clubbed to death. St Sebastian was said to have been tended by St Irene and a surgeon after he had been shot by arrows. The symbolic removal of the arrows (often used as a metaphor for the plague) and the subsequent treatment using nursing and medical techniques was reproduced in a number of scenes from St Sebastian's life [Plate 11]. Sts Roch and Sebastian remained a focus for public devotion throughout the early modern period and across Europe in times of plague.[91]

In Venice, the association with St Roch was particularly close. Benedetti recorded an episode which, he said, inspired laughter on the one hand and compassion on the other: a madman went through the city streets one Sunday after lunch. At each quarantined house, the man took down the planks of wood and said to those inside: 'Brothers and sisters, come out! The city has been declared free of the plague! Praise God!' Those inside the houses, thinking that this message had come from the Health Office, gladly left their quarantine and went quickly to the Church of St Roch, to give thanks to God for the saving of the city.[92] The tragedy, though, was that only a madman could have thought the health of the city was restored. In this story, the choice of location to give thanks was significant: the body of St Roch had been brought to Venice in 1485 and housed in the grand setting of the Scuola Grande di San Rocco, constructed between 1517 and 1549 and famously decorated by Tintoretto between 1564 and 1588. Venetians identified with this plague saint in a way that was entirely complementary with the tie between St Mark and the state.

The fight against disease necessitated a religious response on behalf of individuals and cities alike. By utilising and reshaping the figures of Sts Roch and Sebastian and subordinating them to an image of a saint considered to be synonymous with Venice, the city ensured that it was projected as powerful and pious in the face of disease. The carving was a reminder to patients of the forces they could rely on in times of plague: the Republic of Venice, the charitable giving of the city's inhabitants, filtered through its institutions, and the direct intercession of the saints who, as contemporaries were so often reminded, took a particular interest in the most serene Republic.

---

[91]   For an excellent discussion of imagery see Louise Marshall, 'Manipulating the sacred: image and plague in Renaissance Italy', *Renaissance Quarterly*, 47:3 (1994), pp. 485–532 and Gavin A. Bailey, Pamela M. Jones, Franco Mormando and Thomas W. Worcester (eds), *Hope and healing: painting in Italy in a time of plague, 1500–1800* (Worcester MA, 2005), particularly the essays by Pamela Jones and Sheila Barker.

[92]   Rocco Benedetti, *Relatione d'alcuni casi*, p. 18.

A second carving from the *lazaretto vecchio* also survives from this period [Plate 12]. It remains *in situ* on the island and is likely to be one of those described by John Howard during the eighteenth century as 'the images of three saints (*San Sebastiano, San Marco and San Rocco*) reckoned the patrons of this lazaretto ... over the gateways of two large rooms of warehouses'. This carving stood above an inscription, also still in place, which is documented in the archives of the Procurators of St Mark. Here, it was noted for posterity, that when the long-standing hospital had been in a state of collapse, the Procurators had intervened and given generously.[93] As with the first carving, the placement on the island was significant. Here it was near the Prior's house and faced a thoroughfare for the movement of individuals and goods. The depiction of the islands as religious structures articulated a specific but valid form of defence against disease. It drew upon early modern theories of causation which saw disease as divinely instigated and used the rhetoric of piety to present the institutions as charitable responses to the plague.

The carvings are two of the few fragments from Venice's plague hospitals to have survived the minimalist redesign of the islands undertaken by Napoleonic troops at the end of the eighteenth century. They provide a stark contrast with the depressing, Dantean welcome sign for a plague hospital, suggested by contemporaries elsewhere on the Italian peninsula, which read: 'Abandon hope, all you who enter here.'[94] This is an idea which will be returned to in Chapter 3 but the representations of these hospitals as places which should inspire genuine piety or utter despair complement the different metaphors applied to the sites in the contemporary publications considered earlier in the chapter.

Other important ideas about fighting the plague, beyond the religious, are visible in the development of the *lazaretto vecchio*. In the *lazaretto vecchio*, distance was kept between the Prior and the sick. The *Priorado* (Prior's house) and garden were connected by a small bridge to the rest of the *lazaretto vecchio*. The *Priorado* was a two-storey, balconied structure. The layout was designed to limit contact between the sick and merchandise. The issue of separation was of concern throughout the history of the *lazaretto vecchio*. As will be seen in following chapters, this concern about separation became increasingly prominent during the seventeenth and eighteenth centuries. In 1702, the four rooms known as *la cavana*, which literally means an underground stream – so it may have been a particularly boggy part of the island – were said to be of concern because two of the rooms faced out onto the courtyard of the *lazaretto* and the other two onto the Prior's garden. The balconies of the rooms, onto which the patients ventured to receive light, were so positioned that it was possible for the patients to throw items into the garden or into the section of *la cavana* as, it was said,

---

[93]   ASV, PSMc b. 361 D6, 15r 'Hospitale vetustate collapsum/ Divi Marci Procuratores de Citra/ Veri Pii, ac soli Gubernatores/ ut qui a languoribui cruciantur/ comodicii libernetur;/ summa cura instaurari iusserunt/ anno salutis nostre 1565/ mense maii'.

[94]   Dante, *The Divine Comedy* (Oxford, 2008), p. 56.

had happened during the past few months. Two of the rooms were turned over to use by the Priors. The other two had the balconies and doorways in question walled up.[95] The Health Office officials continued to be concerned about the secret movement of individuals and communication between the sick. In 1732, officials ordered that a wooden staircase within the *lazaretto vecchio*, which led from the portico of the Prior into the *lazaretto*, should be destroyed because the passageway was said to be *occulta* (hidden).[96] A month later this staircase must have been continuing to cause problems – it had earned the label of the scandalous staircase (*scandalosa scala*)![97]

At the beginning of the sixteenth century, the *lazaretto vecchio* consisted of the earlier monastic complex of the church, well and double-stored, porticoed building, with a *Priorado* and Prior's garden. The complex was surrounded by a perimeter wall and only used part of the space on the island. In 1506, a separate area was developed for the disinfection of goods: one of the courtyards was closed off using walls of a convenient height and width, without windows and with a single doorway. Within this courtyard, a house was built with a portico, rooms and windows.[98] On the island, there was also a public gun powder deposit known as a *casello di polvere*. Its structure was that of a rectangular base topped by a pyramid roof. The *caselli* were built on various islands of the lagoon, including both *lazaretti*, as well as in cities of the *terraferma* during the sixteenth century.[99] They were developed in the aftermath of the fire at the Arsenal in 1569 to store the dangerous but essential gun powder out of the city on the separate and yet conveniently located islands of the lagoon. The *casello* in the *lazaretto vecchio* no longer survives. The two examples in the *lazaretto nuovo* remain with later, replacement roofs. In the *lazaretto nuovo*, both were built in white Istrian stone and on one a carving of the lion of St Mark survives.

During the sixteenth century, the *lazaretto vecchio* had separate hospitals for men and women. Men and women were separated, it was said, in order to avoid issues of dishonesty and disorder. We will see in the next chapter that, for a while, this division by gender was made between the two islands but evolved into division between hospital buildings. The two hospitals had their own, separate wells.[100] Various wells were constructed in the *lazaretti* and can be helpful indications of the ways in which the hospital structures were subdivided. In the *lazaretto vecchio* the sick were cared for in hospital wards. Although this may be surprising for

---

[95]   ASV, Sanità 745 169r (11 July 1702).

[96]   ASV, Sanità 751 146r (10 June 1732).

[97]   ASV, Sanità 751 149r (11 July 1732).

[98]   ASV, Sanità reg. 12 13r (13 October 1506).

[99]   Others were built on San Lazaro, San Clemente, Santo Spirito, San Giorgio in Alga and San Secondo. See Gerolamo Fazzini – Giovanni Battista Stefinlongo 'I "caselli da polvere"' in Gerolamo Fazzini (ed.), *Venezia: isola del lazzaretto nuovo*, pp. 67–70.

[100]   ASV, PSMc b. 361 D6 9r (10 marzo 1533) and ASV, PSMc b. 360 book 5 *poliza* 91 (28 February 1587).

patients infected with infectious disease, this was done in order to enable high quality care for patients.

In his discussion of the *lazaretto* in Genoa, Father Antero Maria wrote that large wards were supposed to enable high quality temporal and spiritual care. In terms of temporal remedies, he wrote, what the eyes do not see, the heart does not feel (*occhio non vede, cuor non duole*). Even a staff member with a heart of stone, would eventually be entreated to help the sick in need in a ward but not, he says in a separate rooms. In terms of spiritual remedies, scandals were said to occur in private rooms – particularly when you put three or four vile people together (which, he notes, most of the patients in the *lazaretti* were). In large infirmaries, however, there are not these dangers because of the number of witnesses in other patients and staff. It is also possible to celebrate Mass, pray and administer the sacraments whenever there is need – whereas if someone wants to do that in every room, they would lose their voice and breath before finishing the job.[101] He also added that hospital wards needed to be large because otherwise air would corrupt (literally become poisonous) and the intolerable stench of a smaller space would be too much for staff to endure.[102] The debate regarding the best form for hospital architecture regarding the accommodation of patients would endure through the centuries, as architects and administrators attempted to balance issues of infection and the benefits of separation with the ability to supervise behaviour efficiently. In the *lazaretti*, open wards did not give way to private rooms as the dominant space for the sick until the eighteenth century, despite concerns about contagion.

In addition to providing broad indications of the use of space, archival material indicates more than anything else that the hospital buildings were put under particular strain by overcrowding during outbreaks of disease in the city. Various periods of building work were dedicated to securing or repairing the structures.[103] In 1561, work was carried out to rebuild a hospital for the sick in the *lazaretto vecchio* although it is unclear whether this was the hospital for women, for men or both.[104] In 1575, the women's hospital, the men's hospital and buildings for the doctor and for the body clearers were all noted as being repaired.[105] The final account book of the Procurators of St Mark covers various building projects. Yet again, the women's hospital is noted as being in a poor state of repair. Unfortunately, no information has been found regarding the design of the hospital buildings or their internal decoration, comparable to that for Milan and Florence.[106]

---

[101]　Father Antero Maria da San Bonaventura, *Li lazaretti della città e riviere di Genova*, p. 8.

[102]　Ibid., p. 1.

[103]　See, for example, PSMc b. 360 book 4 17r (24 April 1551).

[104]　Ibid., book 5: 'Conto di la fabrica del ospedal se fa da nuovo al lazaretti vechio'.

[105]　ASV, PSMc b. 334 book 3 227v (8 July 1575).

[106]　Luca Beltrami, 'Il lazzaretto di Milano', pp. 410–11 and John Henderson, *The Renaissance hospital*, part two, chapter five, '"Splendid houses of treatment built at vast expense": wards and the care of the body and soul', pp. 147–85.

A detailed plan of the *lazaretto nuovo* [Plate 13] shows a larger structure than that of the sixteenth-century institution but is a useful starting point from which to identify general features. This can be supplemented by valuable archaeological evidence. The *lazaretto nuovo* was enclosed by a perimeter wall, which was enlarged as the hospital grew. During the sixteenth century, the external wall seems to have been that of the earlier monastic structure. Archaeological work has uncovered foundations of a wall which ran along the western side of the island from the chapel – setting that building into the corner of the original structure. During its time as a monastic site, this area of land around the chapel was the focus for the island, with much of the rest being left as cultivated land. The small cemetery (*campo santo*), also marked on the 1687 plan, was placed near to the early chapel and was a further feature of the original monastery. Later, this area was used for burials, although further archaeological work is required in order to pin down the extent to which it was utilised during the sixteenth-century plague outbreaks.

The early sixteenth-century *lazaretto nuovo* contained the chapel, the cemetery, rooms for quarantine and the *Priorado* (Prior's house). The latter structure was built in the vineyard on the island, at the opposite end of the island from the original centre near to the church. The location was designed to keep the Prior at as safe a distance as possible from those being quarantined. In front of the *Priorado* was the *pontil* (or mooring area) of the island where patients, goods and supplies would arrive.[107] Although kept at a distance from the original centre of the island, the Prior was able to supervise the various movements on and off the island.

The original chapel in the *lazaretto nuovo* was replaced between 1532–33. A fragment of a capital from an external column survives inscribed with the year 1533. Inside the church, Cicogna recorded an inscription on the wall of the chapel dating from 1533 and describing the role of the Prior Cristoforo de' Bartolis in the rebuilding of the church. The other inscriptions dated from the eighteenth century.[108] Archaeological work has found traces of three former chapel structures. The first, undated, had a different orientation from the later two. The second chapel dates from the early sixteenth century. The third structure is said to have been built during the second half of the century. Archival research does not confirm the presence of a new church during the second half of the sixteenth century, however, and neither is such a thesis supported by the survival of inscriptions from 1533 in place in the eighteenth century. Little documentation has been uncovered regarding the rebuilding of the chapel. Neither the motivations for the rebuilding nor the materials and structure of the building are clear. By the eighteenth century, there was a small additional chapel (*oratorio*) with an altar containing a figure of Mary of the seven sorrows near to the entranceway to the island. The depiction of the Virgin of Sorrows (or *Mater Dolorosa*) was one of the two most popular styles of depiction of the Virgin Mary of the seventeenth century – the other being as the

---

[107] ASV, PSMc b. 360 book 5 *polizze* 40 and 41 (16 November 1586).

[108] BMC, Codice Cicogna, 2018 (Iscrizione veneziane inedite), isole, b. 509:2 (Lazzaretto nuovo).

Virgin of the Immaculate Conception. Both modes produced powerful Catholic-Reformation imagery.[109]

As with the *lazaretto vecchio*, there is frustratingly little evidence regarding the interior decoration of the church of the *lazaretto nuovo*. An inventory of the contents of the church survives from 1739.[110] A number of the items are listed as being old and damaged, such as the main altar. Here, the painting on the altarpiece depicted Mary, with the baby Jesus in her arms, St Roch, St Sebastian and St Francis with halo (*zogietta*). The associated equipment for the Mass is described, along with other liturgical items, such as the blanket to cover the altarpiece during Holy Week. The altar displayed a large wooden crucifix along with a further smaller crucifix. Another crucifix was attached to the chapel's wall. Above the doorway a wooden figure of St Roch was prominent. The chapel was also said to include three paintings, showing St Carlo Borromeo, a nativity scene and a paper image of St Antony. By 1700, this chapel was being referred to as the Church of the Madonna and St Roch.[111]

The largest and most prominent building in the *lazaretto nuovo,* unlike the *lazaretto vecchio,* was not the chapel but the *tezon grande* (the warehouse), which was built in 1561. It was pillared and runs the length of the open grass area (*prado*). The warehouse was designed to store the merchandise of incoming merchants and the goods of those undergoing quarantine. The structure is 102 metres long and 22 metres wide and was originally arched. There were seventy archways in total which exposed the goods to wind and to sunshine for disinfection. When the island was taken over as a military site, these were bricked up but are still visible [Plate 14]. The building is divided into two identical sections by an internal wall. The structure is interesting not only for its scale – an indication of the extent to which the island was used to house and disinfect goods – but also for the graffiti uncovered on its internal walls, which will be returned to in Chapter 2. Graffiti in similar buildings also exists in the *lazaretto vecchio* although it has not yet been documented and studied.[112] In scale, the *tezon grande* in the *lazaretto nuovo* was second only to the *corderia* (rope factory) of the Venetian Arsenal. The *tezon*

---

[109]   The seven sorrows of Mary were said to be Simeon's prophecy in Luke 2, 33–5, the flight into Egypt, Jesus taking leave of his mother, their meeting on the road to Calvary, the Passion and the entombment. Increasingly during the Baroque period these sorrows were depicted, echoing Simeon's prophecy, as daggers through Mary's heart. Good examples of this dramatic imagery have been included in two recent exhibitions on art and sculpture and are illustrated and described in the exhibition catalogue. Michael Snodin and Nigel Llewellyn, *Baroque: style in the age of magnificence 1620–1800* (London, 2009), pp. 244–6 provides an engaging discussion in the context of the New World and Xavier Bray, *The sacred made real: Spanish painting and sculpture 1600–1700* (London, 2009), pp. 144–8 in a Spanish context.

[110]   ASV, Sanità b.1009 contains the series of eighteenth-century inventories.

[111]   ASV, Sanità 745, 134v (2 December 1700).

[112]   For a discussion of the graffiti see Chapter 2, p. 96 and Chapter 3, p. 132.

grande shared some architectural features with the *corderia*, including the balcony to allow supervision of disinfection work in the former structure and manufacture in the latter.

For accommodating patients, the *lazaretto nuovo* was notionally divided into four zones, three of which were named *orto*, *pra[do]* and *sanità*. These labels referred to the garden, the grassed open area and a section called 'health'. In 1503 the Prior was instructed to leave the rooms he inhabited and return to those set aside for the Prior so that the *lazaretto nuovo* could be administered using the division into four parts and the sick could change area every ten days. At the end of the forty-day quarantine, the patients could then be licensed to leave with the assurance that they were clean and the inconveniences which could occur as a result of having all of the patients remain together would be avoided.[113] The rooms discovered near the well, which run alongside the perimeter wall between the *Priorado* and the original chapel, were individual cells with fireplaces but it is not clear when they were developed on the island. Three additional rooms were constructed for the *lazaretto nuovo* in 1528.[114] In addition, in 1548–49 building work was carried out in the vineyard of the *lazaretto nuovo* where thirty rooms were built.[115] This building work gradually extended the capacity of the sites rather than altering the way in which the hospitals were administered.

As we have seen, most patients were kept together in the Venetian plague hospitals – in the male and female hospital wards in the *lazaretto vecchio* or in groups in the *lazaretto nuovo*. Originally, in Venice, those in the *lazaretto nuovo* were supposed to sleep in separate rooms (often one per family) but moved round the hospital structure in groups. There was no sense of patients being in strict isolation and this was not seen to cause problems – in fact, as we will see in later chapters, this contact was seen to have a number of collective benefits. During the earlier period, isolation was reserved for the most vulnerable and most dangerous patients in plague hospitals. It was only during the seventeenth century, that the Venetian Health Office acknowledged that various problems could arise from the lack of isolation within the hospitals and that infection could spread quickly hence the architectural changes made to render these hospitals more isolating structures. By the seventeenth century, when greater isolation was desired, the problems of retaining the sick within designated areas of the hospital structure were recognised elsewhere too. In an account which survives from the head of the plague hospital in Genoa, Father Antero Maria da San Bonaventura, he wrote of the great difficulty in governing patients within institutions such as the *lazaretto nuovo* – in fact, he describes them as the most difficult group to govern. They were, for the most part, healthy enough to be able to walk wherever they chose within the hospitals and were affected by the obvious issue of boredom. He also wrote that those convalescing, having beaten death, thought of themselves as immortal

---

113 ASV, Sanità 725 75r (3 June 1503).
114 ASV, Consiglio di Dieci, parti comuni, filza 8 186 (1528).
115 ASV, PSMc b. 360 no 3, 8r (24 October 1549).

and so had little or no interest in being isolated. Father Antero recommended trying to fill the patients' days with *lodevoli esercitii*, as St Carlo Borromeo had done earlier. Perhaps Sansovino's description of prayers and psalms in the plague hospital was right![116]

The Health Office officials were often forced to record the dilapidated state of the islands, particularly following serious outbreaks of plague. From account books, fragments of information can be found in the midst of entries on the materials supplied, noting details such as the raising of the pavement of the *lazaretto nuovo* in 1545.[117] In 1586, for example, the state of the buildings was described as poor (*cattivo*), with holes in the perimeter walls.[118] The strains of the physical environment of the islands and of plague epidemics took their toll on the *lazaretti* buildings, some of which predated the foundation of the hospitals. In Venice, the *lazaretto* sites developed gradually and were extended in times of need. Sites were used to separate the sick from those suspected of having contracted the disease. This contrasts with examples from elsewhere in Europe, where purpose-built *lazaretti* were constructed and single sites could be divided to cater for both sick and healthy. These latter sites were thought to be more prone to spread infection and mortality. Paolo Bellintani, for example, wrote that mortality levels were lower in places where multiple sites were used and compared the low rates suffered in Milan with the higher rates in Brescia and Marseilles.[119] Conversely though, single sites were thought to be more economical structures than the systems which operated with two separate hospitals, not least because they avoided problems of transportation between locations. The variety of plague hospitals was considerable. What follows is intended to give a degree of insight into that variety and sketch out the most common elements of the structures.

The Design of Italian and European *Lazaretti*

Lazaretti were not usually purpose-built. For convenience, existing buildings were often requisitioned; by far the most common sites to be used were either monastic or military. A number of practical considerations shaped the use of these religious and defensive structures. Plague hospitals needed to be a convenient distance from towns and cities – far enough away to minimise the spread of infection and close enough to facilitate the delivery of people, goods and supplies. Both monastic and military sites were often placed on the boundaries of settlements and, indeed, were some of the most common buildings on the outskirts of cities. The demand for quarantine and hospital structures in times of plague was high: a number of

---

[116]   Father Antero Maria da San Bonaventura, *Li lazaretti della città e riviere di Genova*, p. 506.

[117]   ASV, PSMc b. 360 no 1 (13 October 1545).

[118]   ASV, Sanità reg. 3 51v (30 August 1586).

[119]   'La peste é proprio come un fuoco' in Paolo Bellintani, *Dialogo della peste*, p. 149.

buildings were required.[120] The often unexpected strain of epidemics meant that the size and number of sites took precedence over the quality of the architecture. This can be seen in cities and countries across Europe: in Sardinia, convent sites were used for the *lazaretto* and convalescent hospital. A castle was used as the quarantine hospital. Rural churches were said to be needed for individuals and families of rank who had voluntarily left their homes. The sites had to be spacious: the convent of the Magdalen, for example, was used to contain two hundred sick and was sufficiently large to be able to separate the sick from the suspected and the men from the women.[121] In Palermo, a monastic site and a former leper hospital were used as two of the city's *lazaretti*.[122] In Cividale del Friuli four *lazaretti* were used alongside policies of household quarantine.[123] The authorities took over three religious institutions and the members of the religious orders were moved to a private house. The fourth site consisted of wooden structures (*casoni*) built at the side of one of the convents. Three of these sites were used for quarantine and convalescing and the fourth was used for the sick. In the first three, patients were given separate rooms, in the fourth the sick were at least four to a room. The size of at least one of the sites was sufficient to accommodate 150 patients.

An association with defensive and religious structures is appropriate for plague hospitals in a number of respects, including their architectural scale and the quantity of available sites. In addition to their availability, there were qualities of the architectural design of both types of buildings which recommended them as hospitals: high walls and open spaces meant that protection could be offered to those on the inside and outside. Fresh air could circulate freely through the buildings, improving health. In religious sites, cloisters which, on the Continent at least, were not usually glazed, encouraged the movement of fresh air through the buildings and the locations had plenty of open space. *Portici* within the city were described as highly ornamental, an adoption from classical architecture, which provided citizens shelter from the sun, rain and snow and every 'nuisance from the wickedness of the air'. The church was often placed centrally in order to be widely visible. The general characteristics of *lazaretti* buildings can be identified in the plan of the *lazaretto* at Milan [Plate 15]. The sites had prominent (and, indeed, increasingly prominent) chapels, ample space for disinfection (whether it be open ground or warehouses) and finally the space to separate the sick from the suspected and men from women.

Some studies of plague hospital architecture have already been provided by other scholars. In general, however, the designs of institutions have been described in passing. There is extant information about the plague hospital at Ulm, based

---

[120]   See, for example, Father Antero Maria da San Bonaventura, *Li lazaretti della città e riviere di Genova* for the number of institutions used in Genoa and its territory.

[121]   Francesco Manconi, *Castigo de Dios*, pp. 170–71 and p. 174.

[122]   Ingrassia, pp. 213–15.

[123]   Mario Brozzi, *Peste, fede e sanità in una cronaca cividalese del 1598* (Milan, 1982), p. 33.

upon a surviving seventeenth-century ground plan.[124] Here, a single building was used to accommodate the healthy, the infected and some of the hospital's staff. Patients were accommodated in wards, which contained a fireplace and a number of windows to encourage the circulation of air. In her discussion of the structure, Anne Marie Kinzelbach claims that the beds for patients were designed to be placed in rows in the centre of the ward, rather than around the edges, in order to keep patients away from humidity and drafts. The structure also contained a large courtyard, on the south side of the building, with a well and area for bathing. In Ulm, the functions of the plague hospital were combined on a single site.

There is limited information regarding the relationship between architecture and health in the context of plague hospitals; most authors pass brief and general comments on the site and situation of the buildings.[125] The English writer Thomas Lodge [?1558–1625] composed a treatise on the plague and included a chapter dedicated to the appropriate setting for a plague hospital. He writes that the building should be orientated so as to ensure that the northern wind passes through the structure since, of all of the winds, it is the 'most dry and healthfull'. Lodge also advises that the buildings be situated 'in no place that abutteth on dong hils'! He recommended that the building be equipped with separate rooms for patients, which are adjoining, as in religious houses. In Florence in 1630, the *lazaretto* at Badia Fiesolana was established in an elevated position so that the sick could benefit from the excellent air (*aria buonissima*).[126] In Father Antero Maria's account of Genoa, he opened his book by reflecting that there was no more appropriate site for a plague hospital, than that of the convent *Santa Maria della Consolatione.* It was situated on a tall hill (*alto colle*), neither too close to the city, nor excessively close to residential areas. It was exposed to the Aquilonari wind, which he said was the destroyer of pestiferous vapours and adorned with flower beds and gardens (*horti e giardini*) for the pleasure and recreation of those convalescing. The site was served by a good water supply, said to be necessary where a large number of filthy people (*lordure*) congregate. It was also large enough, not only for the significant number of rooms and offices but also for the large church. Above all, it was said to have the enclosed convent adjacent to the Orphan's hospital (*casa delli orfani*) which was built in the form of a hospital with a large infirmary. A large infirmary, he said, was the most important thing in a *lazaretto.*[127] Beyond general

---

[124]   See Anne-Marie Kinzelbach, 'Hospitals, medicine and society: southern German imperial towns in the sixteenth century', *Renaissance studies*, 15:2 (2001), pp. 217–28.

[125]   Very useful ground plans of institutions in seventeenth-century Rome can be found in Cardinal Geronimo Gastaldi, *Tractatus de avertenda et profliganda peste* although they have not be used here because they fall beyond the chronological boundaries of this study.

[126]   John Henderson, '"La schifezza, madre della corruzione". Peste e società nella Firenze della prima età moderna: 1630-1631', *Medicina e storia*, 1:2 (2001), p. 37.

[127]   Father Antero Maria da San Bonaventura, *Li lazaretti della città e riviere di Genova*, p. 1.

observations such as these, however, the theoretical literature on the ideal form for a plague hospital is fairly limited, until the eighteenth century.

A rich and unusual example of architectural description is provided by the physician Giovan Filippo Ingrassia of the *lazaretto* known as Cubba. He includes an image of the site, as well as a detailed description of the function of the space. He noted qualities of the location as being airy, not too far from the city, with an abundant water supply to allow for the thorough washing of infected goods, space to be able to extend the structures if necessary and with a North Easterly aspect.[128] Ingrassia records a female and male hospital, kitchen, store room, chapel and cemetery and rooms for medical personnel. In addition to detailing the division made between the sick – in adjacent, wooden structures – Ingrassia notes the utility of separating men and women as well as those with or without fevers. Finally, the chapel, although not centrally placed within the institution was designed for the administration of Mass and also, Ingrassia emphasises, baptism for babies born within the hospital.[129]

In addition to these descriptions, plague hospital architecture can be considered through a number of case-studies of the best documented purpose-built sites. Verona provides a useful example. Initially, the city authorities made use of religious institutions to serve as plague hospitals. During the Wars of Cambrai on the Venetian mainland, however, the original plague hospital was destroyed, like many of the buildings outside the city walls. In January 1539, the decision was taken to build a permanent *lazaretto*. The preamble to the decision stated that well-instituted cities must care and provide not simply for the present but also for the future and the rebuilding of the *lazaretto* was an important element in this provision.[130] By January 1549, Veronese officials had obtained the permission, site and a model for their *lazaretto*.[131] Unusually for a plague hospital, the Veronese structure has been the focus for a significant number of twentieth-century studies, concerning the original architect of the hospital. Giorgio Vasari [1511–74] attributed the design of the Veronese *lazaretto* to Michele Sanmicheli [1484–1559] and later studies have attempted to prove or disprove this assertion.[132] The thesis of Lionello Puppi has been one of the more recent attempts to attribute the *lazaretto* to Sanmicheli.[133] The unavoidable problem encountered by those who seek to follow through on this attribution, however, is the lack of archival documentation in support of such a claim. The works of more recent authors have

---

[128]   Ingrassia, p. 215.

[129]   Ibid., p. 220.

[130]   'officium est, uno omnis cuiusque bene institutae Republica omni cura et prudentia non solu' presentia verum et futura respicere' ASVer, Sanità, reg. 2 1r (7 January 1539).

[131]   ASVer, ACA, Atti del consiglio, reg. 81 68r (21 January 1549).

[132]   Giorgio Vasari, *Lives of the painters, sculptors and architects* (2 vols, London, 1996), volume two, pp. 395–417 for the entry on Sanmicheli (the reference to his work at the *lazaretto* is on p. 406).

[133]   Lionello Puppi, *Michele Sanmicheli: architetto di Verona* (Padua, 1971), pp. 102–6.

used the ambiguity of the sources to open up the possibility that the design of the *lazaretto* should be attributed elsewhere.[134]

As a consequence of the debate, a number of studies have been produced with the admirable aim of convincing the authorities of the historical importance of the site. These publications, dating from around the mid-twentieth century, are often illustrated with a number of photographs. From these sources, it can be seen that, until the explosion there in 1945, the *lazaretto* consisted of a rectangular structure around a large open courtyard, porticoed on each side.[135] Within the portico, each archway corresponded to a room, of which there were 152.[136] At the centre stood a grand, circular chapel (*tempietto*), which contained an altar at its heart, designed to be visible from each of the rooms within the hospital [Plate 16]. The internal decoration of the chapel is difficult to assess but the dome was topped by a lead statue of St Roch.[137] The hospital as a whole was divided into four zones for quarantine, which were kept separate by two long walls which divided the rectangular space into four irregular trapeziums but which do not survive. Each of these zones was seen as being fairly self-contained, having, for example, its own well to provide a separate supply of water. Since these dividing walls radiate out from the *tempietto*, which was a seventeenth-century addition, it can be assumed that this formal, physical separation of the *lazaretto* into zones did not take shape until this period. This does not, of course, negate the possibility that the *lazaretto* was administered according to a policy within which the structure was divided into four segments, as in the *lazaretto nuovo*, before these walls were constructed.[138]

---

[134]   These debates were summarised by Piero Gazzola, who paid particular attention to the work of Pellegrini and Sancassini on the subject. Sancassini, like Vené before him, worked through this issue by separating the design of the *lazaretto* from the design of the *tempietto*. Whereas, Vené had argued that only the latter installation was executed according to an original design of Sanmicheli's, Sancassini has strong doubts concerning the hand of Sanmicheli on either section of the design, particularly that of the *tempietto* since it was constructed so much later. See Piero Gazzola (ed.), *Michele Sanmicheli* (Venice, 1960); Giulio Sancassini, 'Il lazaretto di Verona è del Sanmicheli?', *Atti e memorie della Accademia di agricoltura scienze e lettere di Verona*, serie vi, vol x (1958–59), pp. 365–77; F. Pellegrini, 'Il lazaretto di Verona', *Studi storici veronese*, 2 (1949–50), pp. 143–93; Armando Vené, 'Il lazaretto vecchio di Verona', *Dedalo* 12 (1932), pp. 253–9.

[135]   On the explosion, see the introduction to Gian Paolo Marchi, *'Il gran contagio di Verona' di Francesco Pona* (Verona, 1972).

[136]   This was measured during the twentieth century as being 238.68 metres long and 117.11 metres wide. The two longest sides consisted of fifty-one archways each and the two smaller contained twenty-four each.

[137]   Eric Langenskiöld, *Michele Sanmicheli: the architect of Verona* (Uppsala, 1938). This statuette is referred to being in the Museo Castelvecchio in A. Vené 'Il lazaretto vecchio di Verona', p. 256.

[138]   For plans of this division see A. Vené, 'Il lazaretto vecchio di Verona', p. 253. For the work carried out 'pro fabrica ecclesia lazareti' see ASVer, SILT, 28, 133r (4 March 1602).

This building occupied the same area as the earlier *lazaretto* structure.[139] This original structure was said to have been split in two by a wall running down the middle and to have had fourteen rooms on each side and twenty-seven running along the longest side. The early *lazaretto* has a strong defensive element to the design, with two bastion-like towers in the corners.[140] This was not the only *lazaretto* used in Verona. Further sites had been established at *Campo Marzo* and at the church of the *Crucifisso*. Both had the function of the *lazaretto nuovo*, as a place for the disinfection of goods and individuals who were suspected rather than infected.[141] Goods were also disinfected at the Castel San Piero. In 1575, the use of sites within the city was described as 'dangerous, infamous and inconvenient' and it was decreed that, in the future, *lazaretti* were not to be set up within the city itself. Instead, all of the infected and suspected patients were to be sent to the *lazaretto* alone, which was to be developed with other rooms.[142] This was part of the motivation for the Baroque development of the structure. The importance of the site was recognised and the experiences of the severe outbreak of 1575–77 prompted the Veronese Council to commit money and energy during the 1590s into developing and enlarging the plague hospital. The specific nature of the redesign was influenced by developing Catholic-Reformation ideas regarding the intensified religious purpose of the sites.

A gradual development of the plague hospital structure is also true of Padua. During the sixteenth century, the *lazaretto* was a practical, pragmatic structure with a notable lack of religious focus to the design [Plate 17]. Three account books survive for the building of the Paduan *lazaretto*, covering the period between 1533 and 1543, although two are more detailed than the third.[143] These offer patchy insights into the building process. The books outline some important elements of the building structure. In 1534, eight rooms were built, followed by a further nineteen later in the year. Each of these later rooms was constructed with fireplaces. By 1536, thirty rooms had been built, along with one large room for the disinfection of goods and a kitchen, although part of the structure was still without

---

[139]   These are reprinted in Lia Camerlengo 'Il lazaretto a San Pancrazio e l'ospedale della Misericordia in Bra: le forme dell'architettura' in Alessandro Pastore, Gian Maria Varanini, Paola Marini and Giorgio Marini (eds), *L'ospedale e la città: cinquecento anni d'arte a Verona* (Verona, 1996), pp. 179–91.

[140]   Similar, military elements of the design can be seen in the instructions regarding the *lazaretto* in Corfu; the building was to have towers built in two corners from which it was possible to see the whole of the site. ASV, Sanità reg. 16 13r (10 September 1588).

[141]   These are described in Alessandro Canobbio, *Il successo della peste occorsa in Padova l'anno MDLXXVI* (Padua, 1576), 3r.

[142]   ASVer, Sanità reg. 2 7r (9 September 1575).

[143]   The three books are ASP, Sanità b. 337, b. 575 and b. 585. Of these, b. 575 only describes entries in 1534 and 1537 in brief. b. 337 concerns the years 1543 and 1544 although in more detail than b. 575. b. 585 covers the full period 1533–43.

a roof.[144] The structure included a portico, sixty *pertiche* (*c.*120 metres) long.[145] It was noted that accommodation was needed for a thousand sick, which was not available at that time. In 1537, a further seven rooms are described. These were placed within a porticoed structure, followed by a further four later in the same year. Thirty-eight rooms are described. The account books also mention a large kitchen, containing seven fireplaces, with rooms above it, which was built facing the river in 1537. Between 1543 and 1544 sums of money were set aside to pay for windows and staircases. Alessandro Canobbio's description of the structure from 1577 is one of the most detailed to survive.[146] It describes the *lazaretto* as a square building complex, with each side being seventy *pertiche* (*c.*140 metres) long. The side facing the river was two storeys high and contained rooms for the sick numbering 300. There was a large warehouse (*gran capanna*) for goods. In total, between the *lazaretto* and the temporary structures that were placed on surrounding land, there was said to be room for 1,000 people at any given time. The *lazaretto* had a central courtyard with a porticoed cloister surrounding it. The structure included wells and bread ovens. As described for Verona, the *lazaretto* in Padua was developed further through the addition of a central chapel in the aftermath of the outbreak of 1630–31.

The plague hospital at Leiden provides a further, excellent example of a purpose-built site [Plate 1], as well as elements of seventeenth-century *lazaretto* developments, albeit within a different confessional context. In 1635, the authorities replaced the earlier institution with a wooden structure to the west of the city.[147] This, in turn, was replaced by a brick building – constructed between 1657 and 1661 under the master builder Huybert Corneliszoon van Duyvenvlucht. The purpose-built site, however, was never used as a plague hospital. It is a representative of the seventeenth-century development in architecture, which was referred to in the Introduction. In place of the Italian Baroque circular chapels, the distinctive feature of the Leiden site is the beautiful order and symmetry of the design. Arranged in a series of squares, the main building of the hospital was split down the middle by a waterway. The building lacks the porticoes of the Italian structures and instead has a number of distinctive small windows and large chimneys. The building is surrounded by two defensive elements: a moat and ring of trees planted two deep. The deliberate design of the site shows an element of the geometric symmetry which would become a hallmark of eighteenth-century *lazaretto* design.[148]

---

[144] ASP, ACA, Atti del consiglio b. 14 248r (31 October 1536).

[145] Ibid. 304v (1 May 1537).

[146] Alessandro Canobbio, *Il successo della peste*, 21v–22v.

[147] For the institution in Leiden see also the Introduction pp. 23–4.

[148] The design of *lazaretto* structures during the eighteenth century is one of the few areas of the subject which has been well-covered. For a reproduction of a number of plans see Nelli-Elena Vanzan Marchini, *Rotte mediterranee e baluardi di sanità: Venezia e i lazzaretti mediterranei: catalogo di una mostra* (Milan, 2004) and for a useful study of

Beyond the general features of plague hospitals in Catholic Italy – prominent chapels, ample space for disinfection of goods and the division of the structure to separate groups of patients – the development of these hospitals was determined by practical, local issues, including the availability of sites, local building materials and the money available to invest in public health. In Venice, existing buildings on the lagoon islands were adapted. As a result, the overall structure was not as coherent as later, purpose-built hospitals. Instead, there was a patchwork development of necessary structures, which combined different architectural styles.

The Venetian *lazaretti* were often described as singular, as institutions shaped by the history and nature of the city; paradoxically, that was the most representative feature about them. In Venice and elsewhere, the *lazaretti* formed part of wider systems of charity and welfare and were shaped by their immediate contexts. The use of space within the Venetian plague hospitals and within the wider city is illustrative of medical and social concerns; so too are the metaphors employed by contemporaries to describe the early modern Venetian *lazaretti*. The two accounts studied at length in this chapter are extreme examples of polarised interpretations of the institutions. Both because of that and in spite of that they can be of use to the historian. They convey something of the desperate attempts to cope with the plague on behalf of the state and the despair felt by contemporaries as their homes and beloved city were transformed by a force over which they seemingly had little direct control. The imagery of Paradise and Hell was pervasive in descriptions of the hospitals and these were powerful ideas. Nevertheless, despite the images of Paradise, Purgatory and Hell, journeys to the plague hospitals were not intended to be Dantean trips to the afterlife. The function of the sites was not to provide antechambers of death – the sheer cost of administering the hospitals is indicative of genuine attempts to cure the plague. The nature of care provided to patients is outlined in chapters that follow. First, however, we need to consider how patients were sent to the plague hospitals and the sort of person who was sent: were they simply sick or did it take something other than the suspicion of infection to make you a patient at the *lazaretto*?

---

the development of structures in the Mediterranean see Daniel Panzac, *Quarantaines et lazarets: l'Europe et la peste d'Oriente (XVIIe–XXe siècles)* (Aix-en-Provence, 1986).

Chapter 2
The Sick-Poor

In March 1555 in Venice, a house in San Nicolò was found to contain four sick people and two dead bodies. The bodies were sent for immediate burial on the *lazaretto vecchio* and the sick were also sent to the plague hospitals, accompanied by the Health Office doctor and *pizzigamorti* (body clearers). A number of the houses within the district were closed up and the inhabitants were sent to the island of San Anzolo de Concordia for quarantine. The houses of the sick were emptied of all items and cleaned by the *pizzigamorti*. The houses were stripped bare – workers were instructed not to leave even a rag in these homes for risk of reinfection when people returned.[1] This brief episode marked the beginning of a plague epidemic in Venice and the measures taken illustrate a number of important points about public health in relation to the plague. Although every individual must have had different experiences during periods of plague, quarantine was, counter-intuitively, often a collective experience. Families, districts and parishes were often quarantined at the same time.[2] Journeys to the plague hospital were made in groups and the departure points differed depending on your area of residence. Venice's layout, with its notable lack of division into neighbourhoods by social status, meant that a cross section of people would have been affected at any given time. Even within the plague hospitals, as we saw in the previous chapter, quarantine was often carried out in zones. Only a few individuals were separated from the crowd, for isolation in its truest sense; these groups included the most dangerous and most vulnerable patients. This chapter will consider the structures by which individuals were sent into quarantine as well as the patients who were sent to the plague hospitals, by social status, age and gender. The identity of the patients will be compared with contemporary ideas about the stereotypes of plague victims.

This chapter will also place introductions to the plague in the context of broader social policies and, in so doing, will illustrate that Ann Carmichael's assertion that 'plague did not create the need for controlling the poor and the propertyless [but rather] the causal relationship may have been the reverse' does not apply to the context of Venice.[3] This may be an appropriate causal relationship in the context of Florence, a city in which permanent responses to the plague in the form of

---

[1] Cucino 5v–12r (31 March–12 April 1555).

[2] For the same situation in Milan see Samuel K. Cohn Jr and Guido Alfani, 'Households and plague in early modern Italy', *Journal of interdisciplinary history*, 38:2 (2007), p. 198 which illustrates that entire families were sent into quarantine.

[3] Ann G. Carmichael, *Plague and the poor in Renaissance Florence* (Cambridge, 1986).

both a *lazaretto* and a Health Board, were made comparatively late. In Venice, however, the *lazaretti* were established almost a century before the introduction of social policies to control the poor and transient. The relationship between plague and poverty was not clear cut and the idea of the vilified poor, in need of control, became more prominent in Venice during the seventeenth century. In earlier centuries, debates abounded about whether it was the nature or lifestyle of the poor that made them predisposed to contract the plague. Poverty was just one of many issues addressed during epidemics and formed part of a multi-causal system of explanation for disease.

Identifying the Sick

Officially, there were two reasons why people were sent to the plague hospitals: they were diagnosed with the plague or they were suspected of having contracted the disease. Once individuals were within the plague hospital system, they could be sent back and forth between institutions for reasons of infection or convalescence. Identifying infection was no easy task. There were two main structures which operated to assess whether or not individuals needed to spend a period of time in quarantine. Outside plague epidemics, the structure was governed by the bureaucracy for trade, centring upon the *Cinque Savi sopra la mercanzia*. During epidemics, the structure was operated by the *Provveditori alla Sanità* (Health Office). It would be too simplistic to portray the structures as entirely separate but there was a shift in the balance of responsibility outside and during epidemics.

The Health Office was situated opposite the customs house [Plate 18] and this was the point within the city around which public health structures were centred. The Health Office scribe (*scrivano*) was a key figure in the bureaucracy of public health for the plague. He worked alongside the notary, captains, *fanti* (runners), *massere* (servants), guards and other employees.[4] All incoming merchandise and vessels were recorded by the scribe and it was he who was responsible for communicating the details of the newly arrived ships to the Priors (heads of hospitals) at the *lazaretti*. Once a vessel had undergone quarantine it was the responsibility of the scribe to record that the vessel had been licensed and to give a note to one of the runners who accompanied the vessels between the customs house and the *lazaretti*. The scribe also sent out the necessary funds to the Priors to accompany individual ships. Incoming merchants would have kept the Priors busy even outside plague years. In 1572, for example, fifty-three ships of varying sizes were sent to the *lazaretti*. The treatment of individuals and their goods onboard these ships was a vital and time consuming task, which will be returned to in Chapter 6.

---

[4]   For the list of workers and salary information see ASV, Sanità reg. 3 39r (16 June 1578).

The sick within the city during epidemics were identified using parish structures and the unit of the household was of paramount importance.[5] Individual heads of households were instructed to report any outbreaks of sickness to the parish priest (*piovano*), who was then responsible for sending daily collated reports to the Health Office regarding the numbers of sick and the numbers of houses which were shut up. Parish priests fulfilled vital roles in plague times. They were given the responsibility for the official *fede* (literally, faith); these *fedi* were passes to allow individuals to travel outside the city.[6] It was often stressed that visitors without a *fede* would not be allowed into cities of mainland Europe.[7] The issuing of passes was stressed as being an important matter of security to which cities should be attentive. This system relied on a culture of mutual trust. Often during periods of infection, cities were perceived to be acting in a self-interested manner and the system of passes entered into difficulties. In 1576, for example, Venetian officials wrote to Padua and to each of the cities within the *terraferma* that 'it was with enormous displeasure' that they had heard of individuals leaving Venice with the required *fedi* who were not being allowed to pass. This was described as a 'terrible prejudice' which was very damaging to the economy of the city.[8] These surviving letters highlight the lack of trust and competing priorities between cities during outbreaks of disease, which partly explained giving the job of issuing passes to parish priests.[9] The priests were also expected to monitor the social status and health of those put into quarantine and if houses of the poor were closed up, the individuals inside were expected to be given alms (*elemosina*).[10]

The use of the parish to administer public health policies was commonplace and the intersection of ecclesiastical and political structures was hardly new; the pulpit was one of the most effective tools for communication within the early modern city, with its partly illiterate society. Poor relief was often administered using the parish as the unit used to assess need and distribute care. In addition to the clergy, one nobleman and one citizen were appointed in Venice in times of plague to the parish in order to aid administration.[11] These individuals were instructed to communicate Health Office decrees, compile statistics and to make

---

[5] For detail on this system see ASV, Sanità reg. 15 445v (18 December 1576). On the sensible decision to base precautions around the household see Samuel K. Cohn Jr and Guido Alfani, 'Households and plague'.

[6] ASV, Secreta MMN 95 17r (13 June 1575) [16]. On the development of such bureaucracy in relation to identification see Valentin Groebner, *Who are you? Identification, deception and surveillance in early modern Europe* (New York, 2007); health passes (*bollette di sanità*) are dealt with in brief on p. 176.

[7] For regulations in Palermo see Ingrassia, p. 332.

[8] ASP, Sanità, b. 27 4r (23 June 1576).

[9] See Jane L. Stevens, 'The *lazaretti* of Venice, Verona and Padua (1520–1580)' (unpublished PhD. Thesis, University of Cambridge, 2008), pp. 67–8.

[10] ASV, Secreta MMN 95 17r (13 June 1575) [8].

[11] ASV, Senato Terra reg. 25 65r (n.d. August 1528).

decisions regarding the transportation of individuals to the *lazaretti*.[12] The use
of parish structures was practical and symbolic – a reflection of the relationship
between individual salvation and the public good.

In order to assist at the parish level, doctors were appointed to serve particular
districts (*sestieri*) to help with the problems of identifying and diagnosing the
plague.[13] Doctors were required to make daily visits and inspect the poor and
sick from doorways and courtyards. Two of the doctors would then take collated
information regarding the state of health of the city to the Health Office on a
daily basis. Individuals were placed into one of three categories by the doctors
within the parish: *libere*, *di rispetto* and *di suspetto*. A Health Office doctor who
worked in Venice and Padua and who had been sent to assist with an outbreak
of plague in Regno di Candia explained these categories in a report he sent back
to Venice. In order to be considered *libere* an individual had to be clear of all
suspicion. *Di rispetto* was the category used for those who may have come into
contact with infected people and goods. *Di suspetto* was used for those who were
known to have come into contact with people or goods infected with the plague.
This group was then further subdivided: *suspetti di breve pratica* for those whose
contact had been momentary or confined to a single incident and *suspetti di longa
pratica*, meaning extended contact (often used for servants and members of the
same household as someone who had died or shown signs of the illness). These
distinctions and categories were important since they determined the nature of
quarantine for individuals.[14]

As considered in the introduction, the forty-day period for quarantine was
symbolic (and literal).[15] Practical considerations meant that alternative periods were
also used. In Venice, during outbreaks, women and children could be confined to
their neighbourhoods for periods of fifteen days.[16] Similar restrictions were placed
on the inhabitants of particular islands, such as Malamocco and the Lido.[17] In
1576, those undergoing individual household quarantine were confined for periods
of eight, fourteen, twenty-two or forty days.[18] Those who had physically entered a
house which was subsequently shut up (classed as *suspetti di breve pratica*) were
quarantined for eight days. Those houses considered to be *de rispetto* because
a quick death had occurred inside (but without signs of contagion) were closed
for fourteen days. In similar cases where the signs were ambiguous houses were

---

[12]   The structure is outlined in ASV, Secreta MMN 95 17r (13 June 1575) and 107v (2
November 1576).

[13]   A list of names is provided in ASV, Secreta MMN 95 10v (22 March 1576).

[14]   ASV, Sanità 737 200r–202r (24 April 1607). Quattrocchi had sent an earlier report
on plague in Candia in ASV, Sanità 736 76r–82v (18 June 1592).

[15]   See the Introduction pp. 7–8.

[16]   ASV, Secreta MMN 95 38r (7 July 1576).

[17]   ASV, Sanità reg. 3 66r (13 January 1593).

[18]   ASV, Sanità 732 149r (13 June 1576) and 156v (1 July 1576).

closed up for twenty-two days.[19] Those unfortunate enough to have entered a house, which was subsequently shut up, more than once were classed as *suspetti di longa pratica* and duly quarantined for twenty-two days. The regulations were extremely specific: if a servant within a household died and they worked downstairs rather than upstairs (*starvia al piano et che non pratichi di sopra*) then only twenty-two rather than forty days quarantine was considered to be necessary.[20] This distinction was also made in Palermo: if a servant showed signs of the plague who worked above stairs (*dalla scala in sù*) then it was necessary to quarantine the whole house; the same was not true if the servant worked below stairs (*dalla scala in giù*).[21] On return from the *lazaretti*, individuals were expected to undergo household quarantine for a further eight days before being licensed, as illustrated in the short list of six individuals contained at the back of the register of baptisms in the parish of San Fantin between 1560 and 1629.[22]

Other factors, including the season, could determine both the length and the location for quarantine. In November 1576 increasing costs and the weather were described by the Health Office officials as making it difficult to use the open sites of the islands for goods and people, which meant that household quarantine was preferred during winter. Elsewhere on the Italian peninsula, it was recognised that a period of forty days could be insufficient for quarantine, particularly during winter. Ingrassia recognised that periods of forty-five days could be more sensible and, in winter, sixty could be more advisable.[23]

Despite the rhetoric of complete confinement and the strong response to epidemic disease that the *lazaretti* were designed to convey, they were often unable to cope with the scale of sickness and infection during periods of disease in Venice. As epidemics became more severe and the number of people in the plague hospitals rose, the complex regulations governing the use of quarantine became even more

---

[19]   ASV, Secreta MMN 95 16v (12 June 1576).

[20]   Ibid., 33v (1 July 1576). It is not entirely clear what this distinction means. The literature on households and servants does not refer to this as an official distinction. See Dennis Romano, *Housecraft and statecraft: domestic service in Renaissance Venice, 1400–1600* (Baltimore MA, 1996). Patricia Fortini Brown, *Private lives in Renaissance Venice* (London, 2004) provides valuable insight into the use of space in households but also stresses the flexibility of the layout of many properties, particularly those owned by Patrician families. In these homes, the *piano terra* often contained the laundry but the kitchen location varied (p. 82). It is difficult, therefore, to associate this distinction with particular household tasks.

[21]   Ingrassia, pp. 260–62. Ingrassia describes the servants above the stairs as normally being male servants, including young page boys. Those below the stairs are those including grooms (*mozzo di stalla*) and footmen (*staffiere*).

[22]   Archivio storico del Patriarcato di Venezia, San Fantino, libro de battizati 1560–1629, final page (unpaginated) (23 January 1576). This list survives from 1576 and details two women and a man returned from the *lazaretti* and three individuals licensed after household quarantine.

[23]   Ingrassia, p. 239 and p. 240.

elaborate. The simple theory of sending the sick and their goods to the *lazaretto vecchio* and the suspected and the convalescing to the *lazaretto nuovo* could not be maintained. Ever-spiralling costs also caused Health Office officials to look to quarantine people within the city to reduce transport and supply costs. In October 1576, four doctors within the city were asked to report on the viability of bringing individuals from the *lazaretto vecchio* directly back into the city without sending them to convalesce on the *lazaretto nuovo*.[24] A change of policy towards the *lazaretto nuovo* is visible in records showing the number of people being sent from the city to the *lazaretti* on a daily basis between August 1576 and July 1577.[25] The use of the *lazaretto nuovo* was high through to the beginning of September and then dropped off suddenly, at a point at which the numbers being sent to the *lazaretto vecchio* and the numbers of suspected plague deaths within the city increased. This change of use may also have been affected by the decision taken in November 1576 that those who had been sick for more than four days would be sent to the *lazaretto vecchio* and the healthy from infected houses or those who had been sick for fewer than four days would be sent to the *lazaretto nuovo*.[26] Concerns regarding the use of the *lazaretti* in winter may have meant that household quarantine was used more readily than the *lazaretto nuovo* for the least severe cases.

Other islands within and beyond the city were utilised as overflow sites in attempts to cope with the large numbers of sick. Sites within the city which were circumvented by water were used for quarantine and treatment. The part of San Nicolò which was surrounded by water housed those suspected of the disease from Dorsoduro in 1576.[27] This same area had been quarantined during the outbreak of 1555 between March and May. In 1576, the monastery and island of Sant'Elena was used.[28] Lagoon islands were also used to supplement the two *lazaretti*. Each was given a specific function as extensions of either the *lazaretto vecchio* or *lazaretto nuovo*. In 1575–77, for example, the *lazaretto vecchio*, San Clemente and San Lazaro were given similar functions. San Clemente was adopted when, according to the Health Office archive, there was not a free corner left in either of the two *lazaretti*.[29] San Andrea della Certosa, San Secondo, San Giacomo di Paludo and San Francesco del Deserto were all used as overflow sites for the *lazaretto nuovo* during the same outbreak.[30] A Prior was appointed to oversee the administration of most of these islands. In effect, these islands became temporary *lazaretti*. Separate islands were also required as cemeteries.[31] It was not only the inhabitants of Venice and their goods that made use of these lagoon islands. In 1576

[24]   ASV, Secreta MMN 95 127v–131r (11 February 1576).

[25]   ASV, Sanità, Necrologi 810.

[26]   ASV, Secreta MMN 95 116r (16 November 1576).

[27]   ASV, Sanità, reg. 14 378r (21 September 1576).

[28]   ASV, Senato Terra, reg. 51 90r (9 July 1576).

[29]   ASV, Secreta MMN 95 75v (22 August 1576).

[30]   ASV, Secreta MMN 95 113v (10 November 1577).

[31]   See the discussion in Chapter 5 pp. 193–4.

it was said that infected goods from Murano needed to be disinfected to the benefit of the Venetian state (*quella terra nostra*). The site of the Abbey of Borgognoni on Torcello (presumably the Abbey of San Tommaso dei Borgognoni), which had been recently sealed off, was to be used. The various extensions of the Venetian *lazaretti* significantly enlarged the capacity of the public health structures.

As described in the previous chapter, monastic islands were perfectly suited to public health use because of their clearly structured sites. Often, Health Office officials would stipulate that only parts of the islands should be used in the first instance. On Sant'Andrea della Certosa, for example, the part of the island outside the church was considered to be apt and suited to the quarantine of the sick and the disinfection of goods. Structures for disinfection were erected using supplies given by the Armouries Office (*Provveditori alle fortezze*) and Water Board (SEA).[32] Less than three weeks later it was decided that the *prado* (grassed area) was no longer sufficient and it was necessary to use the whole of the island.[33] These sites were quickly filled to capacity. In November 1576, it was said that goods could no longer be shipped for disinfection to San Francesco del Deserto, San Giacomo di Paludo, the *chiovere* (open sites in the city for disinfection), Sacagnana or San Secondo and so goods would instead be burned on San Giacomo di Paludo and San Marco Bocalama.[34]

Although the islands adopted for a public health function were often smaller islands and homes of religious communities because of the practical, existing structures and the relative ease of adoption, Venice also made use of other, larger sites, from Sacagnana to Tre porti.[35] When, in July 1576, the *lazaretto nuovo* was said to be full, the island of Mazzorbo was used to house those suspected of the disease. The island's permanent inhabitants were to be shipped out and split between Torcello and Burano.[36] This was to be done whilst Sant'Erasmo was prepared for use. The plan was to build temporary wooden structures with part of the island divided into six *sestieri*, to replicate the structure of Venice, with space divided up according to the size of each *sestiere* and the number of sick poor.[37] In August 1576, it was proposed that healthy people from the city could be housed in small and narrow homes at Lizzafusina (Fusina) on the mainland. The location was felt to be very comfortable and large with space for more than 10,000 people and with a nearby river (the Brenta) which would provide clean water for drinking, cleaning and any other use, although the plan was not put into action.[38] Outside plague times, Health Office officials were keen to restrict the quarantine

---

[32]   ASV, Secreta, MMN 95 34r (2 July 1576).

[33]   Ibid. 53v (22 July 1576).

[34]   ASV, Secreta MMN 95 113v (10 November 1576). For the *chiovere* see Chapter 6, p. 213 especially note 44.

[35]   ASV, Secreta MMN, 95 77v (30 August 1576) and ibid., 113v (10 November 1576).

[36]   ASV, Senato Terra, reg. 51 85v (9 July 1576).

[37]   ASV, Senato Terra, reg. 51 89v (9 July 1576).

[38]   ASV, Sanità reg. 3 30r (8 August 1576).

of individuals and goods to the *lazaretti* islands and avoid the use of other lagoon sites.[39] During epidemics, this was a luxury which they could not afford.

The use of lagoon islands as plague hospitals highlights the relationship between the environment and health in Venice. The *lazaretti* were the first islands of the lagoon to be set apart for permanent public health functions. Their introduction formalised a policy which was already in place by the time of the Black Death [1347–52], when bodies were sent to two outlying islands, San Leonardo Fossalama and San Marco Bocalama, which have now been submerged by the lagoon. Although it was previously thought that ships were sent out to these islands packed full of bodies and then sunk so as to dispose of the corpses in the lagoon itself, archaeological work has not found evidence of this.[40] By the thirteenth century, Venice had already banned certain trades, such as tanners, within the city and relocated them to lagoon islands for health reasons.[41] This policy was extended to other trades during the following centuries.[42] The use of the islands for these trades, however, still required the movement of raw materials, persons and finished goods. Venice wanted the benefits of the products of these trades but sought disassociation from the process of production. As with all institutions and areas that officially represent a closed or isolated community or area, the separation or isolation was never, nor was it ever intended to be, complete.

Within the city, once the decision had been taken about where individuals would carry out their periods of quarantine, infected houses were closed up using wooden planks (*tavole*) and any individuals inside were forbidden from entering, leaving, receiving or giving goods of any kind.[43] Visitors were instructed to remain at two arms' length from the sick and could not visit within the first ten days of illness. If patients were to be taken to the *lazaretti*, a number of practical problems relating to the transportation of patients still remained. The hospitals were sites to which people often had to be made to go by force, using Health Office employees and legal threats. When Venetian Health Office documents describe the problems of convincing people to go to the *lazaretto*, they quickly introduce the threat of making people do one of the few things thought to be worse than being sent as a patient: working there.[44] In 1576, the Health Office officials wrote that those

---

[39]   ASV, Sanità 740 60v (9 December 1646).

[40]   Graziano Arici et al, *La galea ritrovata: origine delle cose di Venezia* (Venice, 2002).

[41]   In 1271 for example the *conciatori di pelli* were sent to the Giudecca. See Niccolò Spada, 'Leggi veneziane sulle industrie chimiche a tutela della salute pubblica dal secolo XIII al XVIII', *Archivio veneto*, 5th series, vol. 7 (1930), pp. 126–56.

[42]   In 1413, for example, dyeing was banned within the city. For the development of the use of islands and civic hygiene measures see, for example, *Venezia e la peste 1348–1797* (Venice, 1980), p. 118.

[43]   ASV, Secreta MMN 95 2r (10 November 1575).

[44]   This is reiterated at various points. See, for example, ASV, Secreta MMN 95 79v (1 September 1576).

people who did not leave their houses on request to go to the *lazaretti* would be removed forcibly by the body clearers from their homes, with the threat of being hanged. Those suspected of infection would be sent to the *lazaretto vecchio* and made to stay for the duration of the plague epidemic.[45] Households were expected to report any outbreaks of disease or thefts of goods but individuals employed tactics such as abandoning the sick in their homes and failing to advise the Health Office of cases of infection to avoid being sent to the *lazaretti*.[46] The Veronese doctor Donzellini wrote that the vile and poor people (*vil plebe et gente povera*) try to hide the disease for three reasons: first, out of greed and fear that their possessions will be burned; second out of fear of being abandoned by doctors and their family; third out of fear of being taken to the *lazaretti*, where, it was felt, most people died.[47] The *lazaretti* elsewhere were also unpopular. Giulia Calvi records that in 1633 popular pressure meant that the *lazaretto* in Florence was closed in favour of the use of household quarantine, although the high costs of the decentralised system soon meant that the institution was reopened.[48] As we will see in subsequent chapters, it was both difficult to persuade individuals to go to the *lazaretti* in the first place and to ensure that they remained within the institutions once they had arrived.

The Health Office officials were reliant on individuals being forthcoming with information regarding the spread of disease and issued instructions demanding honest and truthful reports. Severe threats were placed regarding lies: those convicted would have their tongues cut out. These punishments would hardly have made the institutions seem more palatable. It was not only concern about the nature of the institutions to which they were being taken which may have concerned contemporaries but also worries about the sites they were leaving behind. In Chapter 6 the thefts that took place during plague epidemics will be considered. Contemporaries may rightly have been concerned about the security of their properties and possessions. In addition, some individual homes were temporarily requisitioned for use by the Health Office. Information regarding the use of these sites survives in petitions written after outbreaks complaining about the poor state in which houses were left, very similar to those sent about the monastic sites which were requisitioned.[49]

The Health Office officials attempted to convince contemporaries to go to the hospitals using legislative carrots as well as sticks. In recognition of the

---

[45]   ASV, Secreta MMN 95 49v (16 July 1576).

[46]   Cini, Mantova, carteggio di inviati e diversi b. 1489 bb. 62 (5 September 1556).

[47]   Hieronimo Donzellini, *Discorso nobilissimo e dottissimo preservative et curative della peste* (Venice, 1577) [unpaginated].

[48]   Giulia Calvi, *Histories of a plague year: the social and the imaginary in Baroque Florence* (Oxford, 1989), p. 196.

[49]   See, for example, BMC, MSS Dandolo Pr.div.C.941 (26 July 1577), ASV, Secreta MMN 95 133r (29 March 1577), 134v (30 March 1577), 140v (23 June 1577) and 141r (30 June 1577).

unpopular nature of the hospitals, Health Office workers were instructed to treat patients with charity and respect and to do their best to convince individuals to go to the hospitals voluntarily and calmly. Those in charge of the public health of the individual *sestiere* were informed that they should tell the officials in each parish to use diligence in finding out the locations of the sick and to persuade and quickly and efficiently urge individuals to go voluntarily to the sites set aside for their treatment, where they would be well looked after and well treated.[50] It would seem, however, that a number of contemporaries remained unconvinced. In the previous chapter, various examples of confinement being used for early modern social, medical and religious groups were described. It is important to remember that this was a common enough strategy but it was rare that it would be applied to many of the Christians living in their native city. This idea may also have gone some way to informing resistance to compulsory enclosure in early modern convents. In periods of plague, people resisted attempts to remove them from their homes, which seemed to be safe spaces in contrast with the unfamiliar hospital islands.

Those who did go to the *lazaretti* were taken on boats from different sites within the city, depending on the *sestiere* in which individuals lived, during the night (*a hore xxiii in circa*).[51] During the plague of 1468, boats departed from Rialto and *terra nova* (the site of the large, public granary on the *bacino*, close to both the Health Office and St Mark's Square).[52] In one description of the city during plague time, thousands are described as being taken with horror-stricken faces on white rafts to the 'island of death', from which few were said to return.[53] In Venice, *pizzigamorti* (body clearers) and boatmen rowed boats to and from the islands. The boats were of two types and were colour-coded. The white boats were chalked and disinfected and were used to transport individuals and goods which were either considered to be suspect or which had already undergone quarantine and were therefore considered clean.[54] These worked alongside the black boats which served the hospitals for the transportation of the dead. Benedetti wrote that the lack of *pizzigamorti* during the severe outbreak of 1575–77 meant that the clearly defined system broke down and people were taken to the *lazaretti* in the black boats, alongside corpses. These unfortunate passengers were said to die of

---

[50]   ASV, Secreta MMN 95 113v (9 November 1576).

[51]   ASV, Secreta, MMN 95, 5v (24 November 1575) and 35r (3 July 1576). For more information on the references to time in medieval and early modern Europe, see p. 137 note 143.

[52]   ASV, Sanità reg. 17 18r (17 April 1468).

[53]   'Quinci e quindi varcar veggonsi ogn'ora/Mille c'hanno d'horrore i volti impressi/ ne'bianchi legni a' l'Isola di Morte:/de' quai pochi escon poi da' legni stessi/per l'onde stigie a' le funeree porte.' Benedetti Leoni, *Canzone fatta intorno allo stato calamitoso dell'inclita città di Vinetia nel colmo de' maggiori suoi passati travagli per la peste* (Padua, 1577).

[54]   ASV, Sanità 734 130v (9 July 1579).

nausea and anguish even before arriving on the islands.[55] He also described the distressing number of boats moving constantly to and from the islands. He wrote that it was a terrifying thing to see the thousands of houses within the city closed up with the cross of planks as a sign of infection but it was much more horrible to see the large number of boats serving the *lazaretto nuovo*.

The potential threat of infection from the transportation of individuals and their goods to the *lazaretti* meant that other boats were banned from carrying out these tasks.[56] During the outbreak of 1576 the number of boats used by the Health Office was increased because of the high demand for their service: the Arsenal was ordered to create up to sixty barges (*burchielle*).[57] In particular, these barges were to be used into order to transport the *poveri sani* (literally healthy poor) to the *lazaretto nuovo* with the least possible cost to the public purse. By July, the variety of boats being used to transport people to the *lazaretti* meant that Health Office officials were forced to construct a new list of payments for transportation.[58] Elsewhere individuals were transported by cart or on foot. Canobbio describes the journey for those going to the Paduan *lazaretto* on foot, which he claims to have been able to see from his window. The patients were accompanied by a guard and he writes emotively of the families divided physically, at the crossroads by his home, as the sick went one way and the suspected another. He described the scene as inhumane and cruel.[59]

Once the patients had disembarked at the Venetian *lazaretti*, individuals were interviewed and their names, parishes and other personal details were recorded.[60] They were then inspected for signs of infection. Doctors separated individuals and took particular and minute accounts of background and also investigated for signs of the plague – which the statutes referred to as *giandusse, carboni* or *(pe)tacche*.[61] The sick were immediately given confession and the sacrament.[62] Those who were sent to the *lazaretti* in Venice were allowed to retain only their bedclothes. All

---

[55] Rocco Benedetti, *Relatione d'alcuni casi occorsi in Venetia al tempo della peste l'anno 1576 et 1577 con le provisioni, rimedii et orationi fatte à Dio Benedetti per la sua liberatione* (Bologna, 1630), p. 22.

[56] ASV, Secreta MMN 95 12r (5 April 1576).

[57] Ibid., 30r (25 June 1576).

[58] Ibid., 47v (13 July 1576).

[59] Alessandro Canobbio, *Il successo della peste occorsa in Padova l'anno MDLXXVI* (Padua, 1576), 15v–16r.

[60] By the seventeenth century in Rome, the details included the age of the individual, their stature, skin colour, their face (whether it was long or round), any identifiable marks and whether of good or bad appearance. Cardinal Geronimo Gastaldi, *Tractatus de avertenda et profliganda peste politico = legalis. Eo lucubratus tempore, quo ipse Leomocomiorum primo, mox Sanitatis Commissarius Generalis fuit, peste urbem invadente Anno MDCLVI et LVII* (Bologna, 1684), pp. 585–8.

[61] For a full description of symptoms for the plague see the Introduction, pp. 29–30.

[62] ASV, Sanità 725 132r–134r (26 April 1486) [28].

other pieces of clothing were given over to employees, with a minimum of three witnesses. These objects were sent for disinfection in the warehouses, although, as will be seen in Chapter 6, many were eventually burned. All valuables were supposed to be handed over in the company of the Prior and his assistants and the objects were placed in a lockable chest – which had three keys, held by three different people. From the first moments on the island, the three strands of cleansing: medical, spiritual and physical were obvious.

For those paying for the stay at the *lazaretti* themselves this was the point at which their accounts would be opened.[63] Merchants paid some money directly to the guards of individuals and their boats.[64] For Venetians, those who were able to pay for their own quarantine or treatment were expected to but the majority of those within the hospitals were funded by the Republic.[65] For those individuals who were quarantined within the *lazaretti* from other islands of the lagoon, the Communes had some obligation to cover the costs of their stays. In 1576 there were 400 people from Murano within the *lazaretti* and the deputies in charge of health for the island were described as being in debt to the Prior of the *lazaretto nuovo* to the sum of 300 ducats.[66]

The hospitals received a large number of patients – although it is not clear what their maximum capacities were thought to be. The two Venetian hospitals had originally twenty-four rooms in the *lazaretto vecchio* and eighty rooms in the *lazaretto nuovo*. Even were we to know how many beds there were on the islands, patients shared beds within the hospitals, so that would not help us very much. In Palermo, Ingrassia noted that beds were sufficiently large to accommodate two adults or three or four children.[67] Outside periods of infection in Venice the structures of the hospitals are not noted as having been stretched by the arrival of galley ships, which would have had crews of approximately 200 people.[68] The number of people sent was far greater during periods of plague within the city. In 1555, when the area of San Nicolò was infected, 350 people were said to have been sent to the *lazaretti* and San Anzolo de Concordia from this area alone.[69] In

---

[63]   In 1522, the patron of an infected galley ship was instructed to deposit three hundred ducats in order to cover the costs of quarantine. See ASV, Sanità 726 38r (7 June 1522).

[64]   In 1554, Sebastian Moro was said to have been licensed without having paid his guard. In December of that year a trial was referred to in which Sebastian was obligated to pay the master of the boat and all of the costs of the guard. ASV, Sanità 729 287v (4 December 1554).

[65]   Little information survives within Venetian Health Office documentation as to the process by which payments would have been made.

[66]   ASV, Sanità reg. 14 274v (13 August 1576).

[67]   Ingrassia, p. 218.

[68]   Frederic Lane writes that the number of crew on a merchant galley was fixed by the Republic in 1412 at 212 plus passengers in Frederic C. Lane, *Venice and history: the collected papers of Frederic C. Lane* (Baltimore MD, 1966), p. 5.

[69]   ASV, Sanità reg. 13 3r (23 June 1555).

addition, temporary structures were used to enlarge the hospitals during periods of particular strain. In 1576, the capacity of the *lazaretto nuovo* was enlarged to that of 2,000 people through the use of temporary structures built by the employees of the Arsenal. What is particularly remarkable about this expansion of the *lazaretto* is not only the scale and speed but the ease with which it was said this could be done. The Prior was said to have communicated to the Health Office that the rooms at the *lazaretto nuovo* could be enlarged and equipped at minimal cost to enable these 2,000 people to be housed.[70] In 1630 a large number of beds were added to the hospitals: the Arsenal was instructed to build quickly 1,000 pairs of trestles with planks which were to be used as beds at the *lazaretti* and other hospital islands.[71] They were also instructed to build fifty *burchielle* to transport corpses to burial. These boats were also used to accommodate the poor, along with old galley ships which were used for those convalescing after a period of sickness in the *lazaretto vecchio*.[72] At the *lazaretto nuovo*, quarantine could also be facilitated using boats around the island.

It is clear that a cross section of society continued to be affected by the plague in Venice and that contemporaries were aware of this. Samuel Cohn has written that after 1400 the plague became a disease associated with the poor.[73] During periods of infection in Venice many of the patients were indeed described as poor; during the sixteenth century, this description could be qualitative – a reflection of the state in which individuals found themselves – as well as a more quantitative description of their socio-economic status. The Venetian *lazaretti* in this period were designed for those infected with the disease, not specifically those in poverty. Elsewhere, for example in Genoa, during the late sixteenth century, the *lazaretto* was used specifically to accommodate the poor. This policy was gradually defined so that the *lazaretto* was used to care for those who were thought to be most the most vulnerable, including the disabled, elderly and the young.[74] In many cities, there was a shift, in the seventeenth century, as the institutions became described increasingly as sites for the care of the poor – and in some cases, it was added that they were designed for the disgusting and vile.[75]

---

[70] ASV, Secreta MMN 95 56v (28 July 1576).

[71] BMC, Codice Cicogna 1509 21v (26 October 1630).

[72] Rocco Benedetti, *Relatione d'alcuni casi*, p. 21.

[73] Samuel K. Cohn Jr, *Cultures of plague: medical thought at the end of the Renaissance* (Oxford, 2010), p. 10.

[74] For a discussion of welfare structures in Genoa see R. Savelli, 'Dalle confraternite allo stato: il sistema assistenziale Genovese nel Cinquecento', *Atti della società ligure di storia patria,* nuova serie, XXIV (1984), pp. 171–216. The use of the *lazaretto* to care for the disabled is discussed on p. 198 when Savelli writes that the site was used for 'gli impotenti o debilitate della persona o dell'intelletto o per estrema vecchiezza o per ettà puerile'.

[75] For the *lazaretto* in Rome in 1656 as an institution caring for the poor see Cardinal Geronimo Gastaldi, *Tractatus de avertenda et profliganda peste*, p. 344. For the vile persons associated with the hospital in Genoa see Chapter 1, p. 66.

Studies of 'the patient' within medical history have become increasingly prominent, an important part of survey volumes as well as a subject of monographs. Gianna Pomata's work on early modern Bologna, for example, describes a system within which patients and healers were equal partners in contracting cures.[76] Considerations of patients have also become an important facet of institutional studies, including those of hospitals. John Henderson's work on Florentine hospitals dedicates some attention to the numbers of sick admitted, the length of their stay, the gender breakdown and their mortality rates.[77] In studies of the plague, however, the patient is less frequently studied owing to the difficulty of source material – very few records survive which record the patients in the plague hospitals; only fragments have been uncovered in Venice. Instead, individuals tend to be included as part of mortality statistics in demographic studies. This wider issue is discussed in more detail in Chapter 5. This chapter will address both individual cases and general trends in social status, gender and age, drawing attention to the variety of patients brought to the hospitals where possible.

In the previous chapter, some of the parallels between charitable institutions and the *lazaretti* were described. The establishment of the *lazaretti* predated these institutions by more than a century. A number of studies have been informed by interpretations which have seen plague predominantly as a social problem, even going so far as to claim that 'plague did not create the need for controlling the poor and the propertyless [but rather] the causal relationship may have been the reverse'.[78] This is an oversimplification. The foundation of the *lazaretti* was not motivated by ideas about the treatment of the poor. Instead, contemporary views of poverty took their place alongside the importance of reputation and protection of the trade economy and the emerging role and responsibilities of the state to shape the early modern *lazaretti*.

---

[76] Pioneering works include Roy Porter (ed.), *Patients and practitioners: lay perceptions of medicine in pre-industrial society* (Cambridge, 1985); Barbara Duden, *The woman beneath the skin: a doctor's patients in eighteenth-century Germany* (London, 1991); see also Colin Jones, 'The construction of the hospital patient in early modern France' in Norbert Finzsch and Robert Jütte (eds), *Institutions of confinement: hospitals, asylums and prisons in Western Europe and North America 1500–1950* (Cambridge, 1996), pp. 55–75; Gianna Pomata, *Contracting a cure: patients, healers and the law in early modern Bologna* (London, 1998).

[77] John Henderson, *The Renaissance hospital: healing the body and healing the soul* (London, 2006), chapter eight, 'Antechambers of death?', pp. 251–86.

[78] Ann G. Carmichael cited in Michelle A. Laughran, 'The body, public health and social control in sixteenth century Venice' (unpublished PhD. thesis, University of Connecticut, 1998), p. 125.

The Patients

Various terms were used to refer to the patients at the *lazaretti*. Sometimes they are simply referred to as 'persons' (*persone*), sometimes 'poor and miserable persons' (*persone povere et miserabili*) or 'plague-infected persons' (*poveri apestate*). Most commonly, the term 'the poor' (*poveri*) was used with various adjectives: 'miserable', 'injured' (*feriti*) or 'sick' (*infermi*) and, in some lucky cases, 'healthy' (*sani*). In the decision regarding payments for the 400 people sent from Murano to the *lazaretti* in 1576, the individuals are described as poor people (*povera gente*).[79] We have already seen that notions of poverty were not formulated solely on an economic basis and could reflect the miserable state of these individuals. Benedetti, for example, wrote of poor 'widows and orphans' returning from quarantine but only as a heart-wrenching reminder of social strain. Sansovino commented more directly that 'the vast majority of these people [in the *lazaretti*] were poor who, deprived of all their infected worldly goods left back in Venice, were maintained at public expense for twenty-two days (although there were also various nobles and citizens who paid for their own upkeep)'. This was recorded as part of an effort to praise the charity of the Republic, however, rather than necessarily reflecting the reality within the institutions. The social status of patients varied, depending on whether or not cities were infected. When cities were free from infection, those within the structures were generally those arriving from trading centres – either foreign or returning merchants. At other times, when cities were infected, the social makeup changed so that the *lazaretti* predominantly reflected the social divisions of the wider cities that they served.[80] In Cividale del Friuli, it was said that the *lazaretto* for the sick received patients regardless of status: nobles, artisans, peasants of different statuses and of each sex from the city and wider territory up to its capacity of 150 patients.[81] We will consider the presence of each level of society within the hospitals, although the lack of surviving entry records for the hospitals means that we are reliant, in the main, on contemporary observations.

It is well known that the Venetian nobility was active within the mercantile structures of the Republic, particularly during the medieval period. From the mid-fifteenth century, the nobility spread its economic exposure to include investments on the mainland but maintained trading interests.[82] Noblemen were sent with their galley ships to quarantine but this was not always on the *lazaretti*. In 1522, for

---

[79] ASV, Senato Terra reg. 51 101v (13 August 1576).

[80] For a discussion of the use of the terms 'poor' and 'poverty' in this context, see the Introduction, pp. 16–17. For the social status of those affected in Venice by the plague see Paolo Preto, *Peste e società a Venezia* (Vicenza, 1978), pp. 120–30.

[81] Mario Brozzi, *Peste, fede e sanità in una cronaca cividalese del 1598* (Milan, 1982), pp. 33–4.

[82] See Brian Pullan (ed.), *Crisis and change in the Venetian economy in the sixteenth and seventeenth centuries* (London, 1968) for a discussion of key aspects of the debate.

example, three noblemen were sent with their servants to San Clemente.[83] Nobles were not always sent to the *lazaretti* during periods of plague within the city either. An ambassador's report which wrote that nobles and the poor were both sent to the *lazaretti* also recounted that a nobleman who lived next door to a woman who had died of plague was sent to the Giudecca with his family for quarantine and not to the *lazaretto nuovo*.[84] Those who were allowed to undergo quarantine in their own homes were given permission only if their homes were sufficiently spacious and airy.[85] It was also possible to carry out quarantine in the countryside. In 1522, for example, several noblemen were sent to San Clemente and others to the villa Ronchade (possibly the villa Giustinian built by Tulio Lombardo between 1511 and 1513) in the Trevisano.[86] In 1576, Francesco Zeno, one of the *Avogaria di Comun*, sent a supplication to the government of the Republic, requesting permission to join his family on the mainland at Padua. His family had been in household quarantine for twenty-two days at the point of writing and he had remained in the city with one male and one female servant. Both of these individuals had been infected with the plague: the male servant had died and the female had been sent to the *lazaretto*. He cited human compassion and his familial obligations of care in order to request permission to return to his family in Padua for twenty days, which he was granted.[87] The requirement for spacious homes inevitably meant that the wealthy were granted permission for quarantine outside the *lazaretti* more frequently than the poor. This may also have played some part in affecting the lower mortality amongst nobles during epidemics.[88] In the epidemic of 1575–77, 329 nobles were recorded as having been killed out of a total mortality figure of 50,721 – a low statistic given that nobles made up approximately one per cent of the city's population.[89] In Sardinia, there was a similar differentiation in terms of flexibility of locations for quarantine: the poor were transported to institutions of care and quarantine whereas the rich were given the privilege of choosing their own preferred sites of quarantine.[90]

The account of the *lazaretto nuovo* by Francesco Sansovino, considered in the previous chapter, was said to have been based upon his experience of the institution. This may have been a rhetorical device. What is useful to remember, however, is the expectation of Sansovino that this claim would have added authenticity to his account: in other words contemporaries would have accepted that both rich

---

[83]   ASV, Sanità 726 37r (22 May 1522).

[84]   Cini, Mantua, b. 1489 (2 June 1556).

[85]   ASV, Senato Terra reg. 51 91v (18 July 1576).

[86]   ASV, Sanità 726 38v (20 June 1522).

[87]   ASV, Sanità reg 14 260v (6 August 1576).

[88]   Paolo Preto, *Peste e società*, p. 113.

[89]   The names of the nobles who were killed is given in BMC, Codice Gradenigo 43, at the end of the section 'Notitia delle pesti seguite nella città di Venetia'.

[90]   Francesco Manconi, *Castigo de Dios: la grande peste barocca nella Sardegna di Filippo IV* (Rome, 1994), p. 172.

and poor would have been accommodated within these hospitals. Some nobles were sent to the *lazaretti*. The Paduan physician Gerolamo Mercuriale wrote that it was not fair (*non aequum*) that nobles were sent to the *lazaretto* but instead recommended that they should be quarantined within the city or in towns outside.[91] The physician Frigimelega advised that cities should have two *lazaretti* in order to separate men of quality from the poor, rather than the sick from the suspected.[92] Although during the fifteenth century, the two structures in Venice were used to separate men from women, the division by social status was not made.[93] It is clear, however, that those with the available means could carry out quarantine beyond the *lazaretto* in a boat or within cities. During and outside periods when cities were infected, these institutions served more than just the urban poor but experiences of the sites differed: for the rich, there was distinction of separate zones and more sophisticated sustenance available.[94]

In 1561, the secretary to the ambassador of France arrived in Venice from Constantinople. He was sent to the *lazaretto vecchio* with his company in order to undergo forty days' quarantine because one of his party was sick. The Prior was said to have spent large sums of money for supplies during their stay.[95] Similarly, in 1571 a Turkish ambassador travelling to France arrived in Venice without a *fede*. He was not allowed to disembark within the city but was instead sent to the *lazaretto nuovo* and maintained at public expense for fifteen days.[96] These were institutions to which both foreigners and diplomats were sent. Incoming dignitaries would often have been taken to islands of the Venetian lagoon: to Santo Spirito, to Murano to see several gardens and the glassworks, San Giorgio Maggiore and Santa Maria di Gratia. Particular islands were often the meeting place for such dignitaries and so the lagoon acted as a gateway into the city.[97] The traditional location for meeting state visitors was in front of San Nicolò on the Lido – the location discussed in the previous chapter for the ceremonial welcome for the

---

[91] Gerolamo Mercuriale cited in Paolo Preto, *Peste e società*, p. 127.

[92] Francesco Frigimelega, *Consiglio ... sopra la peste in Padoa dell'anno MDLV* (Padua, 1555) [unfoliated].

[93] ASV, Sal b. 6 reg. 3 15v (2 March 1485).

[94] This can be seen in many different aspects of care. In Palermo, different soap was used for rich and poor: the former used *sapone moscade* (perfumed soap), whereas the the poor used *sapone commune* (ordinary soap). On different types of soap, James Shaw very kindly shared information from his co-authored book with me before publication, which illustrates that a number of different types of soap were used in the Giglio in Florence, sometimes for wholesale distribution, sometimes as part payment for workers and only occasionally for retail sale. He listed *sapone da barba, sapone empolese, sapone ghaetano, sapone moschadato fine* and *sapone nero*. See James E. Shaw and Evelyn Welch, *Making and Marketing Medicine in Renaissance Florence* (Amsterdam, 2011).

[95] ASV, Sanità 730 310r (22 December 1561).

[96] ASV, Collegio, cerimoniali 105r (14 October 1571).

[97] See ibid. for a list of itineraries.

King of France in 1574. For this event, the site was decorated with a ceremonial, triumphal archway designed by Andrea Palladio [1508–80].[98] The *lazaretti* must have provided a sharp contrast with the ceremonial sites on islands usually encountered by these dignitaries.

A large number of merchants were sent to the *lazaretti*, particularly the *lazaretto nuovo*, outside periods of plague within Venice, as attested to by payments for the quarantine of ships which were made to the Salt Office.[99] The merchants are also recorded in evidence of a more unusual kind: the graffiti from the walls of the *tezon grande* (the main warehouse on the island). Here, various inscriptions and designs were rediscovered beneath layers of chalk, which had been applied to disinfect the walls.[100] These were first published in the exhibition catalogue *Venezia e la peste* and were further highlighted in the guide to the *lazaretto nuovo* edited by Gerolamo Fazzini. A variety of designs survive. Many consist simply of merchants' symbols and these would originally have had the practical function of distinguishing sections of goods from one another. The graffiti also shows illustrations of galley ships and armed soldiers, almost life sized. The depictions of soldiers were drawn on the walls of the warehouse beside the open archways. They may have been portrayals of the armed employees of the Arsenal who guarded the *caselli da polvere* (structures for the storage of gun powder) in the *lazaretti*. In addition to the images, some inscriptions survive. These describe the journeys of individual merchants, their places of origin and their lengths of stay. Some are extremely basic and others more intricate in their design. The simplest designs give information regarding places of origins, dates of arrival and names of merchants. More detailed examples mention individuals who worked in the *lazaretti* and give information about the condition of the people staying on the islands and some of the background to the period of quarantine. The inscriptions are a physical testament to the presence of these merchants as a prominent group within the *lazaretto* structure.[101]

Very few of those people who were sent to the *lazaretti* were able to record a description of their quarantine. Surviving supplications from merchants express a number of complaints regarding their experiences within the institutions. Their issues related to the openness of the sites in use – in a number of different ways. One complaint was that the institutions were too open to outsiders, meaning that

---

[98]   For a description in translation see David S. Chambers and Brian Pullan (eds), *Venice: a documentary history, 1450–1630* (Oxford, 1992), pp. 64–5.

[99]   ASV, Sanità 726 38r (7 June 1522).

[100]   Ample scope for comparison for this graffiti should be provided by Giandomenico Romanelli, director of the Musei Civici Veneziani, when he publishes his work on 500 years of graffiti in prisons, which is referenced in Guy Geltner, *The medieval prison*, Chapter Three, note 79, p. 156.

[101]   Images of the graffiti are reprinted in Dorina Petronio, 'Le testimonianze pittoriche conservate lungo le pareti del Tezon Grando: aspetti artistici' in Gerolamo Fazzini (ed.), *Venezia: isola del lazzaretto nuovo* (Venice, 2004), pp. 47–51.

the security of the islands was compromised and the merchandise was vulnerable to thieves. The openness of the architectural structures of the *lazaretti* was also thought to cause physical damage to merchandise, as a result of the wind and rain in winter and overexposure to the sun, presumably in summer. Finally, the openness of the sites affected the merchants themselves. They complained that the lack of cover meant that merchants became sick.[102]

Personal letters from individual patients are rare. A few letters remain from the second half of the seventeenth century, written by Michiel Giovanni.[103] Giovanni's first two letters were sent in October 1675 from Constantinople where, he recorded, he and his party were in good health. By December, however, he was in the Venetian *lazaretto vecchio*. He described his symptoms and noted that he was in bed as a result of a vile and constant fever accompanied by pain all over the body. He wrote of not being able to eat anything. His biggest complaint, though, related to his inability to stomach the very good wine on offer (a Ribuola from Zante) and he requested that he be sent some mature wine – not too sweet and not too sour. By his fourth letter, he was on the mend – saying that the only remaining symptom was weakness, which, he said, he hoped to restore with a healthy regime (*la buona regola di vivere*). Giovanni's ability to keep in contact with those beyond the institution and his expectation that he would receive supplies directly from them are indications of the contact with the outside world that patients at the Venetian *lazaretti* could have in non-plague years of the seventeenth century.

In addition to those patients sent through the institutions for trade, people were sent to the *lazaretti* from other institutions. In 1576 two women were sent to the *lazaretti* from the hospital of San Antonio.[104] Jews were also sent to the *lazaretti*. Despite restriction within the Ghetto, Jews were also accommodated within the plague hospitals.[105] They must also have worked there, since in 1652 it was decreed that Jews were no longer able to be employed as disinfectors on the islands.[106] Elsewhere, in Spalato, it was noted that the individuals arriving for quarantine in the *lazaretto* were Ponentine Jews. There are hints that a strict separation may have been maintained between Jewish and Christian patients and staff. Four Jewish disinfectors were appointed to the hospitals to serve alongside fourteen Christians.[107] There was a division made within the *lazaretto* structure which enabled Christian, Turkish and Jewish merchants to be accommodated separately, in line with the separation of merchandise.[108]

---

[102] Examples from the end of the 1580s can be found in ASV, Sanità reg. 16 16v–19r.

[103] ASV, Scuola Grade di San Marco b. 101 [9]. I am very grateful to Jonathan Glixon for bringing these letters to my attention.

[104] ASV, Sanità 732 147r (22 March 1576).

[105] ASV, Sanità 737 30r (17 October 1597).

[106] ASV, Sanità 741 15r (22 January 1652).

[107] ASV, Sanità 742 178v (27 August 1670).

[108] ASV, Sanità reg. 3 88v (6 December 1609).

It is interesting to note the way in which enclosed institutions were used in times of plague; only some were suitable to be used as substitute *lazaretti*. A document survives from Padua detailing ordinances during the outbreak of 1576 when the religious institution of Sant'Antonio Confessore became infected.[109] The orders contain instructions regarding the use of doors and contact between individuals, which was to be limited as much as possible and, if necessary, was to be carried out with the individuals in question standing a minimum of six feet apart. The sick were to be kept separate in the infirmary under lock and key and those who had contact with the sick were to be kept quarantined in their rooms. Particular restrictions were placed on the passage of cloth and linen from the institution to outside. This is an example of an already closed institution being utilised as a structure for quarantine. The separate, purified image of these institutions made this function possible in times of disease. Antonio Glisente, for example, noted that monasteries and hospitals were not badly affected by the disease because of the comfortable accommodation and the frugality of the subsistence which were said to be of great help in times of plague.[110] In addition to the architectural form of the institutions, the identity of patients could determine which institution was used for quarantine; the *lazaretti* were considered to be interchangeable with other sites for the poor and sick in a way that was not true for religious orders. This was also illustrated by the ways in which *lazaretti* could be used beyond plague epidemics. In the 1580s in Genoa, for example, the *lazaretto* was used to care for the city's disabled.[111] In seventeenth-century Venice the *lazaretto* was used as a temporary prison for criminals, who were thought to pose a risk of absconding.[112] Manlio Brusatin records that the hospital in Milan was used for beggars and the poor in the aftermath of the famine of 1629.[113]

Despite the variety of patients cared for within the *lazaretti*, a sustained conceptual link was made between the plague and the poor. Paul Slack in his study of the plague in early modern England observes that by the seventeenth century, plague was seen as a disease of certain social groups and localities, spread by beggars, migrants and strangers. From these origins it was seen to hold the potential to threaten respectable society.[114] Contemporaries continued to observe that the plague was a disease which affected both rich and poor and yet concurrently developed assessments of the disease as one with a social bias. Medical explanations of health and disease set factors such as diet and lifestyle,

---

[109]   ASP, Sanità, b. 27 87r (24 October 1576).

[110]   Antonio Glisente, *Il summario delle cause che dispongono I corpi de gli huomi a patire la corrottione pestilente del presente anno MDLXXVI.*

[111]   See note 74.

[112]   ASV, Sanità 740 149v (10 November 1648). For a further discussion see p. 106.

[113]   Manlio Brusatin, *Il muro della peste: spazio della pietà e governo del lazaretto* (Venice, 1981), pp. 32–3.

[114]   Paul Slack, *The impact of plague in Tudor and Stuart England* (London, 1985), part III 'The social response', pp. 197–310.

good air and overcrowding high amongst those which affected predisposition to infection. Those with poor diets and poor housing were thought to be most vulnerable but responses to the plague were not simply attempts at social control. They had an important charitable element and the poor may have been seen as the most dangerous because they were the most in need; to neglect this group was to invite the wrath of God.

An association between the poor and plague developed from the fifteenth century.[115] Contemporaries explained the association in different ways: on the basis of the nature of the bodies of the poor, their actions and environments. These ideas affected not only the treatment of the poor but also their goods. This confirms the important points made by scholars working as part of the material turn in recent years, who have emphasised the necessity of considering objects in conjunction with the ways in which they were used.[116] In 1535, for example, it was noted that the poor with debts to creditors were thought to be more likely to risk concealing their goods in infected houses and then reclaiming them when they returned from the *lazaretti*, posing considerable danger to the health of the city.[117] The goods owned by the poor were also thought to be more dangerous because items in the homes of the rich could sit for years without being handled whereas the poor owned less and, therefore, used things more. In 1576, it was said that items from the houses of nobles, citizens or merchants should be divided into those from the room or site where the person had died and those from the rest of the house. The former should be disinfected at a site away from the city and the rest could be brought to the *chiovere* because the objects in these homes would not have been handled by all and sundry. In contrast, the goods of the poor should all be taken away from the city because they would have been, for the most part, handed by everyone within the house and were therefore more dangerous.[118] The way in which the objects were handled, as well as the size of individual rooms and the overall home of the poor, meant that objects owned by the poor were considered to be more dangerous than those of the rich.

Low social status did not always carry a stigma. In discussing the issue of why more poor people die than rich during plague, Father Antero Maria concluded that the rich were privileged in the context of plague when they were healthy, because they were less likely to contract the plague in the first place, but that the poor were privileged in sickness because they were more likely to recover.[119] The poor had the advantage in recovering because their bodies were more accustomed to discomfort

---

[115]   See Samuel K. Cohn Jr, *Cultures of plague.*

[116]   Useful articles can be found in Michelle O'Malley and Evelyn Welch (eds), *The material Renaissance* (Manchester, 2007). For Venice, pioneering work on material culture has been done by Tricia Allerston.

[117]   ASV, Sanità 727 306v (24 July 1535).

[118]   ASV, Secreta MMN 95, 72r (15 August 1576).

[119]   Father Antero Maria da San Bonaventura, *Li lazaretti della città e riviere di Genova del MDCLVII ne quali oltre à successi particolari del contagio si narrano l'opere*

and distress, so they did not feel so oppressed by the sickness as the more delicate and noble rich. This was why, in his opinion, of all of the different types of people, soldiers were most likely to recover from plague. This is an important reflection, which emphasises the role of attitude and emotion in contemporary accounts of plague and which we will return to in Chapter 4.

The poor were not the only group to be thought of as dangerous in the context of plague. At the beginning of outbreaks, discussions of the source of infection were often recorded.[120] Children, women and foreigners were frequently identified as problem cases, as causes for alarm and vehicles for the spread of disease.[121] From the medieval period, children had been seen as particularly vulnerable to plague. Even beyond the famous children's epidemic of 1361, because of the frequency with which the disease affected Europe (approximately once a decade until the end of the fifteenth century), much of the population developed immunity but the young were left exposed.[122] During the sixteenth century, when outbreaks hit less frequently, however, this trend was altered so that it was often only the eldest within the population with previous exposure to the disease. Nevertheless, the young continued to be perceived as more susceptible to plague because their bodies were naturally warmer and wetter than those of adults in contemporary humoural theory. We will consider in Chapter 5 that many of the mortality statistics do not allow us to identify children separately from adults. An exception to this is the series of mortality statistics from the plague of 1630–31 for Venice, Murano, Malamocco and Chioggia, which are partially broken down by age and in which children are differentiated. Here, children (ages 0–7) represent over a fifth of overall mortality.[123]

There are only occasional mentions of children in archival material.[124] Various orphans are mentioned as being cared for after the death of their parents within

---

virtuose di quelli che sacrificorno se stessi alla salute del prossimo e si danno le regole di ben governare un popolo flagellato dalla peste (Genoa, 1658), pp. 294–5.

[120]   For examples of investigations see ASVer, Sanità, reg. 33 24r and 25r (28–29 August 1575) and ASP, Sanità b. 295 (3 August 1575).

[121]   For a comparative discussion of the moral aspect of accusations made for the plague see Andrew Wear, *Knowledge and practice in English medicine*, 'Plague and medical knowledge', pp. 275–313.

[122]   Samuel K. Cohn Jr, 'Changing pathology of plague' in Simonetta Cavaciocchi (ed.), *XLI Settimana di Studi: Le Interazioni fra Economia e Ambiente Biologico Nell'Europa Preindustriale, Secc. XIII–XVIII (Prato, 26–30 Aprile 2009)* (Florence, 2010), p. 45; see also his *Black Death Transformed: disease and culture in early Renaissance Europe* (London, 2002) particularly pp. 212–19.

[123]   ASV, Sanità b. 17 408r ('Morti in Venezia, Murano, Malamocco e Chiozza').

[124]   Andrea Gratiolo, *Discorso di peste ... nel quale si contengono utilissime speculationi intorno alla natura, cagioni e curatione della peste, con un catalogo di tutte le pesti piu notabili de' tempi passati* (Venice, 1576), chapter sixteen.

the *lazaretti*.[125] It is clear from a number of *lazaretto* records that orphans were felt to be at particular risk – especially babies who would be unable to survive without milk after the death of their mothers. As a result a number of wet nurses were employed at the *lazaretti* in Sardinia.[126] In Padua, Canobbio records eight wet nurses (*baile*) being employed and a number of goats being kept, because the wet nurses were unable to supply all of the infants with sufficient quantities of milk.[127] Staying close to a goat was recommended as a preventative measure by the French surgeon Ambroise Paré so this may have been a smart way of supplementing milk supplies in times of plague![128] Children were kept separate from others for care. During the outbreak of 1555, the children from the hospital of San Giovanni e Paolo were sent to Sant'Anzolo di Concordia instead of to the *lazaretti* and the Health Office doctor was sent to administer treatment.[129] Attempts to separate children within the *lazaretti* can be seen from the instructions sent to the Prioresses via Ludovico Cucino.[130] In one instance Donna Marietta is asked to ensure that the children of the head of the hospital (the Prior), for whom she has responsibility, are not allowed to mix with any other children.[131] There are also indications of the number of children in the ordering of supplies: in 1576 1,000 blankets and mattresses were ordered, in varying sizes: two-thirds large and one third small.[132] If this is a true reflection of the make-up of the hospitals, then children comprise a significant but almost silent group within the records of the *lazaretti*.

As with the poor, it was not only the bodies but also the behaviour of children that made them a cause for concern. In Genoa, Father Antero described the role of wet nurses as the busiest and most difficult of the jobs in the *lazaretti*.[133] He wrote that just one young child was enough to occupy a wet nurse all day and for a large part of the night too. It was necessary to hold the children all of the time, except when they were sleeping. Where there were hundreds of children, they needed not only to be kept clean and swaddled many times a day but also to be fed on an industrial scale (*nutricarli industriosamente*). The children wanted food in abundance, because they did not know how to stand hunger for a moment. Imagine

---

[125] ASV, Sanità 732 77r (3 January 1575) and 79r (5 January 1575).

[126] Francesco Manconi, *Castigo de Dios*, p. 176.

[127] Alessandro Canobbio, *Il successo della peste*, 17v. The use of goats seems to have been common: in Brescia in 1580 it was noted that twelve goats and twelve wet nurses were needed to care for nineteen infants. See Brian Pullan, 'Orphans and foundlings in early modern Europe' in *Poverty and charity: Europe, Italy, Venice, 1400–1700* (Aldershot, 1994), III, p. 9.

[128] Ambroise Paré, *A Treatise of the Plague* (London, 1630 [1568]), p. 14

[129] Cucino 58v (31 October 1555).

[130] Cucino 12r (15 April 1555).

[131] Cucino 34v (16 May 1555).

[132] ASV, Secreta MMN 95 91r (23 September 1576).

[133] Father Antero Maria da San Bonaventura, *Li lazaretti della città e riviere di Genova*, pp. 476–7.

the work, he wrote, involved in finding sufficient swaddling clothes and smocks and other necessary things; if you gave one of the children a clean cloth, by the evening it was filthy, not least because the vast majority of the children could not be given any guidance, training or instruction in the hospitals. Every fifteen days it was necessary to cut all of the children's hair, otherwise head lice would nest in such a way that they 'devour[ed] the scalp'. He also asked a number of rhetorical questions: How could the wet nurses sleep amongst the crying, moaning and shrieking? Amongst the filth and the stench? How were they supposed to always be on hand to keep watch on those who, like the adults, are subject to madness? Father Antero noted that the children, if not watched, would leap from their beds, run off naked, and hide themselves so well that it was hard to find them again. Between themselves they shouted and knocked one another down because children aged just one were mixed together with those of five and six. The women knew all this, Father Antero noted, and tried to avoid the job. He advised getting ten- to twelve-year-olds to assist and having a large number of cots and blankets. He also suggested that the head of the hospitals should visit the children regularly since, in his experience, there was always a tremendous amount to sort out in that part of the hospital.

Some contemporaries felt that women's bodies, like those of the young, were predisposed to contracting the disease because they had similar characteristics to those of children, particularly young virgins and those who were pregnant.[134] During the Black Death, it was said that two-thirds of the population of Venice died but, within this, all of the pregnant women of the city were killed.[135] Samuel Cohn has written that plague became a disease to which women were particularly vulnerable and that this is reflected in public health measures, such as the quarantining of women and children in the parish.[136] It may have been, however, that this was done to minimise movement around the city by those not involved in trades. Some information is available regarding the gender breakdown of patients within the hospitals in the mortality statistics. On the issue of whether women or men were more susceptible to the disease, contemporaries were divided.[137]

A strong gender bias is visible in the statistics for Venice from the outbreak of 1555–58 recorded by the Mantuan ambassador. Between March and September 1556, 23,000 people were said to have died within the city and in the *lazaretti*. Of these, 17,000 were said to be women and just 4,000 men and 2,000 children.[138] The statistics that survive for Venice during the outbreak of 1575–77 have been widely

---

[134]   Andrea Gratiolo, *Discorso di peste*, chapter sixteen.

[135]   See ASV, Sanità reg. 17 4r and also Samuel K. Cohn Jr, *The Black Death transformed: disease and culture in early Renaissance Europe* (London, 2002), for example pp. 210–12.

[136]   Samuel K. Cohn Jr, 'Changing pathology of plague', p. 50.

[137]   Bernardino Tomitano, *De le cause et origine de la peste vinitiana* (Venice, 1556) chapter eleven.

[138]   Cini, Mantova b. 1489 bb. 62 (5 September 1556).

reproduced from a variety of copies of the records of the Health Office scribe Cornelio Morello. His statistics also divided up mortality according to gender but not according to age; we may presume that children are included in his totals of deaths within the city between 1575 and 1577 as a result of the plague but he, like many of his contemporaries, is not explicit about this. Morello's statistics are interesting. Bucking the trend of sixteenth-century accounts, his statistics provide an almost identical gender breakdown, with women making up 50.2 per cent and men 49.8 per cent of the total mortality within the city and *lazaretti*. This can be looked at more closely, in the light of the breakdown of the city's population more broadly. Jean Delumeau has shown that Venice and Rome were exceptional in terms of early modern cities because they were made up of a larger percentage of males.[139] As a result, women do seem to have shown a higher vulnerability to the disease during the epidemic. Morello's statistics are broken down further, however, into deaths within the *lazaretti* and deaths within the city. Morello states that overall fewer women than men died in the *lazaretti* – they make up 46 per cent of the mortality there. This indicates that fewer women than men may have been sent to the hospital islands. This, in turn, may have been true of early modern institutional cultures more generally.[140] The lack of surviving detailed records of entries into the hospital and deaths there makes quantification difficult. Only tentative conclusions can be drawn on the makeup of the hospitals in terms of gender, although this was an area of frequent contemporary discussion.[141]

The lack of clear imbalance in terms of the gender of mortality is in parallel with some seventeenth-century statistics for the English village of Eyam and Nonantola in Italy.[142] Elsewhere, however, the issue of gender is more marked.

---

[139] See Jean Delumeau, *Vie economique et sociale de Rome* (Paris, 1957–59), I, pp. 422–3. Delumeau compares Rome and Venice with Palermo, Messina, Florence, Bologna and Bergamo.

[140] Morello's two periods have different mortality rates. In the first, 1,682 men and 1,699 women were said to have died within the city and 143 men and 172 women within the *lazaretti*. In the second, in contrast, the figures are 11,240 men and 12,925 women within the city and 10,213 men and 8,647 women within the *lazaretti*. In total, 23,278 men and 23,443 women were thought to have died during the epidemic, with 12,922 men in the city, 14,624 women in the city, 10,356 men in the *lazaretti* and 8,819 women in the *lazaretti*. ASV, Secreta, MMN 95 164r. These statistics form the basis for the discussion in Daniele Beltrami, *Storia della popolazione di Venezia dalla fine del secolo XVI alla caduta della Repubblica* (Padua, 1954), p. 57. For the same issue of a greater number of men being sent to the *Incurabili* hospital in Venice see Laura J. McGough, *Gender, sexuality and syphilis in early modern Venice* (Basingstoke, 2011), pp. 102–35.

[141] See also ASV, Secreta, MMN 55bis 2r (13 July 1576) for the report of Capo di Vacca and Mercuriale which also addresses this issue.

[142] Samuel K. Cohn Jr, 'Changing pathology of plague', pp. 50–51. The material for Nonantola can be found in Guido Alfani and Samuel K. Cohn Jr, 'Nonantola 1630. Anatomia di una pestilenza e meccanismi del contagio con riflessioni a partire dale epidemie milanesi della prima età moderna', *Popolazione e storia*, 2 (2007), 99–138. On Eyam and issues

Samuel Cohn has illustrated that in surviving records for Milan between 1452 and 1523 women died at a higher rate to men. He claims that this is unlikely to have been caused by biological differences but instead by the greater number of women living in difficult and poor conditions.[143] The statistics recorded by Canobbio for Padua show similarity with those of Milan. Of the total mortality, 3,017 men and 3,800 women were said to have died. Of deaths within the *lazaretto*, 1,964 were men and 1,013 were women.[144] In Milan, Cohn has calculated that female exceeded male plague deaths by 1.78 times in 1468 and 1.76 times in 1483. In Padua, in 1575–77, that ratio was 1.23 in the city and 0.52 in the *lazaretto*. In Venice, for the same outbreak, Morello records ratios of 1.41 in the city and 0.85 in the *lazaretto*. Overall, therefore, the ratios in Venice and Padua in terms of mortality within the city are broadly comparable with the statistics available from elsewhere on the Italian peninsula and illustrate that women were dying at a greater rate than men. In the *lazaretto*, however, the reverse is true – suggesting that women (and possibly children) were more likely to have been placed in household quarantine than sent to the *lazaretti*. Despite the contemporary perception of plague as a disease to which women were more vulnerable, the *lazaretti* may have been male-dominated spaces. In the *lazaretto vecchio* this would have meant that the hospital for men was in greater demand than that for women since patients were divided by gender on this site.

A cultural stereotype emerged during the early modern period of the plague as old and female. The sculpted altarpiece, for example, in the church of Santa Maria della Salute shows the Virgin and Child enthroned, with Venice at their feet pleading for protection. On the right of the scene the plague – shown as a poor, elderly hag – is being driven away into the west by a cherub [Plate 19]. This altarpiece was said to have been imitated in a reproduction sent to the chapel of the *lazaretto vecchio* in the early eighteenth century.[145] Although this piece by Josse de Corte [1627–79] was not finished until the end of the seventeenth century, it expresses similar traits to those described by Cesare Ripa [1560–1623] in his *Iconologia*, first published in 1593. He describes plague as 'a woman … with a pallid, terrifying face. Her dress is open on the side and through the opening one can see a stained and soiled shirt; one can also see her dirty breasts.'[146] This was an image reproduced elsewhere but is an interesting one within the Venetian

---

of story-telling and myth-making in the context of plague see Patrick Wallis, 'A dreadful heritage: interpreting epidemic disease at Eyam, 1666–2000', *History workshop journal* 61:1 (2006), 31–56.

[143]   Samuel K. Cohn Jr, 'Changing pathology of plague', p. 50.

[144]   Alessandro Canobbio, *Il successo della peste*, 34r.

[145]   Giorgio and Maurizio Crovato, *Isole abbandonate della Laguna: com'erano e come sono* (Padua, 1978), p. 117.

[146]   Cesare Ripa, *Iconologia* (Padua, 1611), pp. 421–2. Women personify the majority of subjects described by Ripa.

context.[147] The city projected itself as a Virgin, with strong Marian overtones. The disease was portrayed in opposition to the nature of the Republic.[148] It is this characterisation which informs the image of the disease as an elderly woman, rather than the reality of infection.

The final consideration regarding the patients at the *lazaretti* is the percentage of those within the hospitals who were actually sick. This is the most difficult aspect to assess. For Venice, fragmentary records which detail the number of people being sent to the hospitals during the epidemic of 1575–77, considered in more detail in Chapter 5, show dramatically different numbers of people being sent directly to the *lazaretto vecchio* and *lazaretto nuovo*. Eighty-one per cent of those being sent to the *lazaretti* during this year went directly to the *lazaretto vecchio*: in other words, they had been diagnosed as sick with the plague. It is important to recognise, however, that many of these statistics were recorded after a decision had been taken to limit the number of those sent to the *lazaretto nuovo* from the city and so the percentage may be unrepresentative. Some fragments survive of lists of people within the hospitals beyond Venice which provide snapshots of the *lazaretti* in action. In Verona, for example, in September 1575 there were forty-five people in the hospital and sixteen of them were described as sick.[149] For Padua, licensing and mortality statistics survive for the period from 20 August until 21 November 1576. Combined totals range from 41 to 560 people giving a broad indication of the capacity of the institution there of approximately 1,000 once the sick and suspected are taken into account. This is also the capacity given by the chronicler Canobbio.[150] Just one record from the Paduan *lazaretto* during the outbreak of 1555 survives, which contains three lists of the names of those within the *lazaretto* between 18 August and 26 August. Across this ten-day period, between 14 and 17 per cent of those within the Paduan *lazaretto* were sick, which seems low for a plague hospital during an outbreak but reflects the combined function of the Paduan *lazaretto* on a single site.

Again, in this context, there is a clear need to distinguish between plague and non-plague years. By the beginning of the seventeenth century, the *lazaretti* were put to use for the housing of others beyond the plague sick, including soldiers as well as merchants and this was a policy which increased during the century and beyond. In 1617, for example, in Venice, it was necessary to buy extra mattresses and bed covers, along with other supplies for the treatment of soldiers arriving from Holland.[151] These individuals were also given different foodstuffs. By the

---

[147] See, for example, the image created in Vienna, reproduced in Harold Avery, 'Plague churches, monuments and memorials', *Proceedings of the Royal Society of Medicine*, 59:1 (1966), p. 113.

[148] See, for example, David Rosand, *Myths of Venice: the figuration of a state* (Chapel Hill NC, 2001).

[149] ASVer, Sanità reg. 33 42r (11 September 1575).

[150] Alessandro Canobbio, *Il successo della peste*, 22r.

[151] ASV, Sanità reg. 3 104r (18 November 1617).

second half of the seventeenth century, when the *lazaretti* were used as quarantine centres, the individuals being served were often soldiers and oarsmen (*galeoti*) and they received rice, wine and oil.[152] By 1648, the number of soldiers within the hospitals was so great that it was felt necessary to create orders relating to the care and treatment of the soldiers.[153] The hospitals were to be equipped with sufficient provisions for three days at a time, including bread, meat, wine, eggs, wood and coal, and money was sent to ensure both the quality and quantity of the goods. There was one nurse appointed to every sixteen patients. The governance of the soldiers was under the control of sergeant Pietro Gianella, who was given the title of overseer and held the keys for the hospital as well as keeping records of the sick. Later the same month, it was ordered that a specific hospital in the *lazaretto vecchio* needed to be erected to care for the sick soldiers. The hospital was assigned a doctor, surgeon, assistant, dispenser, four nurses, a cook and an assistant cook.[154] By April, the number of sick had increased and so the number of nurses was augmented and two women were sent out to wash the clothes.[155]

In a similar period, criminals were sent to the *lazaretti*, accompanied by officials, often from the Consiglio di Dieci.[156] In 1651, Andrea Trevisan was in the *lazaretto vecchio* and specific orders were issued to the Prior, guards and officials regarding his care. He was felt to be a particularly dangerous individual, at risk of flight. He was to be placed in cuffs and leg shackles. He was to be free of these irons only when the three doors of the tower (*torre*) were closed. Under no circumstances was Trevisan to be allowed to leave the tower. The guards were to be armed and alert at all times to ensure that Trevisan did not escape and that any attempt to flee would be paid for with his life.[157] Although these examples for Venice date from the middle of the seventeenth century, earlier authors recognised the utility of a few rooms set aside for the purposes of a prison, which could be guarded at eight or ten arms' length from the prisoners.[158]

Certain areas of the *lazaretti* offered space for isolation within isolation. Separate sites could be used for those individuals thought to be most dangerous or most vulnerable in times of plague. The interesting thing about the use of space within the *lazaretti* is to notice that there was a differentiation of zones, for particular groups of people (children, soldiers and criminals) and also for certain, dangerous goods; in 1689, it was said that two potentially infectious bundles of

[152]   ASV, Sanità b. 203 (10 January 1659).

[153]   ASV, Sanità 740 120r (19 February 1648).

[154]   ASV, Sanità 740 122r (28 February 1648).

[155]   Ibid. 125v (23 April 1649).

[156]   ASV, Sanità 740 149v (10 November 1648). For a discussion of the treatment of infectious prisoners in Palermo see Ingrassia, pp. 388–9.

[157]   ASV, Sanità 740 182v (21 April 1651).

[158]   Paolo Bellintani, *Dialogo della peste*, Ermanno Paccagnini (ed.) (Milan, 2001), p. 151.

silk should be opened in the 'most remote part' of the *lazaretto*.[159] Most patients, though, were kept together – in the male and female hospitals in the *lazaretto vecchio* and in groups in the *lazaretto nuovo*. The distinction of zones within institutions was an important part of the administration of these sites and was part of the overall system of allowing interaction between these sites and the city, whilst enabling them to have a degree of separation. A number of individuals moved around the hospital structures, including both patients and staff and it is this latter group which forms the focus for the next chapter, alongside the daily routine of the patients within the *lazaretti*.

---

[159] ASV, Sanità b. 203 (letter dated 6 April 1689).

Chapter 3

'Abandon hope, all you who enter here': Experiences of Staff and the Patients' Daily Routine

In his account of the plague epidemic of 1576–77, Benedetti wrote that the disease hit with a force fiercer than ever before and threw the city into utter confusion.[1] The Venetian *lazaretti*, carefully designed as they were, were put under considerable strain during the worst of the early modern plague epidemics. This chapter will contrast the administration of the hospitals and instructions as laid down in theory with the surviving evidence regarding conditions and care during times of plague. The chapter begins by outlining the staffing structure of the hospitals, describing some of the ways in which roles and responsibilities changed over time. *Lazaretto* workers have been grouped together with Health Office workers in previous studies.[2] This chapter will consider the workers and the specific *lazaretto* structures in their own right. The *lazaretti* employed natives and foreigners across a wide social spectrum. The chapter will consider the *capitolari* (statutes), which determined the number of people working in the hospitals and the roles they undertook. It is worth asking why individuals were willing to work in a plague hospital, considering the nature of available jobs. We will look in detail at the role of the Prior, who headed the hospitals' structures, and at the Prioress, who served initially alongside the Prior but whose position was marginalised at the end of the fifteenth century. During the fifteenth century, the Prior and Prioress were often a married couple, emphasising the important unit of the family in shaping men and women's involvement in medicine,

---

[1]   Rocco Benedetti, *Relatione d'alcuni casi occorsi in Venetia al tempo della peste l'anno 1576 et 1577 con le provisioni, rimedii et orationi fatte à Dio Benedetti per la sua liberatione* (Bologna, 1630), p. 18.

[2]   Workers of Health Offices were particularly considered in the works of Jean-Noël Biraben and Carlo Cipolla. For Venice, Richard Palmer outlined the variety of roles in which people were employed in response to disease and their salaries. He also drew attention to many of the principal roles within the *lazaretti*: the Priors, the doctors, the chaplains and the body clearers. Finally, he also documented some of the most significant trials and criminal cases involving *lazaretti* employees. See Richard J. Palmer, 'The control of plague in Venice and Northern Italy 1348–1600' (unpublished PhD. thesis, University of Kent, 1978). A study of the Netherlands in the seventeenth century highlighted body clearers, boatmen and midwives employed in response to the plague see Martinus A. van Andel, 'Plague regulations in the Netherlands', *Janus*, 21 (1916), pp. 410–44.

even beyond the home. The structure also echoed that of a number of other different social and medical institutions in the early modern city.[3] The significance of the family unit endured but by the end of the sixteenth century, the Prior had become the figure of responsibility on the island and there was little sense of a significant female by his side. Alongside the employment structure, stories of individuals employed in these roles help us to understand that the rules and regulations of the Health Office were obeyed, ignored and altered by individuals according to their will; the descriptions of workers' roles in statutes have to be considered with this in mind. The chapter will then discuss other workers of the *lazaretti*: the chaplain, the *pizzigamorti* (body clearers) and the disinfectors, amongst others, exploring the representations and roles of these figures.

Plague produced extraordinary conditions within cities and it is easy to forget that life would have continued in time of widespread death: this can be seen in the episodes of birth and marriage which took place alongside burials within the hospitals. In the second half of the chapter, episodes like these will be considered as part of the study of the daily life of patients. The care provided was designed to minimise fear, regulate morality and extend Christian charity to those in need. Although the reputation of the hospitals was as hellish, frightening places, this sense of fear would have created an atmosphere as dangerous, choking and potentially infectious as the clouds of smoke generated by the burning of bodies. As a result, early modern public health included a number of strategies surprising to modern sensibilities, such as allowing visitors to the plague hospitals. The idea of somatisation in early modern medical thought, that mental and emotional states had physical effects, and the converse idea, that physical states could shape mental and emotional ones, was actively addressed in the administration of the hospitals.[4] These efforts add substantially to our understanding of what early modern isolation meant in practice as the surviving statutes for the hospitals and the material from the Health Office archive are used to piece together daily life in the *lazaretti*.

The Employment Structure

Various studies have been made of workers within institutions in early modern Europe.[5] John Henderson's work on Florentine hospitals, for example, drew

---

[3]   See Merry Wiesner, *Working women in Renaissance Germany* (New Brunswick NJ, 1986) pp. 75–7 for the roles taken on by married couples in public institutions.

[4]   On the wider social significance of the relationship between the body and the emotions see Ulinka Rublack, 'Fluxes: the early modern body and the emotions', *History Workshop Journal* 53 (2002), pp. 1–16. For discussions of medical understandings see Fay Bound Alberti, 'Emotions in the Early Modern Medical Tradition' in Fay Bound Alberti (ed.), *Medicine, Emotion and Disease, 1700–1950* (Basingstoke, 2006), pp. 1–21.

[5]   Artisans have been studied by James Farr in *Artisans in Europe 1300–1914* (Cambridge, 2000). An interest in the link between work and identity has developed out of

attention to a Prior and Prioress, *commesse* (comparable with religious tertiaries), priests, cooks, servants, nursing staff, gardeners and women employed for the laundry.[6] Other studies of early modern hospitals have been undertaken by gender historians.[7] For women, hospitals offered important opportunities for work because of the domestic and 'motherly' associations of the tasks involved. Women's roles have often been said to be flexible within institutions, in order to be easily adapted to any family obligations. In Augsburg, the staffing structure was headed by the plague house 'caretaker' and consisted of the hospital father and his wife, alongside medical personnel, midwives, nurses and 'other men and women' for the lazaret.[8] Merry Wiesner's book on working women in Renaissance Germany describes women's work within hospitals as day-to-day tasks, such as the purchasing of supplies, the preparation of food and the laundry.[9] Her work also considered women working within the pesthouses of Renaissance Germany where they undertook administrative and maintenance roles. This, Wiesner writes, was because 'actual medical treatment was minimal; the best they could offer was probably a more pleasant place to die'.[10] Finally, recent studies have linked early modern work with identity, an idea which is prominent in Kathy Stuart's book on 'dishonourable trades' in early modern Germany.[11] The contemporary interest in the relationship between work and identity caused the propagation of two stereotypes of *lazaretto* workers, which will be considered before the nature of specific roles in detail.

---

work on the institutions of guilds and *scuole*. For example, Richard Mackenney, *Tradesmen and traders: the world of the guilds in Venice and Europe, c.1250–c.1650* (London, 1987) and Brian Pullan, *Rich and poor in Renaissance Venice: the social institutions of a Catholic state, to 1620* (Oxford, 1971), Part One, pp. 33–196. For Venice, an important work which explores this link in context is Robert C. Davis, *Shipbuilders of the Venetian Arsenal: workers and workplace in the pre-industrial city* (London, 1991).

[6]   John Henderson, *The Renaissance Hospital: healing the body and healing the soul* (London, 2006), chapter six, 'Serving the poor: the nursing community', pp. 186–224. Religious tertiaries were third order nuns, who lived outside formal religious communities.

[7]   For women in Venetian institutions see Monica Chojnacka, *Working women of early modern Venice* (London, 2001) and 'Women, charity and community in early modern Venice: the casa delle Zitelle', *Renaissance quarterly*, 51 (1998), pp. 68–91.

[8]   Anne-Marie Kinzelbach, 'Hospitals, medicine and society: southern German Imperial towns in the sixteenth century', *Renaissance studies*, 15:2 (2001), p. 223.

[9]   See Merry Wiesner, *Working women in Renaissance Germany* and the work of Margaret Pelling, in particular, her useful chapter on 'Nurses and nursekeepers: problems of identification' in *The common lot: sickness, medical occupations and the urban poor in early modern England* (London, 1998), pp. 179–202.

[10]   Merry Wiesner, *Working women in Renaissance Germany*, pp. 43–5.

[11]   Kathy Stuart, *Defiled trades and social outcasts: honor and ritual pollution in early modern Germany* (Cambridge, 1999).

A number of contemporaries mentioned the high mortality amongst *lazaretto* staff.[12] Given the obvious dangers involved in the work, contemporaries explained service as motivated either by extreme piety or extreme desperation. The first idea, about serving the poor or sick out of charity, is often visible in presentations made by individual workers about themselves.[13] The service of religious orders within hospitals and *lazaretti* further underscores this point. In many *lazaretti*, the clergy ran the show, administering both spiritual and physical medicine. In Venice, the chaplain had control only over spiritual and bureaucratic matters.[14] This did not mean, however, that religious ideas and instruction were any less important in these hospitals than elsewhere.[15] The self-sacrificing piety of medical work was familiar to contemporaries because of the image of the doctor as *Christus medicus*.[16] Brian Pullan cites a memorable account of a volunteer working within the Venetian *Incurabili* hospital to emphasise the contemporary link between serving the sick and piety:

> a leper, or one suffering from a form of skin disease, covered all over by a kind of pestilential mange, called one of the fathers and asked him to scratch his back. The father diligently performed this service but whilst he was doing so he was suddenly struck with horror and nausea and with the terror of contracting the contagious disease. But since he wanted to master himself and to suppress his own rebellious spirit rather than take thought for the future, he put into his mouth a finger covered with pus and sucked it.[17]

The pious and selfless nature of those working in disgusting conditions was emphasised in images which showed saints working in hospitals. The painting by Adam Elsheimer showing St Elizabeth is characteristically rich in its detail. It is not an image of what hospital care was like but what it was designed to be: clean, with considerate staff in ample number – one of whom is particularly remarkable for her virtues – and religious images designed to bring comfort, including the suffering Christ [Plate 20].

---

[12]   Francesco Manconi, *Castigo de Dios: la grande peste barocca nella Sardegna di Filippo IV* (Rome, 1994), p. 178.

[13]   For example, the supplications sent by doctors, considered in Chapter 4, pp. 158–9.

[14]   This was also the case in one of the Sardinian *lazaretti* see Francesco Manconi, *Castigo de Dios*, p. 179.

[15]   The place of religion in the historiography of healthcare was considered by Ole P. Grell in the review article 'The religious duty of care and the social need for control in early modern Europe', *Historical Journal*, 39 (1996), pp. 257–63.

[16]   Rudolph Arbesmann, 'The concept of "Christus medicus" in St Augustine', *Traditio*, 10 (1954), pp. 1–28.

[17]   Brian Pullan, *Rich and poor in Renaissance Venice*, p. 265.

The other association of the workers' motivation, with desperation induced by poverty, has generally been developed in stereotypes of roles rather than of individuals. Brian Pullan compared periods of the plague to Carnival claiming that it 'inverted the normal world ... by creating a temporary dependence on the unrespectable poor, especially vagrants and criminals, for the performance of essential service'.[18] The drive to work may have been, in part, desperation. There is much more for us to find out about the effects of outbreaks of plague on employment; many accounts record the closure of shops and limiting of services. To staff some roles, for example that of the *pizzigamorti* (bodyclearers), the unrespectable poor had to be enticed by the offer of benefits including lump sum payments. Even more notorious was the opportunity to wipe the slate clean for convicted criminals as parts of recruitment strategies for *pizzigamorti* in Venice.[19] These offers were partly responsible for the aggressive descriptions of these workers, for example, as wild animals.[20] The image of St Roch ministering in a *lazaretto* by Tintoretto [Plate 21] evokes some of the difficulties and unpleasantness of work within a hospital in a time of plague. The patients are shown on low plank beds, of the type ordered for the Venetian *lazaretti* and shown in artistic images of Milan [Plate 2], if in bed at all. The chaotic placement of the sick and the gloomy setting, with the light focused upon the figure of the saint creates an impression of distressing conditions, which stand in stark contrast to those shown in the Elsheimer painting. Whereas the former image expresses a confident sense of comfort and recovery, the latter has images of corpses being taken to burial in the background. Although each is concerned with care of the sick by a saint, it is the extreme nature of the setting which accentuates the saintly nature of St Roch's service in the latter image.

Whatever the motivations of individuals, the staffing structure was carefully regulated. The minimum number and nature of the workers within the *lazaretti* were determined by the *capitolari* governing the institutions. In each *capitolare*, a clause was included to allow the appointment of other workers on an *ad hoc* basis in times of particular need. In Venice, the statutes were issued to each Prior on appointment. The documents were read aloud in the Health Office and then posted in a prominent position within the hospital structures, so as to be available for consultation by all.[21]

---

[18]   Brian Pullan, 'Plague and perceptions of the poor in early modern Italy' in Terence Ranger and Paul Slack (eds), *Epidemics and ideas: essays on the historical perception of pestilence* (Cambridge, 1999), p. 117.

[19]   ASV, Secreta MMN 95 48r (9 July 1575). The same strategy of offering employment to prisoners is used in 1630. For a reprint of the legislation see *Venezia e la peste 1348–1797* (Venice, 1980), p. 370.

[20]   See pp. 129–31 for the *pizzigamorti* and Jane L. Stevens Crawshaw, 'The beasts of burial: *pizzigamorti* and public health for the plague in early modern Venice', *Social history of medicine* (2011).

[21]   See ASV, Sanità 730 139v (28 April 1557) for examples of these being read aloud and ASV, Sal, b. 6 (13 February 1484) for the clause stipulating they should be posted in a public place within the *lazaretto*.

The statutes were then to be read aloud at least once a month so that the largely illiterate patients would have been aware of their contents. Two versions of the *capitolari* survive in the records of the Salt Office and cover the first fifty years of the administration of the *lazaretti*.[22] A copy of one of the early *capitolari* can be found in the Health Office archive along with one dating from 1557.[23] In the surviving Venetian *capitolari* the employment structure does not alter significantly between the fifteenth and seventeenth centuries. These documents continued to be issued to the Priors and to govern the administration of the hospitals; although full transcriptions do not survive, amendments to various points do.[24] The lack of detailed research on the *lazaretti* restricts extended comparison of these documents. *Capitolari* survive from Treviso and Cividale del Friuli. These describe a similar structure of workers as the *capitolari* from Venice but on a smaller scale.[25]

Archive work on the employment structure at the *lazaretto* at Padua reveals that it consisted of a Prior, vice Prior, head of hospital (*capo*) and deputy (*sotto capo*), inventory clerk (*deputato a far inventario*), doctor, surgeon, barber, chaplain, disinfectors, body clearers, boatmen, cartmen and washer women in addition to the serving men and women.[26] In Canobbio's description of the *lazaretto* in Padua he describes a variety of workers during the severe epidemic of 1576, including Priors, vice Priors, eighteen body clearers, thirty guards, four cooks, ten washer women, four barbers, bakers, kitchen porters, eight wet nurses (*baile*) and a number of goats because the wet nurses were unable to supply all of the infants with milk.[27] The particular responsibilities of each are not clearly outlined but the role of the Prior at the Paduan *lazaretto* was comparable to that of the heads of other hospitals within the city – so much so that individuals moved between the posts.[28] In Padua, whilst the Prior was often a member of the clergy, the captain was appointed as a bureaucrat who had responsibility for notifying the Health Office of deaths within the *lazaretto* and of the movement of people in and out of the hospital.

As in early modern Germany, where the pesthouse, orphanages and bathhouses were administered by a married couple, the Venetian *lazaretti* were presided over

---

[22]   For the role of the Salt Office within the administration of the *lazaretti* see the Inroduction pp. 34–5. These documents survive as ASV, Sal, b. 6 (13 February and 31 August 1484).

[23]   ASV, Sanità 730 140v–145r (1 May 1557).

[24]   For examples of amendments see ASV, Sanità 727 199r (13 July 1532) and ASV, Sanità 730 142v (28 April 1557).

[25]   See Mario Brozzi, *Peste, fede e sanità in una cronaca Cividalese del 1598* (Milan, 1982) and Luigi Pesce, 'Gli statuti (1486) del lazaretto di Treviso composti dal Rolandello', *Archivio veneto*, series five, vol. 112 (1979), pp. 33–71.

[26]   ASP, Sanità b. 345, Part Two, which contains an alphabetical list of names, roles and salaries.

[27]   Alessandro Canobbio, *Il successo della peste occorsa in Padova l'anno MDLXXVI* (Padua, 1576), 17v.

[28]   ASP, Sanità b. 607 48r (undated).

by a Prior who was appointed with his wife or, if he was unmarried, a 'good woman' (*buona donna*).[29] The islands which worked as overflow sites during periods of particular strain – as outlined in Chapter 2 – could have their own Priors but not Prioresses. San Clemente and San Giacomo di Paludo, for example, were extensions of the *lazaretto nuovo* and were headed by a vice Prior, who was given the use of a gondola to go between the two islands.[30] Both *lazaretti* also employed a chaplain (*capellano*) and an assistant (*zago*), a doctor (*medico*) and barber and a certain number of serving men and women. In the earliest statutes, three women were appointed to serve the hospitals and they were soon supplemented with male equivalents. Some of the men were specifically employed as body clearers. A baker (*forner*) was appointed at various times and wet nurses (*nene*) were employed.[31] In the *capitolare* from 1557, few of these positions have altered, with the only addition being two boatmen (*barcaruoli*) for times of plague. By 1576, employees working on the islands were listed as *pizzigamorti* (body clearers), dispensers and servants, serving women, guards, and two boatmen for the *barche da mesa*.[32] Rather than illustrating a shift in the number or nature of those employed in the Venetian *lazaretti*, the later *capitolari* pay more attention to bureaucracy and organisation on the islands, outlining detailed obligations for the Priors.

The Prior and Prioress

In the fifteenth century the Priors were appointed with a Prioress. In early statutes, such as in 1436, the relationship between the Prior and Prioress was not stipulated; the only detailed information on the Prioress related to payment: she was to receive subsistence and clothing but no salary.[33] By 1479, there is more information on financial details: the Prioress was salaried in times of plague but not beyond epidemics but interestingly it was stated that the Prioress should be the Prior's wife.[34] By 1484, the statutes allowed for the appointment of unmarried Priors: if that was the case, a 'good woman' (*buona donna*) should be appointed with him. Her salary was permanent.[35]

Much of the material in the Venetian *capitolari* concerns the day-to-day tasks of the Prior and Prioress. Other workers and their salaries are described because of the role of the Prior in administering salary payments and purchasing supplies

---

[29] Merry Wiesner, *Working women in Renaissance Germany*.

[30] ASV, Secreta MMN 95 1r (20 September 1575).

[31] It is not clear whether a distinction was made between *bailie* and *nene*: the terms seem to have been used interchangeably to refer to wet nurses.

[32] ASV, Secreta MMN 95 9v (11 March 1576). It is not entirely clear what this boat is for – whether for the Mass or perhaps a messenger's boat.

[33] ASV, Sal b. 6 78r (14 June 1436).

[34] ASV, Sal b. 6 106v–107r (3 March 1479).

[35] ASV, Sal b. 6 165 r–v (14 February 1481).

for individual workers using funds from the Health Office. The Prior also received money for each patient within the hospital. The Prior was required to visit the sick along with his assistants (and the Prioress with her assistants) three times a day. Beyond Venice, there are examples of Health Office officials and governors of the *terraferma* visiting those in quarantine in their own homes and in the plague hospitals but there are no examples of the nobility illustrating their humility through visits to the infirm in Venice although other Health Office employees did visit the islands as part of their roles.[36] One of the principal responsibilities of the Prior was record-keeping and this aspect of his role became increasingly important during the sixteenth century. The Health Office relied upon accurate and regular communication from the Priors detailing the number of the people in the *lazaretti* and the number of deaths. Fifteenth-century *capitolari* also allocated a scribe to the Prioress to enable her to send similar information regarding the female patients directly to the Health Office. However, later versions placed the responsibility for these reports solely on the Prior. The Prior was also responsible for the security of the sites and was the holder of keys to the gates and warehouses (although there were usually multiple keys with others held by the doctor and chaplain) as well as inventories of any valuable items.

Length of service for the Priors varied considerably during the fifteenth and sixteenth centuries, ranging from less than one year to more than twenty. During the outbreak of 1575–77 six different Priors were needed to staff the two hospitals; the high turnover of Priors was due to one dismissal and three deaths. Outside periods when the plague hit the city of Venice, Priors could head the hospitals for decades. When the job became vacant, election for the position of Prior was announced in St Mark's Square and at Rialto.[37] Citizens of Venice, of good fame and condition were invited to apply.[38] In 1557, elections came in the midst of an outbreak of plague within the city and twenty candidates still presented themselves for election as the Prior at the *lazaretto vecchio*. The surviving lists of candidates for elections illustrate three things: first, that the position of Prior was one aspired to by Health Office officials as a rung on the career ladder; second, that individuals who had been employed in a different context in the *lazaretti*, such as physicians and surgeons, often applied; third, members of specific families, particularly those whose relatives had served as Priors in the past, often presented themselves for election.[39] Service within the Health Office was often a family affair and the role

---

[36] The Rettor of Brescia records visiting those in quarantine in 1631 in *Relazioni dei rettori veneti in terraferma vol. 11: Podestaria e capitanato di Brescia* (Milan, 1978), p. 345.

[37] For examples of elections see ASV, Sanità 729 60r (3 December 1544) and Sanità 730 152r (14 June 1557).

[38] 'bon citadini di questa citta, di bona fama et condition' in ASV, Sanità 729 60r (3 December 1544).

[39] For examples of supplications regarding family employment see ASV, Sanità 737 174r (12 August 1605).

of Prior was no exception. Particular families did retain the position of Prior across generations but this was not inevitable. It is clear that the position of Prior continued to be sought after. The following sections will explore why this may have been.

The salaries of the Prior did not vary considerably during the sixteenth century. At the *lazaretto vecchio* the Prior received 120 ducats with extra money for supplies. The salary at the *lazaretto vecchio* was always higher than at the *lazaretto nuovo* although, until the mid-sixteenth century, the salary of the latter was supplemented by income generated through renting out the vineyard of the island. In 1549, the vineyard was reduced to open grass land (*prado*) to create more space for the disinfection of goods. Thereafter, the Prior at the *lazaretto nuovo* received only the eighty ducats per year. With the role came the use of the Prior's house (*Priorado*) on both islands. The Priors were required, particularly by the latter half of the sixteenth century to be resident on the islands and neither they nor their family were allowed to return to Venice or to leave the city during periods of infection.[40] Priors were expected to remain in the *lazaretti* in order to oversee the good governance of the institution and ensure the appropriate conduct of workers employed in a variety of capacities.

Priors were generally appointed from the middling range of Venetian society – as members of the *cittadini*. Some feature for short periods of service with surnames linked to patrician families, such as Francesco Gritti in 1575 or Sebastian Contarini during the outbreak of 1576. In general, this was a position held by respectable, citizen men. Tasks were predominantly administrative. Daily communication with the Health Office was expected, providing information regarding people and goods in quarantine. Twice a week the Prior attended the Health Office in person – by the seventeenth century it was expressly stated that this would be Tuesday and Friday morning – in order to back up the written communications in person. The only other time at which the Prior was allowed to leave the *lazaretti* without specific permission of the Health Office was to attend Mass on a Sunday. During epidemics they would have received Mass on the islands. By the beginning of the seventeenth century, however, when plague was hitting the city less regularly there may not have been regular services within the chapels. It was stipulated that Mass should be taken in the location nearest to the *lazaretto* and that the Prior should return to the island immediately after the service.[41]

The roles of the Prior and the Prioress endured through the centuries in which the *lazaretti* were used in Venice but they changed significantly over time. This was said to be as a direct result of the behaviour of individuals. In 1485, for example, the dreadful conduct used by the Prior of the *lazaretto* towards the sick was said to be causing many to prefer to die in their own homes.[42] The account of a Prior at the time wrote that individuals within the city capitalised on the bad reputation of the *lazaretto* and went around the city saying, 'You don't want to send your sick to

---

40   ASV, Sanità b. 2 (16 April 1554).
41   ASV, Sanità reg. 3 79r (25 June 1601).
42   ASV, Sal b. 6 15v (2 March 1485) and *Venezia e la peste*, p. 86.

the *lazaretto* to die of hunger! Send them to us: we'll care for them far better!' In this way, they fooled individuals and then stole their goods, threatening to prolong the plague.[43] Theft was an issue which continued to be of concern throughout the history of these hospitals, and was often associated with maladministration by the Priors. In 1486, a new system of reporting was introduced using assistants, who were supposed to keep their own records and comment on the conduct of the Prior, doctor and barbers towards the sick. The assistants also held some of the keys to the site so that the Priors could not leave without their knowledge. This was just part of the system of checks and balance at work within the hospitals.

The behaviour of Health Office employees during the fifteenth and sixteenth centuries increased the concern of the authorities regarding the illicit movement of goods from the *lazaretti*. In 1605 a reviser was appointed in order to oversee the accounts of the *lazaretti*.[44] In 1630 *Sopraprovveditori* were appointed for the *lazaretti* in order to oversee the revision of the responsibilities and administration by the Priors.[45] Of particular concern were fraud and the mismanagement of the sourcing and distribution of food. In 1656, in the midst of a dreadful plague epidemic which affected much of the Italian peninsula, a *sopraintendente* was instructed to visit although not to enter the *lazaretti* to oversee their administration.[46] In the same year, the governing statutes of the *lazaretti* were reissued in response to disorder on the islands.[47] Although these individuals could concern themselves with the bureaucratic records of the Priors, they could not keep an eye on all employees, all of the time. A number of other employees were involved in thefts and could affect the accuracy of hospital records as much as the Priors, as will be seen in Chapter 6.

The Prior's principal responsibilities included keeping accurate records of patients and goods arriving and departing the islands, distributing food supplies and ensuring the security of the island. Food and supplies were ordered by the Prior according to need and paid for by credit which was then satisfied by the Republic, following the presentation of records showing the number of patients.[48] Use of credit in this way was standard within early modern social and economic relations and the sphere of medicine was no exception.[49] In times of severe outbreaks, such as 1575–77, large sums of money were passed from the Salt Office to the Health Office to cover the costs of the *lazaretti* along with other aspects of the public

---

43   ASV, Miscellanea carte non appartenenti ad alcun archivio, b. 16.

44   ASV, Sanità 737 175v (12 August 1605).

45   ASV, Senato Terra reg. 105 74v (15 April 1630).

46   ASV, Sanità reg. 3 150r (14 July 1656).

47   ASV, Sanità reg. 3 153v–164v (31 October 1656) for the new *capitoli*.

48   A number of examples can be found in ASV, Sal b. 8 94r (23 October 1531).

49   The seminal work on credit in early modern society and the economy has been done by Craig Muldrew. For a discussion of credit in the specific context of early modern Italian medicine see James E. Shaw and Evelyn Welch, *Making and Marketing Medicine in Renaissance Florence* (Amsterdam, 2011), pp. 81–122.

health systems.[50] The Priors were allowed to spend a sum of money per head on the hospital. The Priors received money for the sick, practically but ruthlessly excluding the day of death. The day ran from midnight to midnight and twelve *soldi* was given per person for half of the year. Between October and March the Priors received thirteen *soldi* per person for the winter months. The higher costs of operating the hospitals in winter were recognised by Health Office officials and may have contributed to the seasonality of use of the *lazaretti* mentioned in the previous chapter.

We can learn more about the day-to-day work of the Priors from a letter sent to the Health Office by Cristoforo de' Bartolis, who was the Prior at the *lazaretto nuovo* from 1512 until his death in 1544. His long period of service is recorded in a supplication from 1540. At the age of 72, he reviewed his experiences as Prior. De' Bartolis wrote in order to recommend his nephew, Alvise Ansuin, as a potential successor.[51] He provides a partial inventory of items from the *Priorado* in the *lazaretto nuovo* from 1540, detailing the interior furnishings which belonged to the Prior.[52] This inventory was included with his supplication with a promise that these goods would be left to the *lazaretto* if his nephew was appointed as Prior. De' Bartolis recorded notable events during his time at the *lazaretto nuovo*, particularly the arrival of large ships and their cargo. He emphasised the challenges of finding space for the goods and individuals and stressed the enormous amount of work, inherent dangers and intolerable strains of the position of Prior. De' Bartolis claimed to have called upon his nephew Ansuin during the five years previous to writing the supplication to assist with the burden of work and, therefore, recommended him as an individual experienced in the matters of the *lazaretti*.

De' Bartolis is an interesting individual, who, in addition to being Prior at the *lazaretto*, was involved in the mercantile activity of the Republic. He was granted permission in 1517 to leave the *lazaretto* in the hands of his wife and son and to join a galley ship because of his recognised experience of the journey to Flanders.[53] His travel from the *lazaretto* continued in the following decade and he was granted two travel permits for the season of Lent in 1522 and the month of June 1523. His experience reveals a freedom of movement for the Priors beyond epidemics which cuts against the rhetoric of isolation and containment associated with the hospitals as well as emphasising the link between the *lazaretti* and the mercantile structures of the city.

In addition, de' Bartolis promoted himself as having contributed significantly to the building structure of the *lazaretto nuovo*. He described his involvement in the rebuilding of the chapel on the island, said to have been consecrated in 1535. This, he stressed, had been rebuilt to honour God and the city and for the individuals who arrived at the island, providing them with a place to carry out their private

---

[50]   See, for example, ASV, Sal b. 10 reg. 13 (1574–82).

[51]   ASV, Sanità 728 46r–49r (3 January 1540).

[52]   ASV, Sanità 728 50v–51r (3 January 1540).

[53]   ASV, Sanità 726 10r (7 August 1517).

devotions. The work of Cicogna describes the chapel of the *lazaretto nuovo* and its various inscriptions.[54] An inscription marking the consecration of the new chapel was recorded on the wall. The date was 28 August 1533 and it was carried out by a Bishop who seems to have visited the island from the chapel of Santa Maria Elisabetta on the Lido.[55] This is a useful supplement to the archaeological information gathered about the chapel and printed in the guide to the *lazaretto nuovo*.[56] In the catalogue, a surviving plaque from the wall of the chapel, which names an individual called Bartolo is highlighted as significant, given the dedication of the chapel to San Bartolomeo.[57] The catalogue notes that Bartolo ascertained permission for himself and his family to be buried in the chapel and so must have played an important role in its construction. The identification of this figure as Cristoforo de' Bartholis has not been made, nor has his role as Prior at the *lazaretto nuovo* been realised. This connection opens up fascinating questions about the ways in which these early Priors perceived their roles. De' Bartholis' action illustrated a desire for his service to be attested to permanently within the *lazaretto* structure. There is a disappointing lack of information regarding the rebuilding of this chapel. If the role of de' Bartolis was further substantiated, a more detailed discussion of this unusual example of patronage within the service of the state would be possible. De' Bartolis was interred in the chapel – according to the surviving inscriptions he was the only sixteenth-century Prior to choose to be buried in this way.[58]

The position of Prior was considered sufficiently prestigious to act as a reward on behalf of the Venetian Republic, as is clear in the case of the Nassin family, which provided Priors for the *lazaretti* from 1545. Originally from Napoli di Romania (Nauplion in Greece), the Nassins had been citizens and fief-holders who fled after the city fell to the Turks in 1540 and took up residence in Venice.[59] Supplications record that they left holdings worth 3,672 ducats in Napoli di Romania. In return for loyal service during the Venetian occupancy of Napoli di Romania and to compensate for the abandoned wealth, the family were granted the position of Prior of the *lazaretto nuovo* for the lifetime of Nicolò Nassin (who was appointed

[54]   BMC, Codice Cicogna, 2018 (Iscrizione veneziane inedite), isole, b. 509:2 (Lazzaretto nuovo).

[55]   'R. dns. Dionisius. Grecus. episcopus/Gienesis. et Fremiesis. hoc. divu visitationis. beate. Marie. et Elisabet/templum. et. aram. ad. Dei. omnipoten/ tis. laudem. et. Honorem. anno Dni / M.DXXXIII. die. vero. XXVIII. Augusti / consecravit. ac. Dies. indulgentie / xxxx. concessit ' cited in BMC, Codice Cicogna 2018 b. 509:2.

[56]   Gerolamo Fazzini (ed.), *Venezia: isola del lazzaretto nuovo* (Venice, 2004).

[57]   Ibid., p. 100, note 58.

[58]   According to Cicogna's record of the inscription, de' Bartolis died in 1534 at the age of 65, although archival material says 1543.

[59]   Francesco de Nassin is one of the Nauplion citizens mentioned by Diana Wright in her thesis which is published electronically as 'Bartolomeo Minio: Venetian administration in fifteenth-century Nauplion', *Electronic Journal of Oriental Studies*, 3:5 (2000), pp. 1–235.

in 1545) and his son Zorzi (who served between 1555 and 1576).[60] The Nassins were members of the Scuola di San Nicolò dei Greci after 1541 and branches of the family held other positions within the middling ranks of the Venetian Republic.[61] The role of Prior helped to integrate the family into the social structures of the city. Despite deaths from plague within the family, the Nassin family continued to supply Priors for the *lazaretti*. By the mid-seventeenth century it is clear that the involvement of the Nassin family with the *lazaretti* had altered. In 1647 the family was described as invested with the position of Prior at the *lazaretto nuovo* and a substitute, Tommaso Rotta, was appointed to the position of Vice Prior.[62] In the same year, a supplication from Giovanni Domenico Nassin makes clear that a similar system of substitution for the Nassin family had been in place for the *lazaretto vecchio* since at least 1641. The position of the Prior at both *lazaretti* had become a post which a substitute could rent and the bureaucratic, quotidian elements of the role had been separated from the prestige and financial security which the job was thought to bring.[63]

The role of the family was significant in the administration of the *lazaretti* and the family continued to be a significant unit for determining the appointment of Priors through the sixteenth and seventeenth centuries. In seeking to recommend their successors, individual Priors often emphasised the importance of a family unit which had served together and within which young men had gained experience of administration.[64] The role was one which families could pass between relatives or successive generations.[65] The men who undertook the role of Prior in Venice during the fifteenth and sixteenth centuries were generally citizens, often from well-established and well-respected families or from those who sought integration into the city's social structures. The Priors were respected individuals, expected to carry out various administrative and financial tasks and were given a significant amount of responsibility for the running of the hospitals. The position included a

---

[60] Nicolò died during the outbreak of plague of 1555 and Zorzi during that of 1576. During the later outbreak, Zorzi had transferred from the *lazaretto nuovo* to the *lazaretto vecchio* to undertake the role of Prior, leaving the *lazaretto nuovo* in the hands of his son Nicolò. After Zorzi's death, the role of Prior passed to his brother Zuanne. Zuanne continued in the role until into the 1590s and after his death, the position passed to his son Nicolò. Details of the family are available in their various supplications which continue into the seventeenth century and include ASV, Sanità 729 66v (24 January 1544) and 730 188r (19 January 1557).

[61] For example, Francesco Nassin di Nicolò who lived in Candia and Venice was given the position of *capo dei stratioti*. I am very grateful to Ersie Burke for her generosity in sharing her work on the Nassin family with me.

[62] ASV, Sanità 740 69v (2 March 1647).

[63] ASV, Sanità 740 179v (22 February 1650).

[64] See, for example, ASV, Sanità 732 6v–7r (24 April 1574).

[65] A similar case as has been made regarding the Nassins could also be made for the Mauritios. For more information, see J.L. Stevens, 'The lazaretti', pp. 157–8.

decent salary and the use of the *Priorado* on the island. The experiences of these men stand in sharp contrast to those of the Prioresses, whose significance within the plague hospitals saw a significant decline during the period under study.

The Prior's family *in situ* in the *lazaretti* included his wife or, if he was unmarried, a 'good woman' to undertake the role of Prioress. Both were, initially, roles of some importance and it is clear that the Prior and Prioress worked together. One early Prioress, Anzola Mauritio took responsibility for the *lazaretto vecchio* whilst her husband, Hieronimo Mauritio, served in the Venetian fleet under Andrea Loredan. She was appointed in conjunction with her son, Valerio. After Hieronimo's death, Valerio was appointed Prior with Anzola obliged to serve alongside him.[66] Anzola did not receive a salary but Valerio was specifically instructed to support his family – including his mother, four sisters and three brothers. The early sixteenth-century example cited earlier replicated this arrangement when Cristoforo de' Bartolis left the *lazaretto nuovo* in the care of his wife and son.[67]

The fifteenth-century *lazaretti*, like many charitable institutions in early modern Europe, were administered by a married couple. In Ariadne Schmidt's useful article on Dutch orphanages, she refers to orphanages, poorhouses and prisons that had this family structure, headed by a man and a woman termed the 'father' and 'mother' of the sites, although we know that, in the Netherlands, orphanage parents at least were often unrelated and the family structure was symbolic rather than actual.[68] Nicholas Terpstra's studies have illustrated that orphanages in early modern Italy were similarly administered. He has argued that Renaissance society was familiar with the notion of extended families, which began with 'milk parents' then godparents.[69] This idea extended to the upper echelons of spiritual and secular administration. Kinship and family were often at the heart of political and religious metaphors and, in the Republic of Venice, the government was headed by a married couple: the Doge and Dogaressa of the city.[70] There was the idea of family structures emanating out from the natural, nuclear family. Regarding the purpose of this larger family, Terpstra has written that Renaissance parents sent their children into larger families who would help shelter, feed, educate and raise the children better than any single set of parents could. These larger families might be related by blood or marriage but frequently were not. They were created by choice and circumstance, occupation and neighbourhood. People freely used the language of family to strengthen social ties – honorary brothers and sisters were not found only in monasteries and convents, but also in guilds, in political

---

[66]   ASV, Sanità 725 41r (7 July 1498) and 44v (12 August 1498).

[67]   ASV, Sanità 726 10r (7 August 1517).

[68]   Ariadne Schmidt, 'Managing a large household. The gender division of work in orphanages in Dutch towns in the early modern period, 1580–1800', *History of the family* 13 (2008), 42–57.

[69]   Nicholas Terpstra, *Abandoned children of the Italian Renaissance*, p. 2.

[70]   Holly Hurlburt, *The dogaressa of Venice, 1200–1500* (New York, 2006).

assemblies and in the lay religious groups known as confraternities that helped organise much of people's day-to-day worship and charitable activity.[71]

The unit of the family is one which has often been seen in opposition to centralised charitable institutions. Some work has been done to illustrate the continuation of family ties across the boundaries of institutions (most notably on sociability in early modern convents and hospital visiting).[72] The adoption of the structure of the family at the head of centralised institutions has been widely acknowledged but only superficially studied. The most detailed work on the overlap between domestic and institutional ideas has been done in the sphere of architecture. In Saundra Weddle's chapter on nuns at Le Murate in Florence, she illustrates that the idea of the religious family was reflected in convent architecture as well as administrative language.[73] The convent was housed in a domestic dwelling and Agostino Valerio, in his advice to nuns, referred to their cells as the bedchambers of Christ, the spaces in which the celestial spouse descended when invited by prayer and called by meditation.[74] Notions of the family were also used in other terminology, such as the 'brides of Christ', developed by Tertullian as a deliberate attempt to ensure that women felt a part of a family unit within the convent and did not use a life of virginity as an excuse for escaping the natural role of a woman.[75] As mentioned by Terpstra, the nuns and monks in their relationships with one another were described as siblings, as sisters and brothers. Eunice Howe has considered the ways in which the architecture of Renaissance hospitals was modelled on that of the private home, using Alberti's contention that 'every building of this type [hospital] should be laid out according to the requirements of a private home'.[76] This comparison was drawn in the interests of morality, so that in both places the architecture would shape good, moral relationships.

Terpstra's idea of a public family, there to help when the private family could not cope, is relevant to times of plague which, like other periods of economic hardship,

---

[71]   Nicholas Terpstra, *Abandoned children of the Italian Renaissance*, p. 2.

[72]   For life and sociability in the early modern convent see Mary Laven, *Virgins of Venice: broken vows and cloistered lives in the Renaissance convent* (Harmondsworth, 2003) and for a detailed look at hospital visiting, albeit for a later period, see Graham Mooney and Jonathan Reinarz (eds), *Permeable walls: historical perspectives on hospital and asylum visiting* (Amsterdam, 2009). For the permeable walls of early modern Ottoman hospitals see Miri Shefer-Mossensohn, *Ottoman medicine: healing and medical institutions, 1500–1700* (New York, 2009), p. 158.

[73]   Saundra Weddle, '"Women in wolves' mouths": nun's reputations, enclosure and architecture at the convent of Le Murate in Florence' in Helen Hills (ed.), *Architecture and the politics of gender in early modern Europe* (Aldershot, 2003).

[74]   Cited in Marilyn Dunn, 'Spaces shaped for spiritual perfection: convent architecture and nuns in early modern Rome' in ibid., p. 156.

[75]   Merry Wiesner Hanks, *Christianity and sexuality*, p. 30.

[76]   Eunice Howe, 'The architecture of institutionalisation: women's space in Renaissance hospitals' in Helen Hills (ed.), *Architecture and the politics of gender*, p. 66.

strained family units. Poverty was the spark for the establishment of a number of charitable institutions modelled around notions of kinship and these institutions then took on some responsibilities of domestic sphere: arranging work, providing food and heating, and even organising marriages. Some of these spaces for work and charity were specifically referred to as houses (*case*), such as the *Pia Casa del Soccorso* in Venice. The *lazaretti* took responsibility for the provision of supplies for patients in times of plague. Although the *lazaretti* were not described in house-like terms, the family structure was reflected in the original form of the administration.

Merry Wiesner's assessment of a 'masculinization' of work during the period is visible in the structures of the *lazaretti*. The changes included the increasingly patriarchal form of the public family at the *lazaretto* and strongly-worded criticisms against women in authority, based around perceived inabilities in regulation and control of the hospitals structures (maladministration) and of their own sexual behaviour (immorality). The scandal with the Prioress, outlined below, would have been perceived as dangerous throughout the history of the hospitals. The particular changes in the administration of the hospitals, however, were shaped by the context of the late fifteenth century. One effect of the case was that the use of space within the *lazaretti* was altered. Contemporaries believed that quarantine and times of plague could and should be used as opportunities for repentance and reform and public health structures were shaped in order to provide such opportunities. There was concern that the space and structures of the *lazaretti* had allowed scandalous behaviour to take place.

Originally the Prioress had taken almost full responsibility for the care of female patients but her role altered significantly during the fifteenth century. The Prioress was entrusted with the records of female patients; the statutes stated that because women did not know how to write, a scribe was put at her disposal. By the sixteenth century, the responsibilities of the Prioress were restricted to the care of children. She was instructed to ensure that a sufficient number of wet nurses were retained within the hospitals since money was not sent to the Prior to care for young babies. The Prioress also fulfilled an ambiguous medical role, considered in the next chapter.[77] It is not clear whether the Prioress, like women in the Genoese *lazaretto*, were responsible for the education of children in matters of religion. Of Genoa, Father Antero wrote of the great risk that children without parents could grow up without instruction to live a savage existence (*vita brutale*). The provision of necessary instruction within the hospitals was entrusted to women.[78] In Venice, it is not clear whether the structures at the *lazaretti* aimed to provide a moral education.

Although the family continued to be a significant unit in determining the appointment of Priors, the role of individual women within the hospitals declined. In the case of the Venetian *lazaretti*, sexual mores played a significant role in the changing responsibilities of the Prioress, as can be seen from a surviving trial from

---

[77]   See Chapter 4, pp. 161–2.

[78]   Father Antero Maria da San Bonaventura, *Li lazaretti della città e riviere di Genova*, pp. 483–93.

the Venetian Archive series 'material which does not belong to any other archive'. This case records a fifteenth-century Prioress, whose scandalous behaviour affected the status of subsequent women in relation to positions of authority within the *lazaretti*. In 1484 an investigation was undertaken by the Salt Office – the body in control of the *lazaretti* before the permanent introduction of the Health Office – into the behaviour of the woman in charge of the hospital for female patients, who had formerly been the Prioress. The surviving details of the investigation consist of statements from the Prior, a serving woman, a boatman and the doctor.[79] The information from the serving woman and boatman is less detailed than that from the other two employees. The serving woman, called Elena, was employed as a cook at the *lazaretto vecchio* at the time of the incident. She was a *schiavona* (Slav) married and resident in Padua. She confirmed that Donna Cristina and the chaplain, at mealtimes, went to Donna Cristina's room and had sex within one another (*uxaseno insieme carnalmente*) at various times of the day and night. She also stated that this had been going on during the period in which the previous Prior had been in charge. Elena also confirmed details regarding the theft of clothing and fabric from the *lazaretto* by Donna Cristina, in conjunction with her son-in-law. Elena's account was followed by a shorter statement by a boatman, who described seeing Donna Cristina and the chaplain together one night in the dark in a part of the island which was hidden from the rest, rarely frequented by people – creating a fascinating sense of the hidden, isolated areas of the sites.

Both the Prior and the doctor provided lengthier accounts of the transgressions of Donna Cristina. The Prior's letter is a particularly haughty read and reminds us that we should not make too much of the apparently dual role of men and women in administering the hospitals by the end of the fifteenth century. The Prior made clear that he saw himself as the undisputed head of the *lazaretto*, the principal governor. He recalled his appointment and the recommendation by the Salt Office of Donna Cristina as a 'good woman' suitable for providing company and acting as head of the women's hospital – she was the serving Prioress at the time of his election. He noted that he accepted their recommendation in the hope that Donna Cristina was indeed a woman of worth, who would remain obedient to his instruction. He wrote that his first instruction was that she should be obedient and reverent to his person but that he soon found her to be the very opposite. He recorded a catalogue of grievances and complaints regarding Donna Cristina's moral character and her actions. He noted that her duty was to rest, sleep and observe in the hospital, to direct other workers, regulate the administration and report to the Prior. He accused her of theft of goods, the use of the Prior's wood supply (which appears to have particularly vexed him) and the abuse of funds. Above all, however, he wrote, Donna Cristina had turned the *lazaretto* into a brothel (*bordelli se fa qua*) – doing thousands of things which were abominable to God and to the world. He would warn her to stop, only to discover her at it again

---

[79] What follows is taken from ASV, *Miscellanea carte non appartenenti ad alcun archivio*, b. 16.

that very night with the chaplain, he claimed. The Prior urged the Salt Office to act and to remove her immediately from the *lazaretto* since, until that happened, he was convinced that the island would have no order or rule.

The doctor, Zorzi Corso, wrote a report which is particularly detailed and conveys a vivid sense of claustrophobia on the islands. It appears that the doctor and chaplain often ate together and were accommodated close to one another within the *lazaretto*. The first time that the doctor became aware of the relationship between the chaplain and the Prioress, he was said to have been looking for the chaplain. The doctor was on his way to the boatman's room when he found the Prior, who told him about the relationship and invited the doctor to join him in lying in wait in the cavity of the stairs in front of the Prioress's room. The Prior began to shout loudly 'You're turning this place into a brothel' ('*Bordelli se fa qua*') – at which point the Prioress came out of her room, seemingly repentant. The doctor's suspicions continued to be aroused, though, by the chaplain's continued absence at mealtimes. A few days later, the Prior told the doctor in confidence that he had found the chaplain and Donna Cristina at it again – this time up against the wall in the hospital. A boatman provided a further witness and, again, confessions were forthcoming. The doctor records ample detail of the scandalous behaviour of Donna Cristina but, unfortunately, we do not know how this story ended. Nevertheless, an indirect effect of the case was to reshape the roles of men and women within the *lazaretti* and to heighten concerns about the relationship between the sexes.

Good governance of the *lazaretti* was essential for the public health of the city. In the aftermath of the scandal described above, the governance of the hospitals was said to be poor and, as a result, the reputation of the *lazaretto* had become poor. This was said to be down to the lack of separation being made between men and women, which was of great danger to public health. The Salt Office responded to this lack of separation by increasing the distance between the sexes. The *lazaretto vecchio* was adopted for men and the *lazaretto nuovo* for women, with a Prior appointed for the former and a Prioress to head the latter. In so doing the administrative structure shifted from the model of the home to that of the religious institution (or the domestic to religious family). The explicit concern of the authorities in the legislation was contagion and the spread of the disease but it is likely that there were moral dimensions too, given the scandal with the Prioress, which happened just before the switch in administrative practice.[80] This division of the sexes did not last long – by 1489 there was said to be total chaos on the island under the control of the Prioress. After this episode, the Priors were given undisputed authority within the *lazaretti*, alongside the doctors and chaplains.

These three roles– that of the Prior, the doctor and the chaplain – became the most senior and prominent on the islands and represented the three strands of the medicine offered: practical, medical and spiritual. Although each of the roles was well-defined, there was a degree of overlap between them, particularly in terms of bureaucratic responsibilities. Overlap is also a feature of the roles of the other

---

[80]   ASV, Sal, b. 6 15v (2 March 1485).

workers who will be considered in the next section of this chapter. Individuals often undertook more than one job and in the following section will examine the chaplain and body clearers, responsible for burial and religious matters, as well as the disinfectors, boatmen and serving men and women on the island, to build up an understanding of who else worked within the *lazaretti* and what their roles and motivations may have been. Doctors and other medical practitioners will be considered in more detail in the next chapter on medicine within the hospitals.

Chaplains and Other Workers

A chaplain and assistant were appointed to the *lazaretti* almost from the earliest *capitolare*. They are recorded from 1432, with instructions varying as to whether there would be one chaplain for both *lazaretti* or one appointed for each. The chaplains, like the Prior and doctors, were specifically instructed not to return to Venice during periods of infection.[81] Their primary responsibility was naturally the care of the spiritual health of the patients on the islands. The chaplains had been appointed originally to bury the dead. By the sixteenth century, the concern of the Health Office officials was that the chaplains would ensure that all the patients – sick or otherwise – would live as good Christians.[82] On arrival at the *lazaretto vecchio*, the sick were obliged to receive confession and the sacrament.[83] The chaplain was required to say Mass on all of the principal festival days, which the Health Office determined to be every Sunday, Marian feast days, the feast days of the Apostles and that of St Roch.[84] The chaplains could, beyond times of plague, serve both the city and the *lazaretti* and were elected by the clergy of the city and paid by the Procurators of St Mark *de citra*. They were almost always members of religious orders. They could serve for many years, with a Fra Bernardino, for example, serving for over twenty.[85] Their roles compare with that of the Prior and the doctor in terms of length of service, perception of seniority and responsibilities from the Health Office. They were also involved in keeping records, signing inventories of valuables and recording wills which were made on the islands.[86]

The chaplains were involved in the personal landmarks for the patients within the *lazaretti*: the episodes of birth, life and death. Information on birth and marriage within the *lazaretti* is extremely fragmentary but it is still possible to ascertain that both births and marriages did take place within the hospitals. In Padua, in 1589, the lists of those within the hospitals record the presence of a baby boy born within the

---

[81] ASV, Sanità 725 (26 April 1486).
[82] Cucino 21v–22r (24 April 1555).
[83] ASV, Sanità 730 140v–145r (1 May 1557) [21].
[84] ASV, Sanità, 727 308v (14 August 1535).
[85] ASV, Sanità 727 327r (23 November 1546).
[86] These wills are discussed in Chapter 5, pp. 198–204.

lazaretto.[87] There is no further detail regarding special treatment either for pregnant women or new born infants within this context, although pregnant women were thought to be susceptible to the disease, in part because they had a heightened sense of fear of infection.[88] Neither is there detail as to how the traditional forty days of lying-in after childbirth might have intersected with forty days of quarantine. During the seventeenth century, a fragment survives of a baptism within the chapel of the *lazaretto nuovo* in Venice. The chapel was considered to be part of the diocese of Torcello and Sophia Catharina was baptised there.[89]

There is a little more information about a wedding in the *lazaretto*. In 1528, Vicenzo Cortese da Chioggia made his final will and testament within the *lazaretto nuovo*.[90] He made his wife, Lucretia, his heir – a fact which, in itself, is not remarkable. Of more interest is that he records that they had been married by Fra Andrea the Chaplain to the *lazaretto nuovo*, who was also the scribe for their wills. Their marriage had been witnessed by Zuan da Cathoro, Paolo Furlano, a boatman and Donna Helena, one of the serving women within the hospital. Both Vicenzo and Lucretia's wills survive but further information as to their personal circumstances before their periods of quarantine does not. It is unclear as to whether or not their situation was unusual; the record of their marriage within the *lazaretto* survives not because this was considered noteworthy but because of the Health Office's involvement in the execution of their wills. The wills were recorded by the Health Office notary on 16 September 1528 in order that they might be codified, which indicates that one or both of them died in the period between July and September of that year.

The role of the chaplain was recognised as one which brought individuals into close contact with the sick. During the seventeenth century, Father Antero Maria wrote of Genoa that the serving priests obeyed their superiors in matters of public health and undertook protective measures, which did not contradict the strong faith with which the chaplains served. He wrote that the priests wore wax hooded cloaks – like the *pizzigamorti* in Venice – the material of which, because it had a smooth surface, was thought less likely to carry infected air particles. Priests also wore gloves so that they would be unharmed by touching objects or people. They also wore shoes to avoid stepping in anything infected.[91] The priests sometimes took a preservative dose of *theriac* (treacle) or some other antivelenial. They almost always had a sponge soaked in aromatic vinegar at their noses and also, before entering the hospital wards, would set fire to a bundle of juniper in order to

---

[87]   ASP, Sanità reg. 49 77r (2 June 1578).

[88]   Alessandro Canobbio, *Il successo della peste*, 12r.

[89]   Archivio storico del Patriarcato di Venezia, S. Raffaele Baptizatorum liber (24 September 1695).

[90]   ASV, Sanità 726 153v–156r (2 July 1528).

[91]   Since Antero Maria stresses this point, it may have been that they wore shoes rather than sandals.

purify the infected air.[92] In addition to adopting these general methods, they also shaped their daily tasks in light of the risk of infection. They heard confession as quickly as possible (*con la brevita possible*) and administered the Eucharist using a tool (*l'instrumento*). Issues of infection were handled differently across Italy. Borromeo specifically criticised the use of instruments to administer the Mass in spite of the dangers of serving within the plague hospital. In Cividale del Friuli, confession was given to the sick in household quarantine from the window or the door, with the chaplain remaining at least three *passa* (steps) away from the patients. The sick within the *lazaretto* were moved to the doorway by the *pizzigamorti* and the chaplain was advised to remain the same distance as above. If hearing confession, it was said to be wise, if at all possible, to ensure that the wind was blowing towards the patient!

Chaplains worked in conjunction with their assistants and, in the case of a death of a patient, the body clearers. Body clearing was one of the most important roles within the *lazaretti*. In the earliest statutes of the Venetian *lazaretti* two men were detailed to bury corpses. It was stated in these statutes that burying bodies was considered vital to stop them rotting and releasing a dangerous stench (*fettor*) and thereby causing disease.[93] The importance of having enough people to bury corpses was frequently reiterated by Health Offices. Like the work of the chaplain, the basic responsibility of the *pizzigamorti* was religious in nature: an important part of their role involved moving dead bodies to burial sites or pyres. In Tommaso Garzoni's [?1549–89] publication on the jobs of the early modern city *La piazza universale*, the *pizzigamorti* are described in a section dedicated to funeral processions. Garzoni notes that the work of the body clearers was of the vilest nature and would have been on a par with that of the *curadestri* (latrine cleaners) were it not for its pious and religious purpose.[94] The work of the *pizzigamorti*, although recognised as being disgusting, was seen as acceptable outside periods of plague because it provided essential service, of genuine and eternal significance.[95]

---

[92] On smell and deodorization see Richard J. Palmer, 'In bad odour: smell and its significance in medicine from antiquity to the seventeenth century' in William F. Bynum and Roy Porter (eds), *Medicine and the five senses* (Cambridge, 2005), pp. 61–9; and Mark S.R. Jenner, 'Civilization and deodorization? Smell in early modern English culture' in Peter Burke, Brian Harrison and Paul Slack (eds), *Civil histories: essays presented to Sir Keith Thomas* (Oxford, 2000), pp. 127–44.

[93] ASV, Sanità 730 140v–145r (1 May 1555) [25].

[94] Paolo Cherchi and Beatrice Collina (eds), *Tomaso Garzoni 'La piazza universale di tutte le professioni del mondo'* (Turin, 1996), volume one, pp. 718–22. For the *curadestri* see volume two, p. 1358.

[95] There exists a substantial historiography on the subject of death and burial. Bruce Gordon and Peter Marshall (eds), *The place of the dead: death and remembrance in late medieval and early modern Europe* (Cambridge, 2000) is a useful starting point. For this issue of death in the context of plague see Chapter 5.

In addition to burying bodies, the body clearers undertook other responsibilities.[96] The *pizzigamorti* who travelled in the service of the state may have had a medical role. A contemporary described many patients in the *lazaretto* in Cividale del Friuli who were cured by the Venetian *pizzigamorti*, 'men expert in that profession'. When in Venice, they rowed the boats to and from the islands. The skills of the *pizzigamorti* as boatmen were further developed from the mid-sixteenth century when the Health Office's permanent *pizzigamorti*'s salaries were replaced by a ferry station licence (*libertà di traghetto*). A *traghetto* for boatmen was the equivalent of a guild or *scuola* for other occupations and had religious, social and practical purposes.[97] This *libertà* was a guarantee of income and work.[98] This post was provided to the permanent *pizzigamorti* (who, by the sixteenth century, numbered three). These men were expected to serve the Health Office whenever necessary – in Venice or beyond.[99] These workers were described as boatmen deputised to the Health Office and it was the Health Office officials which instructed the chief officer (*gastaldo*) of the *traghetto* to accept the *pizzigamorti* and to register their names in the rule book (*mariegola*).[100] In 1535, the need for boatmen deputised to the Health Office was commented on directly in archive material relating to the *traghetto* at Santa Sophia. Antonio from Brescia, a Health Office boatman, was made a member of the *traghetto* of Santa Sophia with the proviso that he must continue to serve the Health Office on the *lazaretto* boats whenever requested, on pain of losing the post on the *traghetto* and being banished from Venetian territory. It was not only the Health Office which had a boat at Santa Sophia – the Water Board had two boats and the *Provveditori de comun* had one and there was also one set aside for the hospital of the *Pietà*.[101]

This privilege supported the *pizzigamorti* for the duration of their lives and enabled them to rent out the position on the boats and benefit from the income. There is evidence that boatmen who had not become eligible for a *libertà*, perhaps because of age or lack of opportunity, offered to serve as *pizzigamorti* in return for the promise of the first free post.[102] From 1539, a *libertà* was also given to those

---

[96]   For more information on burial, see Chapter 5.

[97]   See Richard Mackenney *Tradesmen and traders: the world of the guilds in Venice and Europe c.1250–c.1650* (London, 1987).

[98]   Horatio F. Brown, *Life on the lagoons* (London, 1900) pp. 85–112. Useful documents are reprinted in David S. Chambers and Brian Pullan with Jennifer Fletcher, *Venice: a documentary history, 1450–1630* (Oxford, 1992) pp. 280–81 and 286–7. The *libertà*, by the turn of the seventeenth century, had become the responsibility of the government to allocate.

[99]   There are numerous examples to be found in the Health Office Notatorio series of *pizzigamorti* being beyond Venice – for workers sent to Cattaro and Spalato, for example, see ASV, Sanità reg. 13 118r (7 June 1572).

[100]   ASV, Sanità 729 92r (4 May 1546).

[101]   ASV, Milizia da Mar, b. 882 (traghetto di Santa Sophia) 108 and 123 (17 November 1535).

[102]   ASV, Sanità 732 50v (29 September 1575).

returning from naval service.[103] In both contexts, the post was a reward for public service, which integrated these men into the social and charitable structures of the city. Although the *traghetti* were akin to guilds, the members became notorious for bad behaviour and immoral characters. Boatmen were described as absolutely vile and indispensible – in other words, in very similar ways to the *pizzigamorti*.[104] There is a fascinating overlap in the language used to describe workers providing essential and basic services within the city.

In Venice, all those who worked in the plague hospitals were identified by a white sign on their clothing.[105] In addition, the *pizzigamorti* were restricted from walking through the city during the day without a guard and were instructed to have brass bells attached to their legs.[106] The *pizzigamorti* were marked out from the crowd using other distinguishing signs, like the distinctive clothing given to social groups that were perceived to be potentially polluting, such as Jews and prostitutes – similar signs had been used traditionally to identify lepers.[107] Searchers of the dead carried red wands when walking through the streets.[108] Particular pieces or styles of clothing were commonly used as an expression of social status and distinguishing signs were also used for the vulnerable as well as the dangerous within society. Cesare Vecellio [*c*.1521–1601], author of the famous costume-book, for example, records that the poor orphans from hospitals were distinguished through their clothing: those from the *Incurabili* wore dark blue (*turchino*), those from the *Pietà* wore red and those from the hospital at Santi Giovanni e Paolo wore white.[109] Distinctive signs were used throughout Europe. In Geneva, body clearers were instructed to carry white wands to indicate that they had been in contact with infection.[110]

---

[103] Brian Pullan, *Rich and poor in Renaissance Venice*, p. 129.

[104] Tommaso Garzoni, *La piazza universale* (Venice, 1665), pp. 636–7.

[105] ASV, Provveditori al Sal, b. 6 (31 August 1484).

[106] ASV, Secreta MMN 95r (5 October 1576) and 'alla guise di mattacini' BMC, Codice Cicogna 1509. In Palermo, the *pizzigamorti* were instructed to be clothed in sky blue, including the cap (*berretta*), so as to be easily identifiable. The accompanying guard was to carry a bell to warn others of their presence. Ingrassia, p. 343. On distinguishing signs, across the social spectrum (including pilgrims, merchants and beggars) see Valentin Groebner, *Who are you? Identification, deception and surveillance in early modern Europe* (New York, 2007), particularly chapter 2 'Images and signs'.

[107] Carole Rawcliffe, *Leprosy in Medieval England* (Woodbridge, 2006), p. 14.

[108] Kevin Siena, 'Searchers of the dead in long eighteenth-century London' in Kim Kippen and Lori Woods (eds), *Worth and repute: valuing gender in late medieval and early modern Europe. Essays in honour of Barbara Todd* (Toronto, 2011) p. 125.

[109] Cesare Vecellio, *Habiti antichi et moderni di tutto il mondo* (Venice, 1598), p. 116 ('Orfanelle de gli spedali di Venetia').

[110] William G. Naphy, *Plagues, poisons and potions: plague spreading conspiracies in the Western Alps, c.1530–1640* (Manchester, 2002), p. 115.

Few public health workers were thought to be as dangerous as the *pizzigamorti*.[111] Disinfectors and guards did not have the same level of contact with individuals within the city, neither were they associated with crimes in the same way. They did, however, carry out an equally important role. The Health Office placed great importance upon the effective disinfection of goods. A variety of methods were used for disinfection, according to the materials of the objects in question, considered in more detail in Chapter 6.[112] Disinfection of goods could be carried out by guards. Guards were hired to oversee incoming ships and boats requiring a period of quarantine. They also worked within the *lazaretti* structures. These guards came from a variety of occupations and were often foreigners.[113] The motivations of those appointed as guards were questioned by the Health Office during the second half of the sixteenth century. In 1574, it was noted that many guards who had been sent to the *lazaretti* and on board ships were not fulfilling these roles personally but sending others in their places and giving them a cut of their daily wage. This substitution did not sit well with the image of devoted service to the Republic, although it was fairly common practice within the wider city.[114] During the outbreak of 1575–77, the Health Office officials felt that too many individuals had been employed in this role and that, for many, the privilege of carrying arms had been the primary motivation behind election. New elections were announced and the total number of guards was limited to seventy, serving both the city and the islands. Of these, the *lazaretti* were allocated two each, with others going to the temporary *lazaretti* islands.[115] It is clear that the role of guard, like that of the *pizzigamorti* involved retaining a connection with the city. A prominent inscription on the walls of the main warehouse in the Venetian *lazaretto nuovo* was written by a Health Office guard responsible for disinfecting the merchandise from Constantinople. It recorded the death of the Doge Nicolò da Ponte and the subsequent election of Pasquale Cicogna in 1585, illustrating that these islands were not isolated from the transmission of news from the city.[116]

The transmission of news was also enabled because some workers were based within the *lazaretti* full-time, whilst others moved between the hospitals and their cities; among the most obvious of these were the boatmen and cart drivers. In Venice, these men and their boats had originally served both *lazaretti* but in

[111]   For the vivid, vicious images used to describe the *pizzigamorti*, see Jane L. Stevens Crawshaw, 'The beasts of burial'.

[112]   For examples of subdivisions see ASVer, Sanità reg. 33 165r (undated) and for methods see ASV, Sanità, reg. 3 1r (1574).

[113]   ASV, Sanità 729 190v (22 March 1550) and 730 6v (2 April 1555).

[114]   ASV, Sanità, Capitolare 3 3r (20 September 1574). For a discussion of substitution see James Shaw, *The justice of Venice: authorities and liberties in the urban economy, 1550-1700* (Oxford, 2006), pp. 49–54.

[115]   ASV, Sanità 732 52r (4 November 1575).

[116]   Images of the graffiti are reprinted in Dorina Petronio, 'Le testimonianze pittoriche conservate lungo le pareti del Tezon Grando: aspetti artistici' in Gerolamo Fazzini (ed.), *Venezia: isola del lazzaretto nuovo*, pp. 47–51.

1495 this was described as impractical because of the long distances involved and because of the threat of infection for the *lazaretto nuovo*. Two separate boatmen were elected to work at the *lazaretto nuovo*.[117] The boatmen were resident in the *lazaretti*. Early in the sixteenth century it was stipulated that these men should sleep in two rooms separated within the hospital buildings and not, as had been the case, in their boats.[118] The boatmen were not allowed within the hospitals themselves.

Other important roles within the hospitals were filled by the serving men and women. In 1432, men were appointed to bury bodies and to serve the sick. The women were divided into those who cooked, made the bread and did the washing and those who served the sick. The bread was expected to be made with unsifted flour or from dough made with good flour (*da masaria over da pasto da bona farina*). Details on washing within the Venetian *lazaretti* are limited but it is significant that these women were appointed in the earliest statutes and were in permanent employment. As has been shown in recent works, medieval and early modern laundresses were often in temporary and marginal occupation.[119] The appointment of these women emphasises the early priority of keeping clothing and bedding clean and explains, in part, the lack of reference to bathing or washing the body in the Venetian *lazaretti*.[120] In Palermo, Ingrassia set down regulations for washing the bedding in the hospitals and recognised the problem of bed-sharing as a source of infection. He stipulated that the sheets, blankets and *frazzata* or other covers should be washed so that only the mattresses remained.[121] Although it was women who were employed in this role of washing within the hospitals, the disinfection of goods was often entrusted to men.

The men and women who served the sick were based in the hospitals for the men and women in the *lazaretto vecchio*. In Padua, too both men and women were employed to serve in the hospitals. They served the food to the sick and administered 'all items pertinent to their health', as detailed by the doctor.[122] Although these roles continued, the *capitolari* of the sixteenth century become increasingly vague, detailing only that there should be four serving people

---

[117] ASV, Sanità 725 27v (31 October 1495).

[118] Ibid. 78r (31 July 1503).

[119] An engaging discussion of laundry women and the importance placed on clean clothes for reasons of hygiene in the medieval period is given in Carole Rawcliffe, 'A marginal occupation? The medieval laundress and her work', *Gender and history*, 21:1 (2009), pp. 147–69. See also Katherine W. Rinne, *The waters of Rome: aqueducts, fountains and the birth of the Baroque city* (London: 2010), chapter seven for information on the laundresses. Ingrassia, p. 343 records that in times of plague, the use of laundresses was not permitted and one person from each household was expected to do the washing.

[120] See Carole Rawcliffe, 'A marginal occupation?'. Ingrassia refers to washing the body in Palermo on p. 242. Hair would be shaved and hot (or *liscia*) water would be used along with herbal extracts.

[121] Ingrassia, p. 258.

[122] ASV, Sanità 730 140v–145r (1 May 1555) [18].

appointed with more employed in times of need. Serving women were also appointed directly to the Prior, Prioress and doctor to provide specific assistance to these individuals.[123] Father Antero Maria noted that, in Genoa, a greater number of women had to be employed at the *lazaretto* because of their physical weakness.[124] Venetian women may have been built of stronger stuff. By 1630, it was being recommended that women who had recovered from the plague should be employed as serving women, since their immunity would be higher. This indicates that a number of serving men and women became infected as a result of their work and close contact with the sick.[125] By the seventeenth century, cleaners were being hired to clear the rubbish from the islands – one was described as able to clean out ditches.[126] Again, however, information about the cleaning of *lazaretti* in Venice is limited when compared with that for other cities.[127]

In addition to the workers who moved between the city and the *lazaretti*, there were also those who were based within the city but spent periods working within the hospital structures. A significant amount of building work was undertaken during the sixteenth century in the *lazaretti*. A variety of workmen had access to and worked on the structures. For Venice, the names of these workmen are contained in the records of the Procurators of St Mark, with a detailed list available for the periods of work in 1549 in the *lazaretto vecchio* and 1548–49 and 1561 in the *lazaretto nuovo*.[128] Those supplying foodstuffs and goods to the *lazaretti* would have been visiting the islands. Gardeners worked in the *lazaretto nuovo*.[129] The Health Office notary and scribe made frequent visits according to their supplications.[130] These structures employed a significant number of staff (at least ten per *lazaretto* even outside periods of the plague within the city) and other individuals attended, supplied and worked in the hospitals in a variety of roles.

[123]   For Nicolò Colochi see ASV, Sanità 727 261v (19 November 1534).

[124]   Father Antero Maria da San Bonaventura, *Li lazaretti della città e riviere di Genova del MDCLVII ne quali oltre à successi particolari del contagio si narrano l'opere virtuose di quelli che sacrificorno se stessi alla salute del prossimo e si danno le regole di ben governare un popolo flagellato dalla peste* (Genoa, 1658), p. 22.

[125]   BMC, Codice Cicogna 3261 ('Ordini del medicare nelli lazaretti presentato alla Serenissima Signoria da Dottor Girolamo Thebaldi medico').

[126]   ASV, Sanità 740 66r (15 February 1646).

[127]   For particularly detailed instructions for Rome see Cardinal Geronimo Gastaldi, *Tractatus de avertenda et profliganda peste politico = legalis. Eo lucubratus tempore, quo ipse Leomocomiorum primo, mox Sanitatis Commissarius Generalis fuit, peste urbem invadente Anno MDCLVI et LVII* (Bologna, 1684), p. 377.

[128]   ASV, PSMc, b. 360.

[129]   ASV, Sanità 726 6v (30 July 1516) and Sanità 729 198v–199r (26 June 1550).

[130]   ASV, Sanità 733 42r (23 October 1576).

Regimen within the Hospitals

A number of the jobs within the *lazaretti* involved the distribution of charity within the hospitals. The *lazaretti* cared for individuals in a variety of ways. Medical treatments will be considered in Chapter 4 but the hospitals also responded to the 'non naturals' (air, food and drink, sleep and waking, retention and evacuation, exercise and rest, and the passions) of early modern theories of causation. Understandings of the passions and their significance for the health of individuals' bodies shaped the attempts within the hospitals to instil charity and assuage fear. In the next section we will consider how care within the hospitals responded to each of the non-naturals.

The quality of the air on the *lazaretti* was regulated in a number of different ways. As was seen in Chapter 1, the location of the hospitals was supposed to be airy.[131] Aromatic herbs and woods were burned during outbreaks to purify the air with fire.[132] The Veronese doctor Donzellini noted that he felt the quality of air during plague epidemics declined, not least because many people left cities or were sent to plague hospitals and as a result fewer fires were burned within cities.[133] This necessitated burning herbs in public squares. Buildings were continuously cleaned and aired during epidemics using aromatic herbs and wood. The disease was actively countered through fumigation and smoke. Within Venice, the seventeenth-century physician Thebaldi recommended fumigating houses, leaving the windows closed for a few days and then whitewashing the walls of the house. In the *lazaretti*, he recommended burning acidic materials (*fumi d'aceto*) in a number of places within the buildings.[134] The cleansing of the air was generally done using herbs and wood, although there were a few extraordinary suggestions. Ambroise Paré, for example, wrote of a Scythian physician, Alexander Benedictus, who was said to have stopped the plague by using the carcases of dogs, cats and other animals. These were dragged up and down the streets, releasing a putrid vapour which was said to force out the corrupted air that had been causing the plague. The idea that the miasmatic air which caused and spread the plague could be cancelled out by substances which were similar or opposite to its nature underpinned these actions, as it did the burning of aromatic wood and herbs. Paré also wrote that the idea of driving out and preventing the plague using similar, stinking smells caused some contemporaries to keep goats in their homes, because they filled the air with such a strong scent!

The Health Office officials also tried to ensure that the patients were not exposed to cold air. This was done in two ways – through medical treatments and the distribution of clothing and blankets. Ambroise Paré felt that keeping the body

---

[131]   See Chapter 1, pp. 71–3.

[132]   Many authors offer their views on appropriate substances for these fires. For Palermo see Ingrassia, p. 419.

[133]   Hieronimo Donzellini, *Discorso nobilissimo e dottissimo preservative et curative della peste* (Venice, 1577) [unpaginated].

[134]   BMC, Codice Cicogna 3261.

warm, particularly after the ingestion of treatments such as *theriac*, was beneficial and recommended moderate exercise. This could simply involve walking around – anything more strenuous ran the risk of more rapid breathing and the inhalation of increased amounts of corrupt air. Paré also wrote that sweating could be beneficial and induced by putting the sick to bed with plenty of clothes and an early modern hot water bottle – either warm brickbats or tiles applied to the soles of the feet or swines' bladders filled with hot water and applied to the groin (grindes) and armpits.[135]

The distribution of clean bedding and clothing was supposed to bring comfort to the patients and make their stays within the hospitals more pleasant.[136] In 1575, it was noted that some of the poor were returning from the *lazaretti* without the means of covering themselves and giving clothing was described as a charitable act.[137] In 1576, whilst additional accommodation was being constructed for the patients being sent to the *lazaretto nuovo*, it was noted as being necessary to provide mattresses to sleep on and blankets for the comfort of the sick poor. One thousand of each were to be purchased – in different sizes.[138] From the fifteenth century, instructions were issued to the Priors to distribute clothing to those within the hospitals. Men were to be given a large shirt, a jacket, a pair of linen stockings and a pair of shoes. The women were to receive items including a pair of shoes, a large shirt and an overgarment.[139] This was considered part of the charitable function of the hospitals. During the sixteenth century, when individuals were being licensed to return from the *lazaretti* without the ability to clothe themselves, a Health Office proclamation instructed that they were to be sold clothing, at as low a price as possible. Those who were judged to be able to pay the cost of the clothes had the sum recorded as a debit with the Health Office, otherwise the clothes were given for free.[140] There were seven items listed for distribution with corresponding prices: overcoats, hats, shoes, socks, shirts, trousers and vests. By October 1576, the Health Office officials were instructing those who were able to make their own provision for clothing to ensure that they did so, presumably to try to keep down costs.[141]

In addition to clean air and warmth, early modern contemporaries recognised the potential benefit to health of good quality food. The daily routine within the *lazaretti* started with inspections of the sick and if appropriate, individuals were sent between sections of the hospitals or, in Venice, between islands depending

---

[135]   Ambroise Paré, *A Treatise of the Plague* (London, 1630 [1568]), p. 47.

[136]   For the laundry in Genoa see Father Antero Maria da San Bonaventura, *Li lazaretti della città e riviere di Genova*, p. 480.

[137]   ASV, Sanità 732 69v (18 December 1575). An entry in the Health Office archive from 1542 offers a possible point of comparison with the charitable giving of clothes by the Republic. It describes 'diabolical persons' within the city who were enticing poor orphans, unable to provide for themselves, with the offer of clothes in ASV, Sanità 729 7r–v (27 July 1542).

[138]   ASV, Secreta MMN 95 91r (23 September 1576).

[139]   ASV, Sanità 725 132r–134r (26 April 1486) [10].

[140]   ASV, Sanità 732 128r (9 April 1576).

[141]   ASV, Secreta MMN 95 106v (30 October 1576).

on their conditions. In theory, boats of supplies would then arrive, so that the food could be distributed at the designated rate per person. Meal times were set down by the Health Office in Venice. In 1503, the Prior of the *lazaretto nuovo* was instructed to ensure that by one hour after *terce* the lunch had been prepared and that by two hours after *terce* everyone had eaten.[142] Dinner was to have been prepared and served before sunset.[143] Across Europe, administrators and observers reported problems of supply – particularly of high quality food and medical supplies. A series of letters survives from 1576 in which the captain in Padua described individuals and their families, the number of people present in the *lazaretto* and the need not only for more supplies but also more horses to enable people, goods and provisions to be moved between the *lazaretto* and the city. The supplies in particular shortage were bread, wine, flour, oil, salt and eggs.[144]

We have already heard about the ideal of the *lazaretti* as lands of plenty, in which food was distributed with order and calm. Such a representation was designed to portray the hospitals as beneficial from the point of view of religious healing. The items distributed were also seen to have medical benefits and the nature of the items did change over the centuries. In the early sixteenth century, good wine and good bread were distributed along with meat or fish according to the season, as instructed in the hospital statutes.[145] The seasonality of the food distributed was an important factor in determining supplies in Venice and beyond.[146] Statutes stated that veal, goat and chicken should be alternated and that, according to individual need, fresh eggs (*uova fresca*) should be given, although without discussing the cases in which this might happen.[147] Eggs were particularly prized as being easy to

---

[142] The period of *terce* was part of the canonical clock, one of five parts of the day which divided the hours of daylight, so the equivalent time in our modern system would have varied depending on the season.

[143] ASV, Sanità 725 78r (31 July 1503). These times are given as xxii hours and xxiii hours in the text. These times seem to have been given in the italian clock (*l'ora italica*) as described by Ernesto Screpanti. These hours consisted of twenty four units of sixty minutes but they were counted from sunset rather than midnight. He makes the point that this means, therefore, that xxiv hours would always have fallen before sunset and it is this assertion that has been used to interpret the dinner times at the *lazaretti*. For a very helpful explanation of what is a complex system of time see Ernesto Screpanti, *L'angelo della liberazione nel tumulto dei Ciompi: Firenze, giugno-agosto 1378* (Siena, 2008). I am grateful to Prof Samuel K. Cohn Jr for drawing this work to my attention.

[144] ASP, Sanità b. 273 covers the period 1576–1736. The sixteenth-century letters can be found on folios 338–56.

[145] ASV, Sanità, 725 78r (31 July 1503).

[146] For the seasonality of foodstuffs, particularly meat, in Florence see Allen J. Grieco, 'Il vitto di un ospedale: pratica, distizioni sociali e teorie mediche alla metà del Quattrocento' in Lucia Sandri (ed.), *Gli Innocenti e Firenze nei secoli: un ospedale, un archivio, una città* (Florence, 1996), p. 90.

[147] ASV, Sanità 725 132r–134r (26 April 1486) [35]. This has been translated as fresh rather than raw since *uove crude* tends to be used to refer to the latter.

digest and as foodstuffs which were entirely nutritious and did not contain anything superfluous.[148] Fresh eggs were more expensive than *uove normali* – in medieval Florence, the former cost double the price of the latter, although it is not clear how the prices may have differed in Venice.[149] Bread was distributed at the rate of four loaves, along with four measures of wine, one *lira* worth of meat and, on Fridays and Saturdays, eleven *soldi* worth of fish, or two eggs per person per day. In 1511, it was noted that large debts were being run up in order to pay for food supplies, particularly wine, bread, meat and eggs, because of the high prices during a period of famine.[150] The Health Office recognised the need to continue with these expensive supplies, particularly for the sick in the *lazaretto vecchio*. Chicken, veal and fresh eggs were all described as restorative foodstuffs (*cose restaurative*).

Food affected the health of the body as a result of its nature, its texture and the way in which it was cooked. Bread was one of the few 'tempered' foods, which was not thought to have a dominant effect on the humours of the body.[151] The other foodstuffs were thought to improve health actively by counteracting humoural imbalances. The value of these foodstuffs can be seen in a particularly interesting example of how appropriate food for treating or preventing the plague might be interwoven with the abstinence of Lent. In Gastaldi's account of plague in seventeenth-century Rome he records a dispensation which was given to allow inhabitants of the city to eat dairy products (*latticinii*), eggs and meat four days a week (Sunday, Monday Tuesday and Thursday). Inhabitants were encouraged to compensate for the dispensation in terms of food by going more frequently to Mass, increasing alms-giving and oration, so that both natural and supernatural treatments could be used to end the plague.[152] Although food is generally considered in relation to the physical health of the body, it was recognised to affect the health of the soul but only hints can be extracted from the records of the *lazaretti* regarding the seasonality of food and the place of food as a religious as well as bodily treatment.

The items distributed in Venice are broadly similar to those of *lazaretti* elsewhere, although sometimes the items intended for staff and the sick are difficult to distinguish. In Padua, bread, wine, cheese, fish, meat, salt, oil, eggs, figs and other items were sent to the *lazaretto*.[153] Allen Grieco's important work on the diet of patients at the Innocenti in Florence during the medieval period has established the difficulty of ascertaining the foodstuffs that were distributed to patients across the social spectrum when using account books – as survive for Padua. He makes clear that distinctions were drawn between different social

---

148   Michele Savonarola cited in Allen J. Grieco, 'Il vitto di un ospedale', p. 91.

149   See Allen J. Grieco, 'Il vitto di un ospedale', pp. 85–92. It is not clear what the dividing line between a 'fresh' and 'normal' egg was.

150   ASV, Sanità reg. 12 19v (6 November 1511).

151   See Ken Albala, *Eating right in the Renaissance* (London, 2002) p. 84.

152   Cardinal Geronimo Gastaldi, *Tractatus de avertenda et profliganda peste*, p. 481.

153   For the accounts see ASP, Sanità b. 345 16 r–v and b. 572.

groups and that some expensive, speciality foods were ordered in small quantities on, for example, feast days; the limited amounts that are ordered are indications that the food was distributed to only a few patients. It is difficult too to know about foodstuffs that may have been produced within institutions (and, therefore, do not appear in account books) and the way in which ingredients were cooked once they arrived at the hospitals. In Venice, the problems with space meant that open land was repeatedly cultivated and then cleared in order to facilitate the effective disinfection of goods. The production of foodstuffs must, therefore, have been sporadic but may have been more extensive elsewhere. Although bread making was carried out within the hospitals, it is unlikely that chickens were kept in order to provide eggs. Even in ordinary hospitals where the birds were kept, the demand for eggs was so great that supplies still had to be ordered in from outside the hospitals. In Venice, the Prior of the *lazaretto vecchio* was not allowed to keep dogs, pigeons or other birds, presumably because of a fear of infection.[154] The keeping of chickens within *lazaretti*, therefore, is unlikely to have been common.

Bellintani wrote that individual portions of food in *lazaretti* elsewhere for patients per day were four bread rolls, three measures of watered down wine, a portion (*una libra*) of beef and two bowls of soup. The sick were given eggs and broth. Women and children received a half portion of bread and wine. The issue of the diet for children is an engaging one but there is no indication for Venice of whether or not children ate more regularly than adults, in line with contemporary medical advice. Those under the age of fourteen were thought to need to eat in abundance, four times per day, whereas adults only needed to eat once or twice.[155] The comments by Father Antero Maria for Genoa that the children in the *lazaretto* were constantly demanding food may indicate that they were fed more frequently than adults but this cannot be proven with any degree of certainty. For Venice, the records refer to general times for the distribution of food and do not mention breakfast for children in addition to the lunches and dinners which were provided for all.

The lists of foodstuffs distributed in Venice correspond to Carlo Cipolla's list of items distributed at the *lazaretto* in Prato (bread, wine, meat, dry grapes, vinegar, eggs, oil, salt and chicken).[156] In Florentine hospitals, John Henderson has noted expenditure within Santa Maria Novella for wheat and other grain for bread, meat, poultry, eggs, fish and wine. Eggs and chickens were also bought by the hospital of San Matteo in order to produce nourishing broth for the sick.[157] At the Innocenti, the diet was based upon bread of differing quality – white bread on special occasions and possibly for the sick and *pane scuro* at other times.[158] This

---

[154]   ASV, Sanità b. 2 73r (16 April 1554).

[155]   The issue of meals for children and adults is discussed in Allen J. Grieco, 'Il vitto di un ospedale', pp. 86–7.

[156]   Carlo Cipolla, *Cristofano and the plague: a study of public health in the age of Galileo* (London, 1973) appendix four, pp. 148–51.

[157]   John Henderson, *The Renaissance Hospital*, p. 65.

[158]   Allen J. Grieco, 'Il vitto di un ospedale', p. 89.

system of supplying food to all patients was extremely costly and could only be achieved by cities. Elsewhere, on the *terraferma* for example, there are examples of families continuing to supply their relatives in the plague hospitals with food.[159]

Food for the sick formed a prominent part of physicians' treatises for the plague. Frigimelega, for example, wrote that the sick should consume bread, chicken broth, fresh eggs, meat and no wine. Patients, in general, were advised to avoid foods which were liable to become corrupt. Massa wrote that corrupting foods included Savoy cabbage, turnips, cucumbers, melon and other moist fruits.[160] Garlic and onions were said to inflame the blood. Patients were advised to partake of food which would assist the body in resisting putrefaction. Massa wrote that bitter foodstuffs helped in this regard. Borgarucci recommended meat broth, made up of good quality capon or cockerel, partridge, pheasant or similar game with lettuce or herbs.

Most physicians agreed that the diet of the sick was to involve footstuffs which were easily digestible, such as poultry, white meat and poached eggs. Other good meats were said to include cockerel, chicken, capon, pigeon, thrush, kid, calf, mutton, hare and venison. In 1630 Thebaldi wrote that it was very difficult to source meat in times of plague but that mutton was a laudable foodstuff and could be given to the sick when better meats were not available. Although fish was classed as easily digested, some physicians, like Ambroise Paré thought that it was best avoided, unless a patient was particularly fond of it. Bad meats from the point of view of digestion were pork, lamb, goat and all brain and sweetmeats.[161] It was not simply the basic foodstuffs which were considered but also the recipes and methods of preparation which could be used to encourage digestion. Meat was thought to be particularly good if served with acidic sauces involving vinegar and citrus fruits, raisins, sour cherries, prunes and caper berries to counter putrefaction. For those with weaker stomachs, the sauces were to include sugar and cinnamon. Meat could also be served in a broth made up with herbs. Particular herbs, such as saffron were thought to engender the spirits and help the body to resist poison. Broths were thought to introduce nutrients to the body in a gentle form and could be used to return patients, gradually, to a normal diet. Legumes, though, were a step too far in encouraging digestion, which threatened to 'engender grosse winds'.[162]

Broadly speaking, the diet of patients at the *lazaretti* followed medical advice, although the lack of information regarding the recipes used to prepare food makes

[159]   Elisabetta Girardi, 'La peste del 1630–1 nell'altopiano dei Sette Comuni', *Archivio Veneto*, 205 (2008), p. 81.

[160]   Nicolò Massa, *Ragionamento ... sopra le infermita che vengono dall'aere pestilentiale del presente anno MDLV* (Venice, 1556). Detailed lists are provided in BMV MISC 2411:2, Eustachio Celebrino, *Reggimento mirabile et verissimo a conservar la sanità in tempo di peste* (Venice, 1527).

[161]   For a long published series of instructions regarding the distinctions between good and bad meat see ASV, Sanità 727 85r–87v.

[162]   Ambroise Paré, *A Treatise of the Plague*, p. 38.

comparisons with the detailed instructions given by contemporaries difficult. In Bartolomeo Scappi's famous cookbook of 1570, in which the sixth book is dedicated to food for convalescence and illness, the recipes which are provided would have been used for a small number of elite individuals.[163] A number of broths, herb soups, preparations for eggs and roast meats are listed, alongside sweet cakes and it is useful to note that the nature of the food would have been similar to that distributed in the hospitals, even if the finer points of preparation and quality and variety of ingredients differed significantly.

The physician Massa stressed that food was an important part of the explanation for the absence of plague amongst the rich and its prevalence in the poor. The rich were able to purchase good food, good quality meat and eggs and avoid the bad humours which were generated as a result of ingesting poor quality foodstuffs. Foodstuffs possessed properties which were related to the four humours of the body, so the effect of food could be to heat, cool, moisten, dry, thicken or thin the humours. Ambroise Paré wrote that food to counter the plague should be cooling and drying. He also wrote that the sick should keep themselves well fed, since hunger could cause venomous matter to be drawn back from the superfluous parts of the body to the internal organs. Dehydration was also thought to be dangerous and so contemporaries paid as much attention to drink as to food in the context of plague.[164]

The distribution of wine was widely discussed by doctors.[165] Galen's observations on wine as an essential nutrient, because of its qualities which made it the closest substance to human blood, had suggested that wine was suited to encouraging the production of blood in medical treatment. Some of the many effects of wine on the body were thought to be the generation of heat as well as the production of gas and urine. Wine's qualities as a hot and moist substance made it most suited to those of a melancholy or saturnine personality (including artists and scholars!) as well as those of a cold and dry complexion. Wine was associated with moisture because it was a liquid. It was noted by a number of observers, though, as a result of their own experience, that the effect of wine could be dehydrating. The compromise position became that wine did not have universal qualities; the effects depended upon the quality and quantity of wine consumed. In relation to the use of wine in medicine, authors were specific about the types which were to be used and it was not thought to be appropriate for all patients, for example Muslims.[166]

---

[163] Bartolomeo Scappi, *Opera* (1570).

[164] Ambroise Paré, *A Treatise of the Plague*, p. 4 and p. 44.

[165] A very useful discussion is provided in Ken Albala, 'To your health: wine as food and medicine in mid sixteenth-century Italy' in Mack P. Holt (ed.), *Alcohol: a social and cultural history* (Oxford, 2006) pp. 11–25 and his *Eating right in the Renaissance* (London, 2002) p. 121.

[166] For a discussion of views of wine as medicine in the early modern Ottoman Empire see Miri Shefer-Mossensohn, *Ottoman medicine:healing and medical institutions, 1500–1700* (New York, 2009), pp. 91–2.

Wine continued to have a role as a preservative and was also part of the rations distributed within the *lazaretti*.

The distribution of wine was a traditional benefit for employees of the state in Venice. For cattle butchers, sailors and the workers of the Arsenal, the distribution of wine had originated in part as a supplement for low wages, as well as being designed to combat the problem of supplies of water for the employees and to provide a safe replacement for water when this was considered unclean.[167] White wine was said to be preferred by the workers and was also favoured for its medicinal properties. Workers at the Arsenal were given *bevanda delle maestranze*, wine diluted by water at the ratio of 1:2, which, Robert Davis has noted, would have produced a drink with 'an alcoholic strength of somewhere between 4.5 and 5.5 per cent, not unlike that of modern beer or ale'.[168] The watered wine was thought to keep people hydrated. Davis cites a contemporary observer who noted that 'only half as much bevanda was consumed in the winter as in the summer, since "the cold of the [winter] season suppresses the thirst"'.[169] Medical writers, such as Antonio Fumanelli, wrote that watered wine would have the effect of cooling bodies.[170]

The best liquids for hydrating the sick were much disputed. Water was distributed in some areas. Prospero Borgarucci did not recommend wine of any sort but encouraged the drinking of fresh water. If wine was consumed, he said, it should be dry and sharp and not sweet. A good drink in times of plague was said to be a mixture of vinegar and water, which would help to purge choler – although, even with this beneficial claim, it does sound like a less than pleasant alternative. In Rome, it was noted to be particularly important to be able to give water to the sick during the summer and it was suggested that each room should have a bell and a hatch in the door of about a palm-sized square through which it was possible to pass jugs and wash basins or fill up vessels with water without opening the door.[171] In Venice, though, it is only the distribution of wine which is detailed in the statutes and the use of the water which was delivered to the *lazaretti* is not explained.

Medical advice as to what could be eaten or drunk in order to improve health must, at times, have seemed overwhelming in its specificity and different recommendations – not unlike today. It would have been impossible to put into practice all of the advice that was given about food and drink in times of plague but the general principles of physicians' treatises are reflected in the foodstuffs distributed within the *lazaretti*. Those suspected of the plague would have eaten differently from the sick. For those suspected of the disease, the staple diet was bread, meat and wine. Regarding food for the sick, the doctor to the Venetian

---

[167] Robert C. Davis, 'Venetian shipbuilders and the fountain of wine', *Past and Present*, 156 (1997), pp. 55–87. Arsenal workers received lumber scraps for firewood and sailcloth along with wine.

[168] Ibid., p. 61.

[169] Ibid., p. 62.

[170] Ken Albala, 'To your health', p. 14.

[171] Cardinal Geronimo Gastaldi, *Tractatus de avertenda et profliganda peste*, pp. 581–4.

lazaretto, Nicolò Colochi's, instructions survive. His medical recipe will be considered in the next chapter in more detail. Colochi's information on food serves as a guide to the light but nutritious meals which would have been provided to patients – particularly meat broth and bread. He prescribed a diet of soup and water and no wine. He wrote that it was important to remain hydrated and ensure moderation of temperature – hence the restriction on wine which, despite the potential advantages, he thought opened up the pores and, therefore, increased the exposure to disease.

Despite attempts to provide nutritious and strengthening meals to patients, the conditions within which this food would have been consumed on the islands during periods of infection had their moments of the horrendous. For all of the charitable giving on the islands, much of what contemporaries record in their accounts consists of details of hellish conditions. During 1575, it was recorded that one of the hospitals in the *lazaretto vecchio* was full of beds on which people had died. They were said to be giving off such a stench that the doctor considered it necessary to evacuate and disinfect the hospital and the beds in question were burned.[172] It should be remembered that the sick would have consumed their meals with any such stench filling their nostrils as they tried to fill their stomachs. Father Antero Maria in Genoa recorded that the sick within the *lazaretti* stank horribly – so much so that a single patient could render a room uninhabitable. He wrote that individuals in the *lazaretti* fled the company of others because of the smell and confessed himself to having hesitated many times before entering rooms – not, he says, for fear of infection but because the smell was so foul. This was made worse by the vomiting brought on by the illness. This, he said, was so disgusting that it turned the stomach. He recorded it as the most difficult aspect of the conditions in the *lazaretto*, too abominable to describe in words.

The hospitals were decidedly overcrowded during epidemics, as attested to by the series of building works and the comments on the state of the overflow islands after plague epidemics, considered in Chapter 1.[173] Although open wards were supposed to improve the care provided by staff, the sheer number of people must have affected treatment.[174] The effect of these conditions and the effects of the disease on patients was said to be to drive them into a state of madness and fear. Benedetti described the sick who were maddened by their illness and leapt from their bed and screamed with the terror of a soul possessed, left the hospital and, lashing out, fell to the ground dead. Some threw themselves into the water or ran mad into the gardens, where they would be found dead, amongst the thorns, covered in blood. Madness in the plague sick was also recognised in the hospital statutes: provision was made in the *lazaretti* for the treatment of what were described as the manic sick (*infermi frenetici*). Such comments were not simply elaborations on the tradition of associating crazed frenzies with the plague, which

---

[172]   ASV, Sanità 732 59v (18 November 1575).
[173]   ASV, Sanità 733 213v (28 September 1577).
[174]   On the effects of layout on care see Chapter 1, p. 66.

Samuel Cohn has written, dated back to early accounts of the Black Death.[175] These patients were to be placed in low barrows with mattresses placed on top. They were to be tied with bands or strips of fabric and not with ropes and were to be supervised day and night so that they did not injure themselves.[176] It is not entirely clear whether this restraint was imposed simply to prevent patients from harm or whether it was also felt that restraining the body would calm the emotions. Patients and the madness of the disease were described in the *lazaretto* at Genoa. Father Antero Maria wrote that the sick were particularly prone to madness. One of the principal reasons for housing the sick in wards rather than individual rooms was the need for guards to be on hand to be able to force down or even chain those enraged by the disease. He wrote that five or six serving men were required to restrain patients in their maddened state from doing themselves harm. They were said to be strengthened by the violence of the illness and would run wild into the forest, hurl themselves through windows or almost drown themselves in the well or even manage an escape from the hospitals by leaping over railings and tall walls.[177] This behaviour was not an excuse for ill-treatment by the staff. Regulations were imposed to ensure that the sick and suspected were treated with respect. In Venice, the *capitolari* set down that workers within the hospitals were forbidden to hit or injure (*bater, ne inzuriar over contrestar*) the sick within the hospital, with threat of losing their job and any credit with the Health Office.[178]

Fear of the plague hospital was widely referred to by contemporaries. Lorenzo Condivi memorably described the *lazaretti* as a slaughter house (*beccaria*) and cited the phrase used in the title to this chapter 'Abandon hope, all you who enter here', suggesting it as an appropriate sign over the main entrance to the hospital.[179] Father Antero wrote that many of those who entered the plague hospitals despaired of their situation. It seemed to some to be Hell, he wrote, deserving of the same welcome sign cited by Condivi. The phrase comes from Dante's *Divine Comedy*, when, in canto 3 of the Inferno, Virgil passes through a gate, beyond which are the 'sad souls of those who lived without occasion for infamy or praise ... the miserable and useless gang of those who please neither God nor his enemies'.[180] These are the people rejected by both Heaven and Hell and are 'without even the hope of death'. The potential futility of time spent in the plague hospital, as people

---

[175]   It is interesting to note that Cohn records a decline in comments on frenzied behaviour as a symptom of the plague in the Milanese *Libri di morti* through the fifteenth century. See Samuel K. Cohn Jr, *Cultures of plague: medical thought at the end of the Renaissance* (Oxford, 2010), p. 68.

[176]   See ASV, Sanità 725 132r–134r (26 April 1486) [36].

[177]   Father Antero Maria da San Bonaventura, *Li lazaretti della città e riviere di Genova*, p. 16.

[178]   ASV, Sanità 725 132r–134r (26 April 1486) [38].

[179]   Lorenzo Condivi cited in Samuel K. Cohn Jr, *Cultures of plague*, pp. 273–4.

[180]   Dante, *The Divine Comedy* (Oxford, 2008), pp. 55–7.

Plates

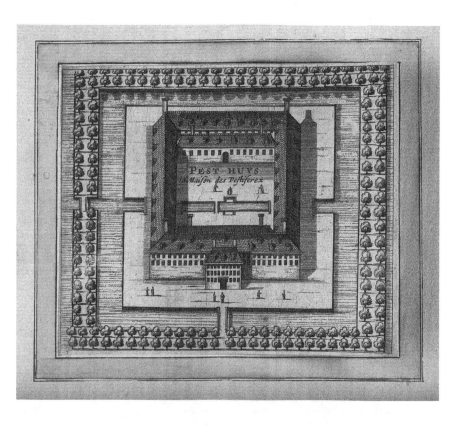

Plate 1   Plague hospital at Leiden, bird's-eye view (Wellcome Library, London)

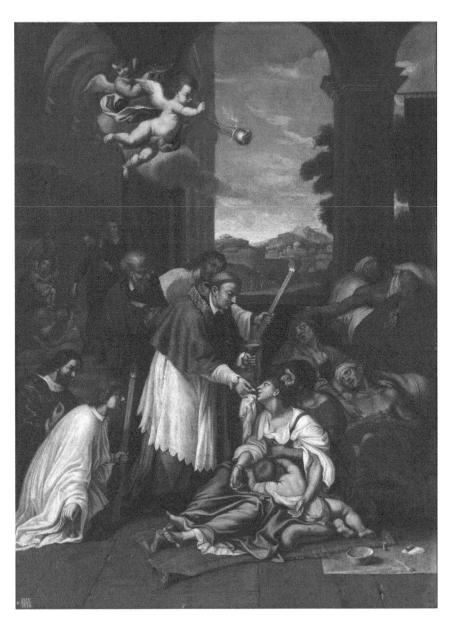

Plate 2   Carlo Borromeo ministering to plague victims in the *lazaretto* (Wellcome Library, London)

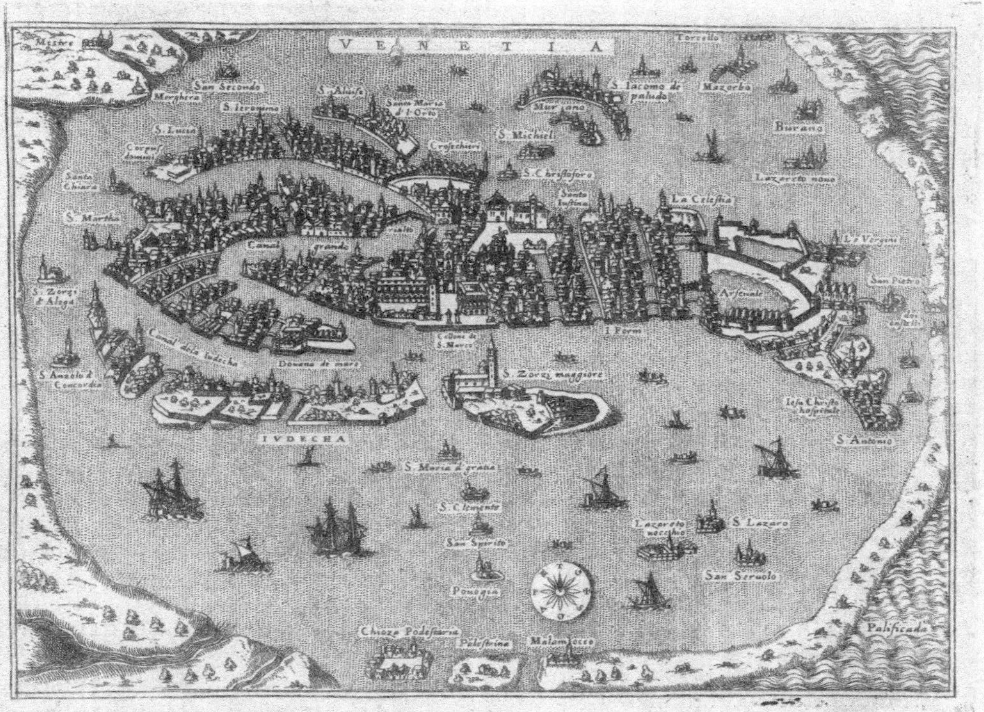

Plate 3   Map of Venice, Tommaso Porcacchi (Wellcome Library, London)

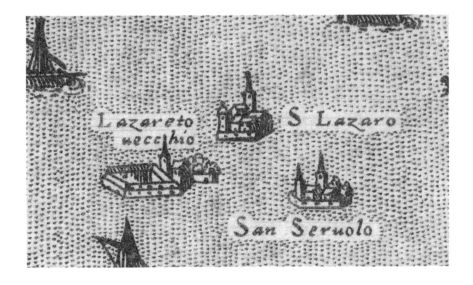

Plate 4   Detail of the *lazaretto vecchio*, Venice from Tommaso Porcacchi's map of the city (Wellcome Library, London)

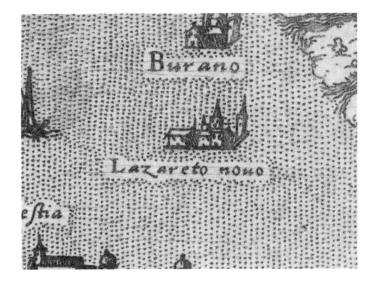

Plate 5   Detail of the *lazaretto nuovo*, Venice from Tommaso Porcacchi's map of the city (Wellcome Library, London)

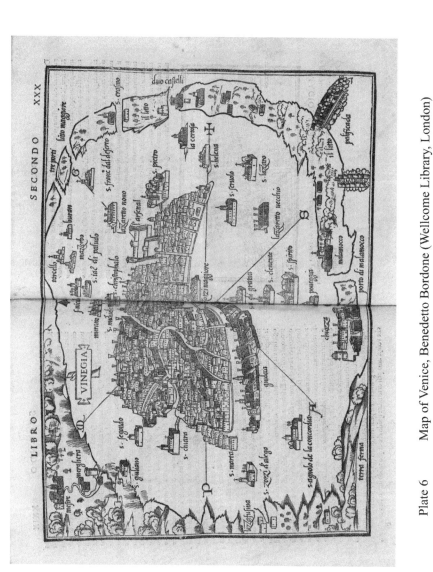

Plate 6   Map of Venice, Benedetto Bordone (Wellcome Library, London)

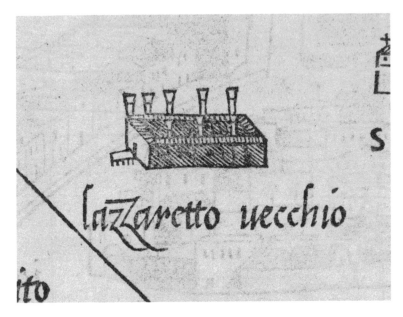

Plate 7   Detail of the *lazaretto vecchio*, Venice from Benedetto Bordone's
            map of the city (Wellcome Library, London)

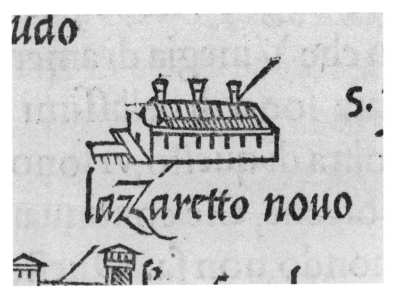

Plate 8   Detail of the *lazaretto nuovo*, Venice from Benedetto Bordone's
            map of the city (Wellcome Library, London)

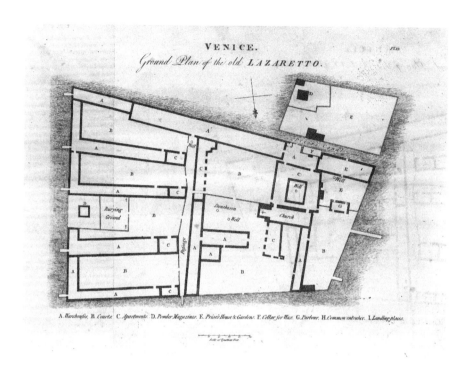

Plate 9   Ground plan of the *lazaretto vecchio*, Venice, John Howard (Wellcome Library, London)

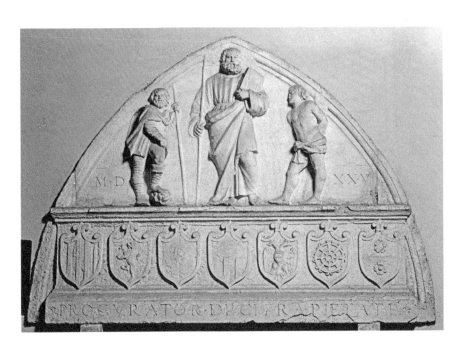

Plate 10   Carving from the *lazaretto vecchio* (Museo Correr, Venice)

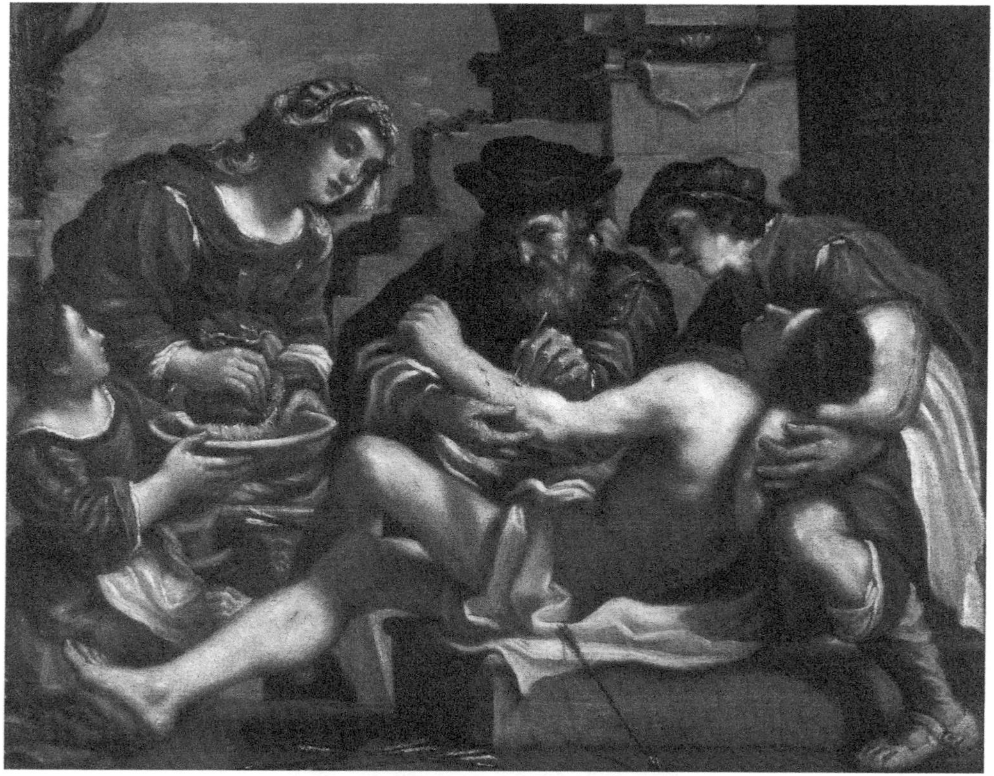

Plate 11   After Giovanni Francesco Barbieri, *Saint Sebastian being succoured by a surgeon and others* (Wellcome Library, London)

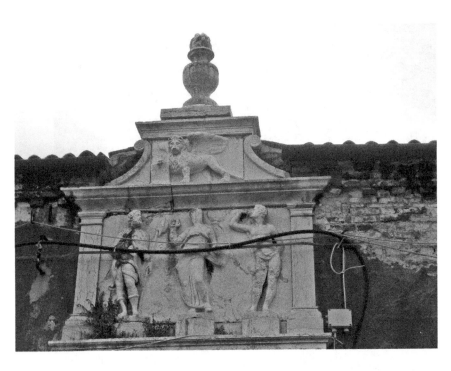

Plate 12   Carving from the *lazaretto vecchio*, from photograph (author's own)

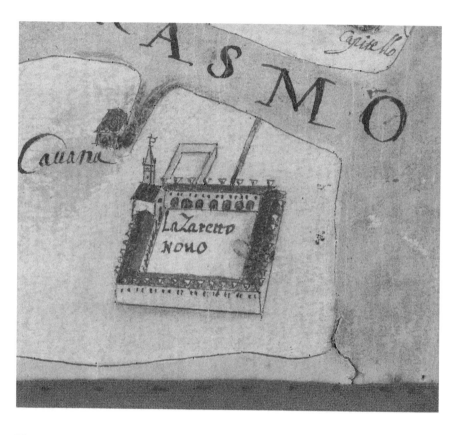

Plate 13   Ground plan of the *lazaretto nuovo* (Archivio di Stato, Venice)

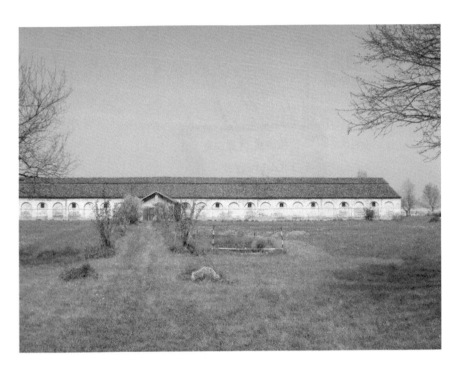

Plate 14   *Tezon grande* in the *lazaretto nuovo*, from photograph (author's own)

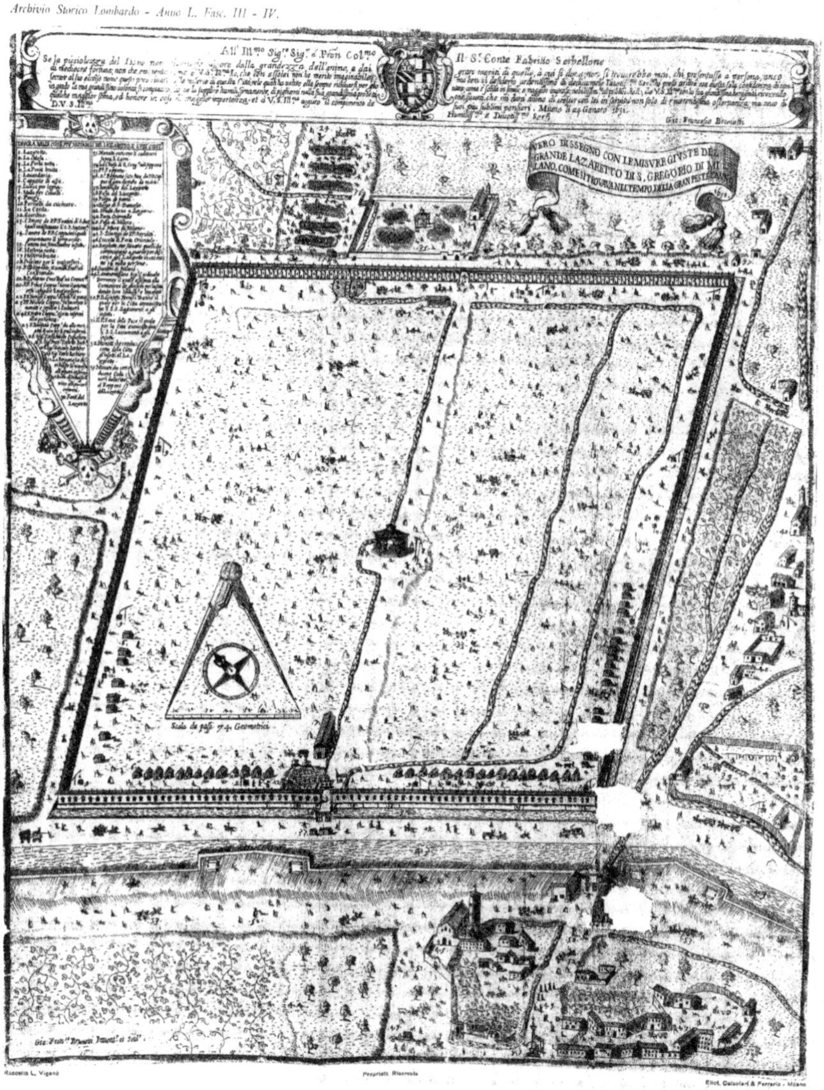

Plate 15   G.P. Bognetti, plan of the *lazaretto* at Milan (Wellcome Library, London)

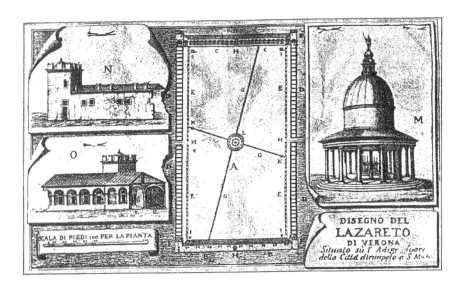

Plate 16   Plan of the *lazaretto* in Verona. E. Langenskiöld, *Michele Sanmicheli: the architect of Verona* (Uppsala, 1938) p. 95.

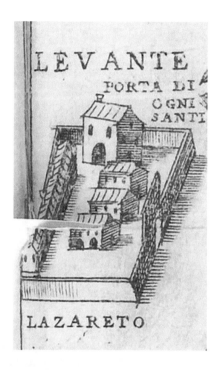

Plate 17   Map of Padua showing the *lazaretto* complex (detail) (Wellcome
Library, London)

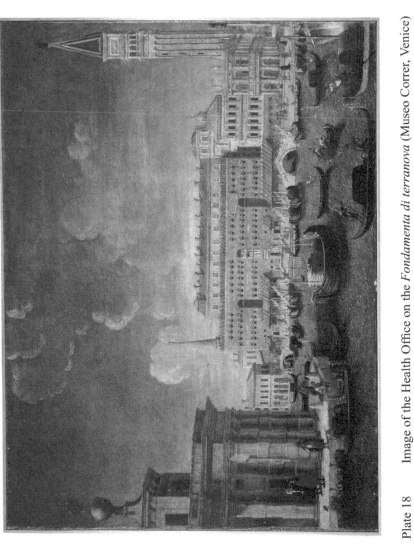

Plate 18   Image of the Health Office on the *Fondamenta di terranova* (Museo Correr, Venice)

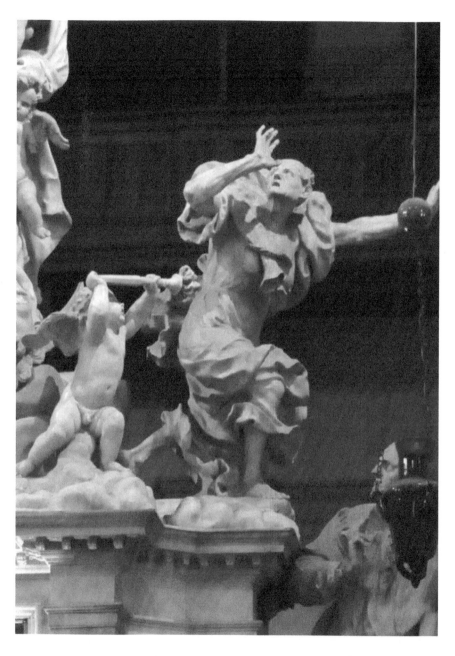

Plate 19   Detail showing the plague from the altarpiece at *Santa Maria della Salute*. © Wolfgang Moroder

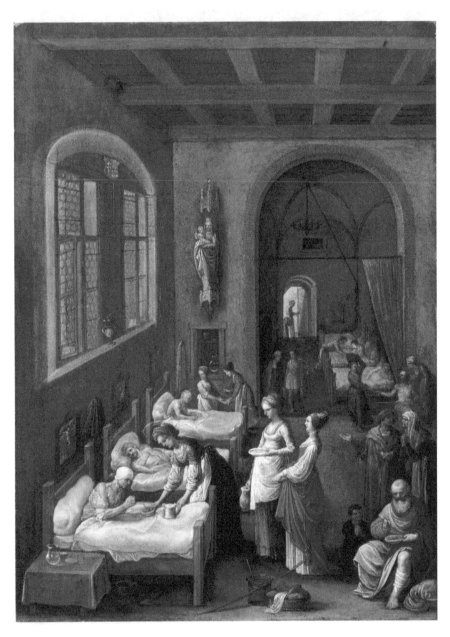

Plate 20 Adam Elsheimer, *St Elizabeth of Hungary bringing food to the sick*,
       (Wellcome Library, London)

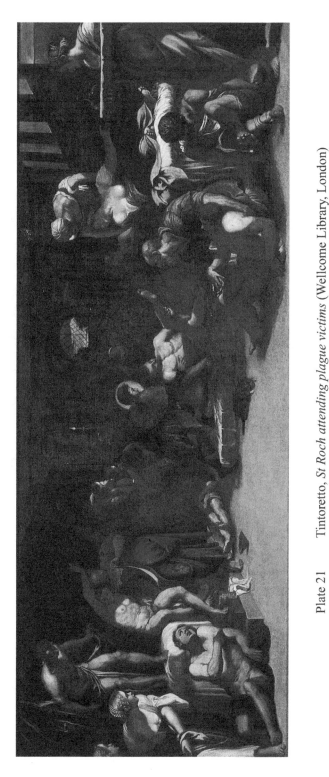

Plate 21   Tintoretto, *St Roch attending plague victims* (Wellcome Library, London)

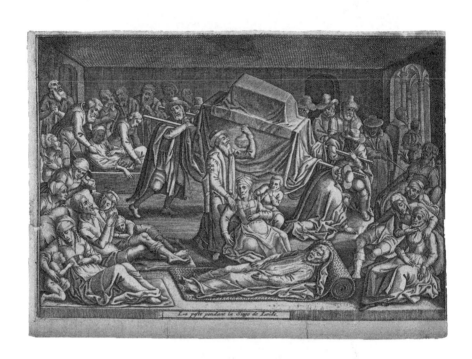

Plate 22   Image of the interior of the plague hospital in Leiden in 1574
(Wellcome Library, London)

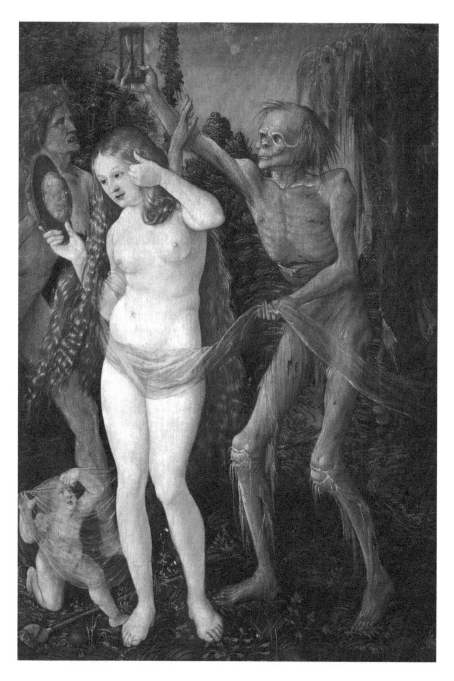

Plate 23   Hans Baldung Grien, *Three ages of man, and death* (Kunsthistorisches Museum, Vienna)

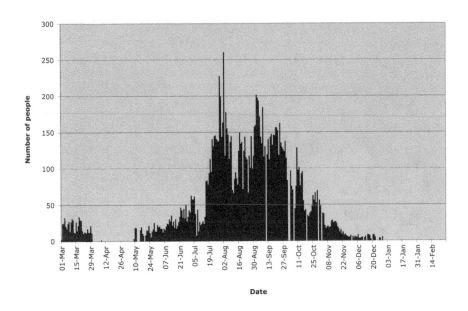

Plate 24   Graph showing suspected plague deaths in Venice (3 March 1576–
28 February 1577)

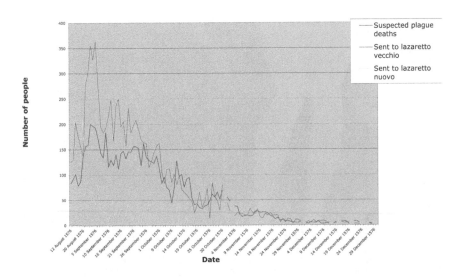

Plate 25   Graph showing suspected plague deaths and people sent to the
Venetian *lazaretti* (12 August–29 December 1576)

Month	Suspected plague deaths in the city	Number to *lazaretto vecchio*	Number to *lazaretto nuovo*
March 1576[a]	594	550[b]	149[b]
April 1576[a]	465	550[b]	149[b]
May 1576[a]	426	550[b]	149[b]
June 1576	796	1,211[c]	883[c]
July 1576	2,516	4,148[d]	1,240[d]
August 1576	3,783	5,187[e]	1,170[e]
September 1576	4,366	6,404	850
October 1576	2,114	1,813	44
November 1576	600	550	149
December 1576	161	112	23
January 1577	0	45	0
February 1577	0	44	0
Total	15,815	21,164	4,806

[a] The records of suspected plague deaths in the city for these three months are not complete. The original statistics have been used to calculate a daily average and the monthly totals have been increased using these averages to fill in the blanks.

[b] For each of these months, the records from November 1576 have been used as a comparative period.

[c] The comparative period from 15–30 October (suspected plague deaths total of 815) has been used.

[d] The comparative period from 12–30 September (suspected plague deaths total of 2,594) has been used.

[e] The comparative period from 5–30 September (suspected plague deaths total of 3,675) has been used for the *lazaretto vecchio* and that of 12 August–6 September for the *lazaretto nuovo* to allow for the changing use of the latter institution. The former period would have produced a statistic of 644 which was too low for this month. The changing use of the *lazaretto nuovo* is discussed in Chapter 2 pp. 83–4.

Plate 26   Chart showing suspected plague deaths and people sent to the Venetian *lazaretti* (March 1576–February 1577)

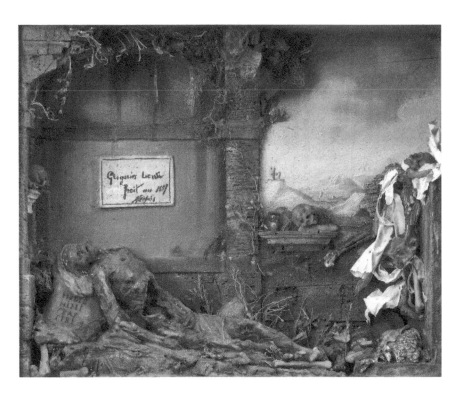

Plate 27   Gregorius Lenti, *Wax model of plague time*, 1657 (Wellcome Library, London)

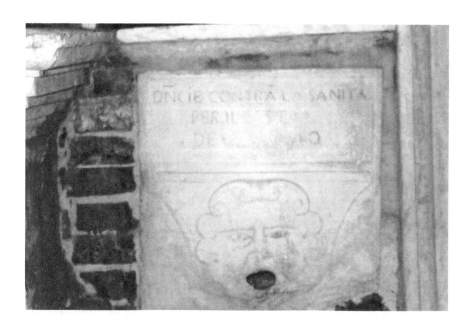

Plate 28   Photograph showing a lion's mouth for denunciations for crimes against health in Dorsoduro, from photograph (author's own)

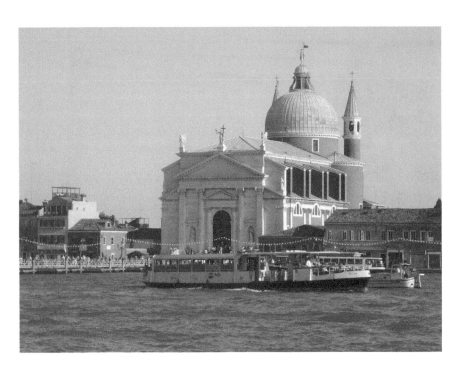

Plate 29   Image of the Redentore, from photograph (author's own)

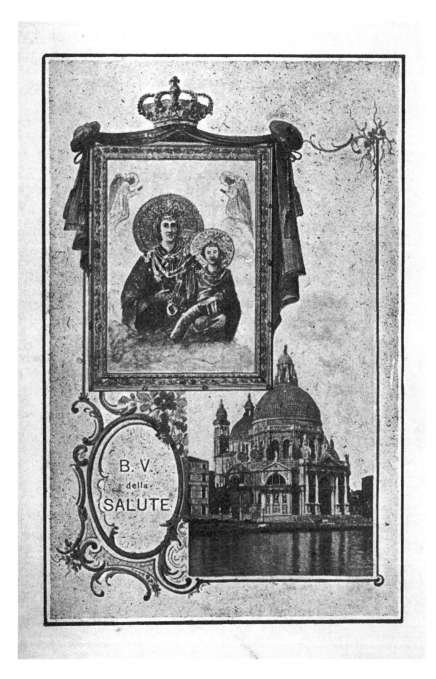

Plate 30   Blessed Virgin of Health at Santa Maria della Salute, Venice
            (Wellcome Library, London)

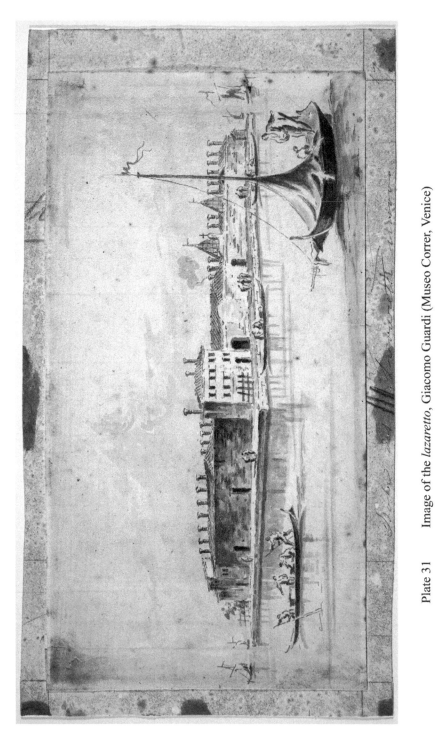

Plate 31   Image of the *lazaretto*, Giacomo Guardi (Museo Correr, Venice)

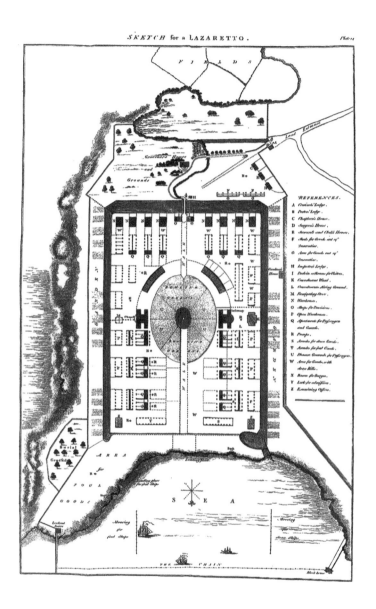

Plate 32   Sketch for a *lazaretto*, John Howard (Wellcome Library, London)

waited without occupation or activity may have resonated with contemporaries who associated the hospitals with this part of Hell.

Father Antero was insistent that entry into the plague hospitals was not tantamount to a death sentence. Nevertheless his book describes two groups of patients who were particularly vulnerable – the *infermi frenetici* and the *infermi agonizanti*. The first group were those enraged by the illness. The second group was those who were terrified by the illness. He was far from alone in recognising the terror instilled by the disease and it seems that staff were no less immune than patients. In Rome in 1656, Gastaldi records, in a fascinating text, which includes copies of Health Office instructions, two proclamations regarding staff who had fled from the *lazaretto*: the first, twenty-five-year-old Jacomo di Francesco Crispiani from Assisi, was described as being of 'mediocre' stature, black-skinned and as someone who had served in the *lazaretto* at Ponte Quattro Capi; the second, Domenico di Giovanni Sabbatino, from Rome, was thirty years old, short with dark hair and a dark beard. He had been serving as a *pizzigamorto* when he fled in November 1656.[181]

Health Office officials recognised that a response to the atmosphere of fear could be an attitude of *carpe diem* and attempts to forget about the conditions in which individuals found themselves. Such behaviour could prove dangerous and a number of contemporary authors agreed that alongside treatments for the body there should be remedies for the soul.[182] Samuel Cohn has noted that the tract written by a Bolognese druggist Pastarino recommended that individuals purge themselves of 'bad blood, evil thoughts and dirty words' in the context of plague.[183] Various attempts were made to regulate behaviour within the *lazaretti*. The threat of punishments was made visible within the structure. Gallows were placed within the *lazaretti* as a threat that anyone caught stealing goods from the hospitals would be hanged.[184] During a period of sickness of the Prior at the *lazaretto vecchio*, a series of unacceptable acts were said to have taken place, which included the sick mixing with people from the *Priorado* (Prior's house) and the *pizzigamorti* forcing their way into the *Priorado*, it was said, to make bread with the serving woman – it is not clear whether that was a euphemism. The doctor Cucino was asked to adopt temporarily the role of Prior and to remind all on the islands that they should remain obedient to official instructions – with the threat of the gallows

---

[181] Cardinal Geronimo Gastaldi, *Tractatus de avertenda et profliganda peste*, p. 339 and p. 453. For an engaging discussion of modes of description and identification in early modern Europe see Valentin Groebner, *Who are you? Identification, deception and surveillance in early modern Europe* (New York, 2007), particularly chapter 5, 'Nature's way: the color of things'.

[182] On fear and the advice to keep one's spirits up in times of plague see Samuel K. Cohn Jr, *Cultures of plague*, pp. 266–77.

[183] Ibid., p. 17.

[184] Cini, Mantua, b. 1489 (21 June 1556).

if they did not.[185] This was reiterated the following day in a proclamation from the Health Office.[186] Cucino was instructed to report all indiscretions by staff and patients to the Health Office and to inform potential transgressors that, if caught, the staff would have their salary stopped in addition to standard punishments and that individuals would be put into wooden blocks, chains or prison.[187] An earlier report from Cucino made clear that some patients were hoarding bread and other foodstuffs – one patient had managed to scurry away forty bread rolls and other items. Clearly not all of the patients were convinced by Sansovino's idea of the island as a land of plenty.[188] The Health Office officials wrote that patients should be reminded to be obedient and sensible, otherwise they would be punished by hanging, although no such events are recorded.[189]

It is worth considering the regulations and restrictions of the *lazaretti* alongside those of the city lest the former appear particularly severe.[190] In 1576, as a response to plague, officials in Venice announced that dances were not to take place within the city and the same was true for the hospitals.[191] This was not confined to Venice. One memorable account from the *lazaretto* in Milan records how one of the members of the religious order in charge of the institution discovered a party in one of the rooms of the hospital, something which had been explicitly forbidden. The brother in question decided to break up the party and frighten the dancers by collecting the corpse of an old woman who had died the previous day. He carried the corpse to the room in question and knocked on the door. To the question, 'Who is it?' he replied, 'People who want to dance.' The door was opened and the brother threw the corpse onto the ground in the middle of the dance and said 'She wants to dance too', reminding them that the avoidance of death relied upon avoiding offending God through their behaviour.[192] This is an extreme example of attempts to control behaviour within the institutions. More will be said about crimes and the regulation of behaviour on the islands in the final chapter. Here, however, it is sufficient to recognise the fine line which was sought in the regulation of behaviour: too lax an approach and individuals threatened to prolong the plague through their sinful behaviour and dangerous actions – this is not a particularly revolutionary idea. What is important to note alongside this, however, was that

---

[185]   'li pizzigamorti per forze sono venuti nel Priorado et hanno voluto fare il pan la insieme con le massare dell'hospitali' in Cucino 12v (14 April 1555).

[186]   Cucino 14r (15 April 1555).

[187]   Cucino 34r (16 May 1555).

[188]   For the idea of the *lazaretto* as a 'land of plenty' see Chapter 1 pp. 46–7.

[189]   Cucino 24r (2 May 1555).

[190]   ASV, Secreta MMN 95 4v (13 November 1575).

[191]   ASV, Secreta MMN 126v (25 January 1576 m.v.).

[192]   Federico Odorici, 'I due Bellintani da Salò ed il dialogo della peste di Fra Paolo' in Giuseppe Mueller (ed.), *Raccolta di cronisti e documenti storici lombardi inediti* (Milan, 1857), p. 288.

too fierce an approach could prove equally damaging because of contemporary understandings of fear and its effects on the human body.

Fear, a common characteristic of the sick within the *lazaretti*, was believed to have medical effects.[193] The passions or emotions were thought to allow poisons into the body, meaning that depressed or melancholic spirits could render an individual more vulnerable to infection. An English physician wrote that fear in those in the pesthouses 'made them an easier Prey to the devouring Enemy'.[194] Although contemporaries observed that, during outbreaks of plague, familial and friendship bonds broke down, visitors were allowed to visit the *lazaretti*. Venetian Health Office decrees from the outbreaks of plague in 1556 and 1576 deal with the issue of visitors to the *lazaretti* and other islands being used as overflow sites. Visiting was seen as standard practice.[195] On application to the Health Office, siblings, children, parents or spouses of the sick would be issued with a permit to visit the islands. They were entitled to visit and speak with the sick, although they were not allowed to disembark onto the islands and no entry was allowed into the hospital complexes.[196] In Cividale del Friuli, Jacopo Strazzolini described a group of individuals who remained within the hospitals for as long as two months without contracting the disease. These were the individuals who entered the *lazaretti* voluntarily, in order to care for their sick parents.[197] In Venice, it was

---

[193] Giovanni Andrea Bellicochi, *Avertimenti di tutto cio che in publico da Signori et in privato da ciascuno si debbe far nel tempo della peste* (Verona, 1577). See William G. Naphy and Penny Roberts (eds), *Fear in early modern society* (Manchester, 1997) particularly the contribution by David Gentilcore, 'The fear of disease and the disease of fear', pp. 184–208. Andrew Wear, 'Fear, anxiety and the plague in early modern England' in John R. Hinnells and Roy Porter (eds), *Religion, health and suffering* (London, 1991), pp. 339–63. More generally on the relationship played by the emotions see the first section of Fay Bound Alberti, 'Emotions in the early modern medical tradition' in Fay Bound Alberti (ed.), *Medicine, emotion and disease, 1700–1950* (Basingstoke, 2006), pp. 1–21. She sets out that the body and soul were indivisible for early modern physicians and the soul influenced emotions as well as the emotions being the mechanisms of the soul within the body. As a result, the emotions could both alter humoural balances and in turn be brought on by humoural changes.

[194] Nathanial Hodges cited in Andrew Wear, 'Fear, anxiety and the plague', pp. 357–8.

[195] For a discussion of hospital visiting between the eighteenth and twentieth centuries see the useful volume by Graham Mooney and Jonathan Reinarz (eds), *Permeable walls: historical perspectives on hospital and asylum visiting* (Amsterdam, 2009). The editors draw a distinction between patient visitors, public visitors, house visitors and official visitors. If these categories are adopted, the early modern *lazaretti* received all types, except public visitors. This category includes entertainers, tourists and clergy. Although spiritual issues were important within the *lazaretti*, these were dealt with by permanent chaplains, as described on pp. 127–9.

[196] ASV, Sanità 725 132r–134r (26 April 1486) [33]. The mechanisms of this are not made clear.

[197] Mario Brozzi, *Peste, fede e sanità*, p. 47.

explicitly stated in the statutes for the hospitals in 1486 that no one could enter the hospital buildings of the *lazaretti* during outbreaks. Visiting was restricted and regulated. This concern about access also caused visiting to be limited during the worst of the early modern epidemics. In September 1556 the practice was suspended because of the 'urgent state' of the health of the city.[198] In 1576, it was noted that the number of people who had been sent to the *lazaretto nuovo* had increased and that the work involved in providing for and governing this number was enormous. The number of people arriving at the Health Office daily to request permissions to visit friends and family in the *lazaretti* was described as large. This was causing great inconvenience to the Prior who needed to be left to carry out his duties. For fifteen days, no one was allowed to visit the *lazaretti*, except in exceptional cases, which were not elaborated upon.[199]

For understandable reasons, this system of visiting was carefully controlled. In 1522 a number of nobles were said to have disembarked at the *lazaretto vecchio* to visit Piero Michiel. Amongst this group was Michiel's wife.[200] The secret entry of the group within the hospitals provoked the Health Office to act in order to make an example to others. Access to the *lazaretto* sites was of widespread concern. In Sardinia, the Health Office was concerned that the *lazaretto* was becoming a meeting point for prostitutes and cleaners or workmen (*gli inservienti*).[201] The Venetian Health Office magistrates were understandably concerned about the issue of access, which was addressed in a number of contexts and attempted to deal with a diverse selection of individuals' apparent lack of concern regarding infection. Repeatedly, officials had to forbid fishermen from fishing in the canal of the *lazaretti*. Reminders were issued that plague-infected goods were being disinfected in lagoon water and that there was a series risk of corruption to food supplies.[202]

In addition to having visitors, individuals also seem to have brought their animals to the *lazaretti*. In 1555, the Health Office issued an instruction to kill the cats and dogs in the *lazaretti*.[203] Similar instructions were issued within cities.[204] In Padua in 1576, the Health Office decided that in order to avoid the various threats to public health, dogs and cats were to be stopped from moving around particular sections of the city centre. The options presented were immediate slaughter of the

---

[198]   ASV, Sanità 730 75r (29 September 1556).

[199]   ASV, Sanità 732 149r (30 March 1576).

[200]   ASV, Sanità 726 38r (11 June 1522).

[201]   Francesco Manconi, *Castigo de Dios*, p. 179. For the problem of prostitution in Palermo see Ingrassia, p. 359 and the restrictions placed on courtesans and prostitutes, p. 366.

[202]   For example see ASV, Sanità, 729 33v (14 July 1544). For concerns more broadly about fishing in corrupted waters and the effect on food supplies see Ken Albala, *Eating right in the Renaissance* (London, 2002) p. 122.

[203]   Cucino 19v (20 April 1555).

[204]   In Milan, Bisciola wrote that the problem with cats and dogs was that they spread the plague as a result of children's play. See Samuel K. Cohn Jr, *Cultures of Plague*, p. 104.

animals, for cats to be kept indoors or for the animals to be sent outside the city.[205] In Verona, cats and dogs were to be killed because they 'carried the plague inside them'. Similarly pigs, pigeons and chickens of all sorts were to be killed because they often carried the disease.[206] For these reasons, the Prior of the *lazaretto vecchio* was not allowed to keep dogs, pigeons or other birds.[207] Such instructions were not restricted to cities of the Veneto. Mark Jenner has noted similar actions on behalf of the authorities in early modern London. Here he claimed that the animals were targeted as visible signs of disorder and that the policy may have been an attempt at a 'ferocious reinstation of magisterial authority'.[208] Jenner's chapter forms part of a wider volume on fear in early modern society. Roaming dogs and cats, like the beggars and rootless, presented a threat to the containment of infection.[209] In addition to their movement around the city, the dangerous potential of fur as a carrier of disease would have heightened the sense of threat. Within cities, the maintenance of segregated areas in order to prevent the transmission of infection was seen as paramount. So too was the effective maintenance of zones of quarantine within the *lazaretti*. The killing of the animals must have been a horrible experience; Benedetti described the killing of the cats and dogs as a *vespero siciliano* – which refers to the slaughter of a French garrison in Sicily in 1282.[210]

The Venetian Health Office officials found it necessary to work hard to regulate the behaviour of staff and patients within the *lazaretti*. For both groups, the temptations to sinful behaviour were great but, in the context of early modern epidemics, so too were the consequences of such actions. In the treatment of patients, there was an attempt to balance the sense of fear and the sense of comfort as a result of charitable giving – the middle line between these two emotions would, it was hoped, produce perfect behaviour to combat the plague. The significance of behaviour and morality in causing and curing the plague meant that these hospitals needed to be monitored and could never be fully separated from the wider city. Further connections between the city and the hospitals were provided through the staff. These hospitals were large, and became even more so during the most serious epidemics. Staff were employed in a number of specific and necessary roles as the institutions attempted to provide holistic care. This can be seen even more clearly when considered alongside the subject of our next chapter: the medical care on offer within the *lazaretti*.

---

[205] ASP, Sanità b. 325, 10r (9 July 1576).

[206] ASVer, Sanità reg. 33 127r (n.d. 1577).

[207] ASV, Sanità b. 2 (16 April 1554).

[208] Mark S. R. Jenner, 'The great dog massacre' in William G. Naphy and Penny Roberts (eds), *Fear in early modern society* (Manchester, 1997), p. 54.

[209] William Empson has stated that canine metaphors were used to describe vagrants and that a policy against these animals was expressive of a developed mindset in relation to this social group, cited in ibid., p. 56. On beggars in Palermo see Ingrassia, p. 358.

[210] Rocco Benedetti, *Relatione d'alcuni casi*, p. 18.

Chapter 4

Syrups and Secrets: Treating the Plague

It was said that the only certain way to survive the plague was to flee quickly, stay long and return slowly ('*cito longe tarde*'). This piece of advice was endorsed by even the most qualified of physicians and reproduced in their treatises.[1] Indeed, many physicians took this advice themselves and fled from cities during epidemics, a move which could attract criticism.[2] The exhortation to escape and the exodus of medical professionals would hardly have inspired confidence in medical treatments to prevent and cure the plague. Given the devastating mortality rates associated with the disease, contemporary criticisms of medicine in the time of plague as misguided at best and non-existent and harmful at worst are understandable. Historians have picked up on these criticisms, which have complemented their own assessments of the false assumptions made by early modern doctors in the face of plague. It would be easy, on the back of these accounts, to characterise the recourse to medical treatments during epidemics as desperate and futile. This chapter will, by contrast, illustrate that genuine attempts were made within the *lazaretti* to cure the plague. In addition, there was innovation and change in treatment over the course of this period.[3] Although early modern contemporaries debated and criticised the use of plague hospitals, the *lazaretti* continued to be used in Venice and across Europe well beyond the period studied in this book because the cost of using the structures appeared to outweigh those of abandoning them.

---

[1]   See, for example, Bernardino Tomitano, *De le cause et origine de la plague vinitiana* (Venice, 1556), 21v.

[2]   For the lively debate regarding the responsibilities of those in authority, doctors and the clergy during plague epidemics. See Ole P. Grell, 'Conflicting duties: plague and the obligations of early modern physicians towards patients and commonwealth in England and the Netherlands' in Andrew Wear, Johanna Geyer-Kordesch and Roger French (eds), *Doctors and ethics: the earlier historical setting of professional ethics* (Atlanta GA, 1993), pp. 131–53 and Patrick Wallis, 'Plagues, morality and the place of medicine in early modern England', *English Historical Review*, 121 (2006), pp. 1–24.

[3]   For important studies that set out the use of experimentation and experience to bring about change in the treatments applied to early modern diseases see William Eamon, *Science and the secrets of nature: books of secrets in medieval and early modern cultures* (Princeton NJ, 1994) and Samuel K. Cohn Jr, *Cultures of plague: medical thought at the end of the Renaissance* (Oxford, 2010).

Despite the devastation and scale of early modern epidemics, genuine attempts were made to provide preservatives and treatments against the disease. Contemporaries believed that, given the right conditions, people could be cured of the plague. In Cividale del Friuli one contemporary wrote that most of the sick were cured by the medicine provided – it is interesting to note that in this case the treatments were administered by the Venetian *pizzigamorti*.[4] Governments invested significant sums of money in public health to fund the employment of staff and the supply of medical provisions. This chapter will focus upon the experiences of those employed to work in medical roles in the Venetian *lazaretti* as well as the medical treatments which were administered to patients.

Early modern medical practitioners included physicians, doctors, surgeons, apothecaries, barbers, female healers and charlatans. Each of these groups worked, in different forms and on differing terms, within the *lazaretti*. Individuals moved between posts in hospitals in the city and the *lazaretti*.[5] Those who served in the *lazaretti* were employed by the Health Office and it is the records of this magisterial body which provide the principal source material for this discussion. Although this chapter is concerned with medical care, it is important to remember that this was provided alongside the practical and spiritual treatments outlined in the previous chapter. The *lazaretti* responded to the contemporary concept of health in all of its various manifestations and meanings. As we saw in the previous chapter in relation to isolation, not all patients were treated identically. Different treatments were provided and children, in particular, were singled out for age-appropriate care.

Remedies for the plague ranged from urine to daffodil essence. For modern readers, the connections between the cures (which go beyond the colour yellow) can be difficult to fathom.[6] This chapter will describe the elements of medical care which were provided within the *lazaretti* and explain why contemporaries believed they would be effective. Many of the medical treatments of the *lazaretti* are similar to those of other early modern hospitals and the medicine available in the early modern city and these will be used as points of comparison. Medicine on the *lazaretti* was specific, however, in terms of the scale on which treatments had to be produced and administered. In addition to standard elements of early modern

---

[4]   Mario Brozzi, *Peste, fede e sanità in una cronaca Cividalese del 1598* (Milan, 1982), p. 34 'la maggior parte guardivano per esser medicate da picigamorti veneziani'.

[5]   For example ASV, Sanità 738 180r (3 July 1624).

[6]   Although underexplored in the existing historiography, the issue of colour was a relevant one in early modern medicine. At the Giglio in Florence, for example, a treatment for the cure of the heart was deliberately made of red ingredients (including rose) and was often applied with a scarlet cloth. See James E. Shaw and Evelyn Welch, *Making and Marketing Medicine in Renaissance Florence* (Amsterdam, 2011), p. 252. The doctrine of signatures was at the heart of interpretations of colour – that an object's visible signs could act as a clue as to the meaning and value of the substance. See Ken Albala, *Eating right in the Renaissance* (London, 2002), pp. 80–81.

medicine, new cures were tried and tested in the *lazaretti*. These cures were marketed as medical secrets. Many were unsuccessful but a few were remarkably effective in responding to the plague.[7] One such success story is the cure which belonged to the doctors to the Venetian *lazaretti* Nicolò Colochi and his son-in-law Ascanio Olivieri. This was sold to the Venetian Republic and adopted as a state secret, used across Venetian territory throughout the sixteenth and seventeenth centuries. Three versions of the secret cure of Nicolò Colochi and Ascanio Olivieri survive in the library of the Museo Correr in Venice. This innovative cure was part of the day-to-day medicine provided in the plague hospitals and it is worth considering the details of the surviving recipe. Secrets were also used in *lazaretti* elsewhere, as illustrated by the case of a more ambiguously placed individual – a charlatan, Giacomo Coppa. Coppa treated the sick in the Paduan *lazaretto* before moving to Venice where his remedies brought him to the attention of the Venetian Health Office. Coppa's recipe does not survive but there are brief comments from patients regarding the effects of the medicine he used.

Although much of the surviving material relates to the treatments which were offered within the hospitals, there are hints that patients could exercise a degree of agency in shaping their care and refusing particular remedies but this is not sufficiently well documented to form a substantial theme in this chapter. As with so many elements of these hospital structures, the information regarding medicine provided is fragmentary. Nevertheless, when viewed as a whole, it is clear that the medical structures of the *lazaretti* were ambitious and varied. That does not mean that the hospitals were necessarily viewed as satisfactory or convincing by contemporaries. The chapter ends by considering views of the efficacy of the *lazaretti* in combating the plague. The utility and cost of the structures were debated by governments and physicians as they attempted to assess the institution's value for money.

Medical Practitioners

The Veronese doctor Hieronimo Donzellini wrote that the *lazaretti* should be staffed by intelligent and able medical practitioners and not imposters, empirics, vagabonds or torturers, as they often were.[8] Of the medical practitioners in the

---

[7]   Jane L. Stevens, *The lazaretti*, pp. 120–44. Paolo Bellintani reflects of the number of contemporaries who promised successful cures for the plague in Paolo Bellintani, *Dialogo della peste*, Ermanno Paccagnini (ed.) (Milan, 2001), p. 174.

[8]   'non ceretani, non empirici, non vagabondi, non carnefici di Christiani' in Hieronimo Donzellini, *Discorso nobilissimo e dottissimo preservative et curative della peste* (Venice, 1577) [unpaginated]. David Gentilcore records a contemporary description of the *cerretani* of Umbria: 'mendicants falsely claiming to beg alms on behalf of the shrine of Cerreto' in *Medical charlatanism in early modern Italy* (Oxford, 2006), p. 15. The label 'empirici' is problematic and may hint at a further association with charlatanism but is a complex and loaded terms. For a discussion see David Gentilcore, *Medical charlatanism*, pp. 61–2.

hospitals, doctors are the best documented. For other workers, the available source material is brief and fragmented; as a result, the discussion here is necessarily limited. The available sources are used to discuss the responsibilities, background, remuneration and treatments of Health Office doctors alongside those of other practitioners.

The Venetian Health Office employed two doctors on a permanent basis during the sixteenth century.[9] In theory, one was responsible for the city and the other for the *lazaretti*. The appointment of a specific doctor for the *lazaretti* is an indication of the importance placed upon treating the plague during the sixteenth and early seventeenth centuries. During the sixteenth century, the division of responsibilities between the two roles was not firmly fixed. Individuals appointed to the *lazaretti* served within the city and *vice versa*. In addition, both doctors were sent to assist and report on outbreaks of plague elsewhere in the Venetian state.[10] The seventeenth century witnessed a significant change to the two roles. By 1617, the doctor to the *lazaretti* was being described as the assistant (*coadiutante*) of the doctor to the city.[11] It was during this period that the figure of the Protomedico was named in Venice, later than elsewhere on the Italian peninsula and Spain.[12] Giovanni Battista Fuoli had been appointed as the doctor to the *lazaretti* in 1623 and was qualified in both surgery and physic. The following year, Fuoli revoked his post at the *lazaretti* in order to take up the job as Protomedico. Amongst his various other duties, the Protomedico assumed responsibility for the day-to-day oversight of the plague hospitals. With the decline of plague in Venice, specific doctors for the *lazaretti* were appointed on a temporary basis, according to need. Giovanni Battista Fuoli's nephew, Cecilio, followed in his uncle's footsteps as Protomedico. He was described as a doctor, physician, surgeon and public anatomist in archive records, indicating the breadth of his skills and his responsibilities.[13] This shift in the roles and responsibilities of the two Health Office doctors was broadly concurrent with the change in the nature of the *lazaretti*, from plague hospitals to quarantine centres over the course of the seventeenth century.

Before this shift, the roles of both Health Office doctors involved visiting, diagnosing and prescribing for the sick in line with the Hippocratic treatment of

---

[9]   For comparative information on permanent state doctors see Andrew W. Russell (ed.), *The town and state physicians in Europe from the Middle Ages to the Enlightenment* (Wolfenbüttel, 1981).

[10]   For example, Alberto Quattrocchi, health office doctor to the city from 1587 until 1624 visited both Padua and Crete during his period of service.

[11]   ASV, Sanità, 738 93v (5 July 1617).

[12]   For comparative material on the Protomedici of Italy see David Gentilcore, '"All that pertains to medicine": protomedici and protomedicati in early modern Italy', *Medical History*, 38 (1994), pp. 121–42.

[13]   ASV, Sanità 740 9v (28 April 1643).

the individual – the traditional method of the early modern physician.[14] Broadly speaking, physicians were responsible for the internal treatment of the sick, meaning that they prescribed medicines which were for internal consumption by patients. This branch of medicine was thought to be the most complex and learned since it required the practitioner to move beyond the superficial and what could be seen by the naked eye. External treatments were manual tasks and the hands-on treatment of surgery was sometimes associated with the work of artisans or labourers. This is a distinction often drawn in other fields as well. Artists, for example, claimed the superiority of their work over that of sculptors on a similar basis. Leonardo da Vinci [1452–1519] wrote of the distinctions between the two arts, emphasising the sweat, dirt and dust involved in sculpture as indications of its less noble nature. For many years, historians of medicine have focused their studies of medical practitioners around the notion of hierarchies of status, education and wealth. The distinctions between medical groups were said to solidify over the course of the early modern period, as the illustrious but belligerent physicians strengthened their hold over the regulation and restriction of other practitioners. Recent studies have done much to blur the boundaries between groups of practitioners but much work still remains to be done. The distinction between physicians and surgeons has often been overstated. Physicians practised surgery and often held degrees in both subjects. Health Office doctors, whether their background was in surgery or physic, prescribed drugs and directed both external and internal medical treatments.[15]

Occupational labels were applied to medical practitioners loosely: those undertaking the role of Health Office doctor were referred to as *medico, physico*, and *cirurgo* interchangeably.[16] Although the titles used to address the *lazaretto*

---

[14] ASV, Sanità 727 30r (10 June 1529). On doctors and their treatments see Richard J. Palmer, 'Physicians and surgeons in sixteenth-century Venice', *Medical history*, 23 (1979), pp. 451–60 and 'Physicians and the state in post-medieval Italy' in Andrew W. Russell (ed.), *The town and state physicians*, pp. 47–61.

[15] For important correctives to the traditional historiography see Vivian Nutton on the learned surgeon in 'Humanist surgery' in Andrew Wear, Roger K. French and Iain M. Lonie (eds), *The medical Renaissance of the sixteenth century* (Cambridge, 1985), pp. 75–100; Richard J. Palmer, 'Physicians and surgeons'; Sandra Cavallo *Artisans of the body in early modern Italy: identities, families and masculinities* (Manchester, 2007), chapter one, 'The view of the body of an ordinary surgeon', pp. 16–37; Samuel K. Cohn Jr, *Cultures of Plague*, particularly p. 14 note 26.

[16] This is a reminder of the difficulty of using fixed categories of healers, which cannot simply be imposed onto the past. See, for example, the use of the term *medico* in Cucino 5v (31 March 1555) and *cirurgo* in ibid., 6v (1 April 1555). Ludovico Cucino's son Battista took a degree at Padua and graduated from the Venetian *studio*. Battista was also referred to as a doctor and surgeon; these terms were used loosely despite his reputable medical qualifications. See Richard J. Palmer, *The studio of Venice and its graduates in the sixteenth century* (Padua, 1983). For similar observations regarding the difficulties of the term 'doctor', see John Henderson, *The Renaissance hospital: healing the body and healing the soul* (London, 2006), pp. 226–30.

doctors are not revealing regarding the background and qualification of these individuals, some information can be gleaned from surviving lists of those who put themselves forward for election to the post. The 1553 election, for example, is a useful example. The surgeon Santo da Salo from Capo d'Istria was elected from a group of three surgeons and a barber. It should be noted that in the sixteenth and early seventeenth century elections, neither the barbers nor the female practitioners who proposed themselves for the role were elected: time and time again a surgeon was successful. The backgrounds of the candidates contrast with those in elections for the doctors for the city, when the majority of candidates were described as *physico* and only a few surgeons applied. In this case, it was generally one of the physicians who was elected. Richard Palmer observed in the course of his work that

> The doctors employed in the lazarettos ... were normally surgeons, since the treatment of plague cases, which might involve the lancing of bubonic swellings, was considered as primarily a surgical operation.[17]

This was partially correct. The doctors were often surgeons but the nature of the medicine did not dictate this. Other surgeons and barbers were appointed in order to cope with these sorts of operations. The background of the *lazaretto* doctors was partly dictated by the salary offered and partly by the nature of the conditions within which these individuals worked.

A further difference in the candidates for the two posts is that most doctors for the city were Venetian whereas those for the *lazaretti* were almost always from outside Venice.[18] Those for the *lazaretti* were predominantly drawn from within the Italian States and France. In Genoa, the same was true of the surgeons in the *lazaretto*: French, Neapolitan, German, Swiss and Genoese surgeons all served during the plague of 1656. Of the ten in total, only two were native to Genoa. The head of the hospital at the time, Father Antero noted that the epidemic was a time of great need, when doctors and surgeons were brought from France, Germany, England and others of the most remote countries.[19]

Most Health Office doctors did not belong to the Venetian College of Physicians and would not have held the reputation or social standing of these men. Membership of this body was not compulsory for those practising medicine within the city.[20] Some of the Health Office doctors for the city did have membership

---

[17]   Richard J. Palmer, 'Physicians and surgeons', p. 455.

[18]   Doctors for hospitals within cities were often natives. For comparative material for Florence see John Henderson, *The Renaissance hospital*, p. 242.

[19]   Father Antero Maria da San Bonaventura, *Li lazaretti della città e riviere di Genova del MDCLVII ne quali oltre à successi particolari del contagio si narrano l'opere virtuose di quelli che sacrificorno se stessi alla salute del prossimo e si danno le regole di ben governare un popolo flagellato dalla peste* (Genoa, 1658), p. 24.

[20]   On the Venetian College see Richard J. Palmer, *The studio of Venice*.

of this corporate body, including Domenico da Castello, who, according to his own supplication, worked in the *lazaretti* in 1555.[21] Other members of the College served in the *lazaretti* of cities of Venetian territory, such as Alessandro Serratico who was appointed to the Veronese *lazaretto* in 1575.[22] The Venetian Health Office also required the service of physicians from the College within the city during epidemics, for example, thirty were sent out to the city's parishes during the plague of 1576. The College was also used as a source of medical advice. Members of the College influenced the hospital structures even when not in permanent posts within the *lazaretti*.

Although the *lazaretto* doctors do not fit obviously within traditional medical hierarchies, the breadth of their responsibilities within the hospitals makes it clear that they were respected and trusted figures. The Cucino letterbook provides insight into the responsibilities of Health Office doctors, recording correspondence between the doctor and the Health Office on an almost daily basis. Cucino's responsibilities for medical treatments extended to the city as well as the two *lazaretti*. He was also told to concern himself with the Priors and their families. Cucino was sent a number of corpses from the city as and when individuals' deaths were considered to be suspected cases of plague. For the most part, the symptoms in these cases were not described; the correspondence refers to bodies being sent and a request for Cucino to report back in the usual way (*al modo solito*). His contract with the Health Office stated that he should go to inspect corpses at a moment's notice. An example of a death causing suspicion was of a woman from San Moise who had been affected by episodes of madness and epilepsy.[23] Cucino conducted his own *post mortems* as well as being a point of information and advice for physicians within the city, who wrote to him with descriptions of corpses and asked for his advice regarding the nature of the disease.[24] Cucino was clearly in charge of the medicine in the *lazaretti* and the Health Office officials sent instructions to two surgeons serving at the *lazaretto vecchio* reminding them that Cucino was to be obeyed as a 'doctor superior to them'.[25]

Cucino's responsibilities within the *lazaretti* were more than medical. Three times during the outbreak of plague in 1555–58, Cucino was asked to adopt temporarily the role of Prior because of the sickness or death of the head of the hospital. Even at other times, however, doctors worked in conjunction with the Prior and the chaplain as the senior figures in the hospitals. The doctors were well paid and shared the responsibility for the safety and security of the island and its inhabitants through the safekeeping of goods and keys as well as the maintenance

---

21   ASV, Sanità b. 730 20r (5 August 1555).

22   Richard J. Palmer, *The studio of Venice*, p. 130.

23   Cucino 37r (26 May 1555).

24   Cucino 97r (26 June 1557).

25   This was just after Cucino had adopted temporarily the role of Prior and so the instruction to the surgeons was to obey Cucino as the Prior and as a doctor superior to them (*ubidirlo come Priore et come Medico superiore a Voi*) in ibid., 13v (15 April 1555).

of bureaucratic records, the interrogation of the sick and the recording of wills. It was important, therefore, that Health Office doctors were capable of fulfilling the bureaucratic aspects of their roles. Those appointed to the position of doctor to the *lazaretti* were examples of what Sandra Cavallo has termed the 'learned doctor-surgeon' and stood on the boundary of medical categories.[26]

The varied backgrounds of *lazaretto* doctors influenced their remuneration. Ludovico Cucino, for example, is one doctor who was remarkably well compensated for his work. He was initially offered a sum, albeit temporarily, of 100 ducats per month for two months at the start of his career with the Venetian Health Office. In his permanent contract, his salary was markedly higher than those of his predecessors. Cucino was to be given 240 ducats per year, although this was later reduced to 200 ducats. However, Cucino did take on his role in the midst of a severe outbreak of the plague. At other times, doctors would have been able to supplement their income with private practice. During epidemics this was not possible since doctors were permanently resident on the *lazaretto* islands. Cucino's higher salary was, in part, recognition of the period of hardship during which he served but also recognised his qualification and experience as a physician. His salary was closer to that of Health Office doctors for the city and more than the *lazaretto* Priors.[27] Despite his experience, it is interesting to note that he too was addressed as a surgeon (*ceroico*) by the Health Office in their correspondence.[28] At the end of the epidemic of 1555–58, Cucino was replaced by Bernardin Verialdo whose contract for treating the sick during times of health as well as of disease offered him seven ducats per month (or eighty-two ducats per year), as did that of Ascanio Olivieri who was appointed as Verialdo's successor. These salaries were in line with those of the period before the outbreak of 1555. In 1528, Nicolò Colochi had been offered five ducats per month for service during times of health, raised to seven ducats in 1531 with 100 ducats per year during outbreaks of disease. The material benefits outlined in contracts for the doctors were generally consistent with a few, exceptional cases during outbreaks when the fame of individuals or treatments could lead to significantly higher salaries for a temporary period. For most, this was a job for life, however, and brought with it other potential benefits.

In Venice and across Europe, the dangers of service in a medical role during plague were recognised. Those who carried out the work emphasised their personal sacrifice in supplications made in the aftermath of epidemics. Requests submitted to city authorities, which emphasised the dangers of service, meant that these jobs could provide more than simply immediate, material benefits. The doctor Ogniben de Ferrari had served in Verona and the *lazaretti* as well as the wider Veronese territory in 1576. In a petition to the Veronese commune, he claimed to have served in

---

[26]   Sandra Cavallo, *Artisans of the body*, p. 16.

[27]   Giovanni Francesco da Burano, for example, was paid one hundred and fifty ducats per year.

[28]   Cucino 40v (22 June 1555).

all manner of conditions, in rain, wind and snow, by day and by night and requested that his faithful and committed service be considered as sufficient to allow him to be made a citizen of the city.[29] Nine months later, Ferrari published a work dedicated to the Veronese College of Physicians and concurrently made an application to be accepted into this body and was duly accepted.[30] His service to the Health Office, within the city, territory and *lazaretti* was the basis upon which he justified his application to become a citizen of the city and his subsequent application to the College. It was the basis for his establishment within the city's social structures and for the formalisation of his position within the medical structures.

For some, the position was a rung on a career ladder and one which (like Cucino) they undertook for a limited period. For most, however, the role was retained for life. Bearing in mind the conditions in which they were working, the service of doctors 'for life' may not be saying much. Although, by the fifteenth century, very few doctors in Milan were dying of plague, whereas barbers continued to die in large number, it is clear that the *lazaretti* doctors in Venice were affected by the disease and some individuals died within days of their appointment.[31] For others, periods of service were considerably longer and individuals often tried to ensure that the job was passed down within families. Nicolò Colochi held the position for twenty-five years and his son-in-law Olivieri served for thirty-five, the longest serving *lazaretto* doctor on record during the early modern period in Venice. Similar periods of service are recorded for the doctors to the city with the (diligent and studiously named) Alberto Quattrocchi serving for thirty-seven years before requesting the termination of his employment.[32] Like other roles within the *lazaretto*, that of the Health Office doctor could be secure, stable and desirable.

As a result of these attractive elements of the role, barbers and female practitioners also applied for the position of *lazaretto* doctor but were not successful in their election. Nevertheless, a number of these individuals worked within the hospitals. Barbers provided a physical branch of medicine, which involved administering balms and medicines according to the needs of the patients, taking blood and carrying out any other operation necessary for the sick. The Health Office in Sardinia emphasised the importance of being able to produce plasters and take blood in discussions of the necessary skills of these workers. As a general rule, barbers had more direct contact with the sick than doctors,

---

[29] 'ne havevano bisogno non riguardato à piogge, à venti à neve ne à qual si voglia altra fattica di di o di notte' in ASVer, ACA, Atti del consiglio, reg. 89 144v (22 June 1576).

[30] Ogniben de Ferrari, *Quorum duo priores de tuenda eorum sanitate posteriores de curandis morbis agunt* (Brescia, 1577). For the College of physicians see ASVer, ACA, Collegio dei Medici, reg. 610–11 56r (18 March 1577).

[31] Samuel K. Cohn Jr, *Cultures of plague*, p. 69. This is likely to be as a result of the contact between the sick and the doctors. In Palermo, Ingrassia categorised physicians as those who have only passing contact with the sick, meaning that they needed to be subject to less rigorous quarantine on p. 256.

[32] ASV, Sanità 738 178v (1624).

whether in the *lazaretti* or the city: in Venice it was recommended that barbers rather than physicians enter spacious houses where individuals were undergoing quarantine.[33] Information in the archives is minimal regarding the experiences and responsibilities of the barbers, although some recent studies have developed our understanding of these practitioners in other contexts.[34] What does survive is prescriptive rather than descriptive material.

Barbers were responsible for one of the most controversial of early modern treatments for the plague: phlebotomy (bloodletting). In early modern medicine, if sickness was being caused by an excess of heat, a physician could apply bloodletting. If the humour could not be so easily removed from the body, medicine could apply a substance either similar or opposite to that causing the sickness or physicians could prescribe a purgation in order to clear the body of corrupt material. Although in keeping with medical thought, bloodletting during the plague was widely debated by physicians. Bloodletting was the first recommendation provided by the Paduan physicians to the Venetian authorities in 1575.[35] Although the plague was associated with an excess of heat within the body, and many physicians observed fevers accompanying the disease, the treatment was acknowledged to weaken the body's constitution if the disease had affected the heart. Ambroise Paré wrote that the physicians who treated the sick in France in 1565 recorded that patients who had blood taken from them waxed and waned and died whereas those who were given internal treatments, for the most part, recovered.[36]

An account of medicine in the *lazaretti* from the physician Thebaldi in 1630 records instructions for barbers in treating fevers by taking blood, so we know that it was part of medical treatment within the hospitals.[37] For Thebaldi, bloodletting could be justified only in specific cases, when patients showed signs of internal or external inflammation (delirium, choking, flushed face, bloodshot eyes and severe headache). In these cases, a small amount of blood could be taken from the feet and patients were to be given a dose of syrup of poppy (opium) to 'moderate' the patient. Thebaldi stressed some general rules of thumb for the treatment by barbers: that blood should not be taken in particularly hot or cold temperatures or from patients showing particular signs of weakness or those who had an obvious lack of appetite, those who had liquid oozing from the body, those who were breathless, had weakness of the stomach or those who vomited continuously. Thebaldi also stressed that if barbers were in doubt regarding the nature of an ailment, they

---

[33]   ASV, Sanità reg. 13 208r (28 June 1576).

[34]   Sandra Cavallo's recent work has blurred the boundaries between doctors and barbers, undermining the clear distinction made between the administration of internal and external medicine. She has emphasised the fluidity of labels used to refer to the two professions. However, this does not appear to be the case in the context of the Venetian *lazaretti*. See Sandra Cavallo, *Artisans of the body*, pp. 50–51.

[35]   ASV, Secreta MMN 55bis 4v (13 July 1576).

[36]   Ambroise Paré, *A Treatise of the Plague* (London, 1630 [1568]), pp. 49–51.

[37]   BMC, Codice Cicogna 3261.

should neither take blood nor administer medicines. The body in its natural state, Thebaldi said, was more likely to fight off a disease than incorrect medical treatment by a barber. His assertion could be an example of medicalisation and an attempt to reduce the independence of other medical practitioners. It could also be the result of genuine concern regarding the potential danger of ill-administered or inappropriate treatments. In spite of the debate, bloodletting was fairly widely applied within the *lazaretti* during the sixteenth century and it was during the seventeenth century that it fell out of favour there as a treatment for the plague.[38]

In addition to barbers, women also served in the *lazaretti* as medical practitioners, beyond their role as serving women discussed in the previous chapter. As has already been seen in Chapter 3, the Prioress had originally taken almost full responsibility for the care of female patients but her role altered significantly during the fifteenth century. The Prior became the individual in sole charge of the *lazaretti* and the responsibilities of the Prioress were restricted to the care of children. Although the bureaucratic responsibilities of the Prioress declined, these women continued to fulfil a medical role. Donna Marieta was the good woman put in charge of the children of the Prior of the *lazaretto vecchio* in 1555.[39] In April, the Health Office officials wrote to the *lazaretto* doctor Cucino expressing concern about a recipe from Donna Marieta, which they had been sent. Marieta was specifically instructed not to medicate or use any remedies without the specific permission and prior knowledge of Cucino.[40] It is very unusual to have this sort of reference to the work of women in a medical role within the *lazaretti*. It is important to highlight the focus of the Health Office's complaint: the use of a remedy which had not been specifically authorised. The fact that this remedy was being administered by this 'good woman' was not even commented upon, a clear indication that this was neither surprising nor controversial. However, the Health Office officials were concerned to ensure that the Health Office doctor remained in a supervisory role of all of the medical treatments administered on the islands. Cucino was instructed to discuss the issue (and presumably the nature of the recipe) with Donna Marieta. Unfortunately further information as to how the issue was resolved does not survive. In 1576, Cecilia Maraveglia, the wife of the Prior Zorzi Nassin, was granted a licence to leave the *lazaretto nuovo* in order to treat the sick in the city, although she was soon recalled to the *lazaretto* because of the great need there.[41] The role of women in providing medical care in the early modern domestic and community spheres has been well-discussed, as have the services of noblewomen within their localities and across European wide

---

[38] For the debate see Samuel K. Cohn Jr, *Cultures of plague*, pp. 16–17.

[39] For further discussion of these 'good women' see pp. 115–16.

[40] Cucino 18v (18 April 1555).

[41] ASV, Sanità 732 143v (10 March 1576). Her will is in ASV, Archivi Notarili, Testamenti, Atti Cavanis b. 193 no. 261 (14 April 1576).

networks.[42] Female healers in the *lazaretti* were of artisan and citizen status and archive material contains hints rather than substantial detail regarding their role but their entry into medical roles within the *lazaretti* came through the institution of the family – either as the Prior's wife or her substitute – as it would often have done within the wider city.

In addition to the appointment of doctors, surgeons, barbers and female practitioners for the *lazaretti*, ties were made with apothecaries. The importance of this branch of medicine is evident in the significant sums of money which were spent by the Health Office in purchasing these materials for the hospitals.[43] Specific shops within Venice were given the contract to supply the *lazaretti* with medicines, balms, plasters, waters and other items.[44] The treatments were ordered by the doctors and collected either by them or one of the Health Office servants.[45] Although individual apothecaries would have had no call to visit the *lazaretti* in person, the medicine they provided was a central part of the care within the hospitals.

The medical practitioners at work in the Venetian *lazaretti* – doctors, surgeons, barbers and female healers – are broadly similar to those of other plague hospitals. The *lazaretto* in Sardinia, for example, employed a doctor, two surgeons and a barber. *Lazaretti* of smaller cities and towns were not in a position to staff their hospitals so fully. This meant that doctors from larger cities were sent to assist within their territorial states – for example individuals were sent from Venice to Padua, Crete and Cividale del Friuli, amongst others. The practitioners in the *lazaretti* can also be compared with the practitioners who made up the pluralist medical structures of other hospitals and the early modern city more generally.[46] Within early modern cities, these practitioners were augmented by 'popular

---

[42]   For general discussion of female practitioners see Margaret Pelling and Frances White, *Medical conflicts in early modern London: patronage, physicians and irregular practitioners, 1550–1640* (Oxford, 2003), chapter six, 'Gender compromises: the female practitioner and her connections', pp. 189–224. See Lucinda M. Beier, 'In sickness and in health: a seventeenth century family's experience' in Roy Porter (ed.), *Patients and practitioners: lay perceptions of medicine in pre-industrial society* (Cambridge, 1985), pp. 101–28. Alisha Rankin, 'Becoming an expert practitioner: court experimentalism and the medical skills of Anna of Saxony (1532–1585)', *Isis*, 98 (2007), pp. 23–53.

[43]   ASV, Secreta, MMN 95 101r (23 October 1576) and 115r–v (16 November 1576).

[44]   See ASV, Sanità 730 87r–v (29 November 1556). This is also discussed in Richard J. Palmer, 'Pharmacy in the Republic of Venice in the sixteenth century' in Andrew Wear, Roger K. French and Iain M. Lonie (eds), *The medical Renaissance of the sixteenth century* (Cambridge, 1985), note 42.

[45]   The supplication in 1571 by Leonardo Sandelli claimed that he went personally to the apothecaries shops to 'pigliar le medicine et a comprar diverse sorte d[i] vittuarie et li portano p[er]sonalmente al lazaretto vecchio'. ASV, Sanità 731 108r (19 September 1570).

[46]   For a discussion of the historiography see the introduction, pp. 32–3.

healers', for example charlatans.[47] These individuals are only occasionally described as providing treatment within *lazaretto* structures, as will be considered in more detail in the final section of the chapter.[48]

There were a number of medical practitioners employed within the hospitals but, as was seen in Chapter 2, diagnosis often took place beyond the hospitals. Leaflets containing information on how to identify the disease and what to do in the case of the plague were circulated. The leaflets are indications of the desire of the state to restrict some medical processes – in this case, diagnosis but sometimes also treatment – within households and parishes in order to prevent the spread of the disease. In the same way that modern governments distribute 'how to' guides on the identification of contagious diseases so that basic treatments can be administered in the home, so too did *lazaretto* doctors get involved, as the experts on the ground, in describing diagnosis and treatment which individuals could then apply themselves. Information on symptoms, in particular, was distributed so that heads of household could not use a lack of medical knowledge as an excuse for not revealing cases of sickness in their homes.[49]

Medical Diagnosis

In 1555, a boatman, Lorenzo, from San Cassian was asked how many people lived in his house and he replied that he, his wife, his five children (ranging from four to thirteen years old) and his sister all lived there. It was his nine-year-old daughter, Catherina, who was the focus of the enquiry. He was asked how long his daughter had been ill for. He replied that last Wednesday she had been out with other children but started burning up. She went into the canal, up to waist deep and stayed there for more than two hours because she was so hot. When she came out of the canal, she said that she felt tired and needed to sleep a little. She went to bed and slept well that night. In the morning, she ate some breakfast and seemed to feel better. By Friday, she seemed to have improved. However, on the night previous to the enquiry, at about six, he said, she had claimed that worms had entered her throat and were drowning her (*li vermini mi vengono alla gola et negomito alquanti*).[50] She died between six and seven. She was not visited by a doctor, he explained, because of the speed with which she had deteriorated.[51]

---

[47]   On the term and the practitioners more generally see David Gentilcore, 'Was there a popular medicine in early modern Europe?', *Folklore*, 115 (2004), pp. 151–66 and *Medical charlatanism*.

[48]   For the case of the charlatan Giacomo Coppa who treated the sick in the *lazaretto* of Padua see pp. 176–7.

[49]   Ingrassia reflects on this on p. 336.

[50]   On worms accompanying the plague, particularly in children, see Samuel K. Cohn Jr, *Cultures of plague*, p. 67.

[51]   Cucino 26r (4 May 1555).

Cucino's letterbook preserves this striking account given by someone close to the sick regarding the progression of the disease. These details were taken by Cucino and submitted to the Health Office. Once a confirmed death or infection had been identified, a patient or next of kin was interrogated to determine potential sources of infection and other areas or individuals which may have been exposed to the disease.[52] After such a diagnosis and investigation, instructions would have been given as to how to proceed, potentially with family and goods being sent to the *lazaretti* and being given preservatives or treatments. On arrival at the *lazaretto*, patients were seen by a doctor and assessed again. During their stays in the hospitals, patients were visited daily by the doctor and the Prior as a way of monitoring care and the condition of the sick. The observations of the Paduan physicians Hieronimo Capo di Vacca and Gerolamo Mercuriale are helpful for assessing diagnosis of the plague by doctors.[53] They offered to visit, observe and treat twelve individuals within the city, not with the aim of curing the city (an idea which they described as 'absurd') but instead of exploring the nature of the disease.[54] In their original supplication, they had offered to touch the sick, test their urine and do all things necessary for the health of the souls and bodies of the individuals.[55] Just a week later, however, they were keen to stress that, in ministering to the city, they did not intend to enter into the houses of the sick but rather to observe and diagnose from the doorways.[56] This is an important element of diagnosis and treatment within the *lazaretti* as well. It is clear from hospital statutes that patients were observed from the balcony or doorway of the hospitals by the Priors. Whether or not the doctors came into closer contact with the sick is unclear but it may have been that they remained at a distance within the hospitals, as they often did within the city.

The techniques which were used for diagnosis within the *lazaretti* are those traditionally associated with physicians, although they differ from those familiar to us today. The full-scale physical examination of patients was a technique which developed from the nineteenth century. In previous centuries, the physician would have been expected to use each of his senses, to varying degrees. Most important for the physician was the use of sight in observing the patient, his urine and his immediate environment. Touch was used to take a pulse, temperature and to assess the texture of the skin. These diagnostic tools can be seen in the image of the plague hospital in Leiden in 1574 [Plate 22]. Here, a physician takes centre stage as he tends a female patient and can be identified by the urine flask that he is holding in

---

[52]   For the charting of plague spread in Milan see Ann G. Carmichael, 'Contagion theory and contagion practice in fifteenth-century Milan', *Renaissance quarterly* 44:2 (1991), pp. 213–56.

[53]   ASV, Sanità reg. 13 204v (27 June 1576).

[54]   ASV, Secreta, MMN 95 40v (July 1576).

[55]   'tocandoli, vedendo l'orina et facendo quanto pensareme esser necessario per la salute delle anime et de i corpi' in ibid.

[56]   ASV, Sanità reg. 13 208r (28 June 1576).

his left hand, although the obvious stretcher immediately behind which is being used to carry out the dead does little to encourage confidence in the doctor's work.

These general features of diagnosis were used by Health Office doctors: Cucino was specifically instructed by the Health Office to '*veder, toccar et medicar*', in other words to observe, touch and treat his patients. There is mention of the use of uroscopy within the *lazaretti*. The patient in question was the Prior of the *lazaretto vecchio*. It was recorded that the Prior's urine and his moderate thirst illustrated that the fever was not very severe, although the combination did point towards a possible weakness of constitution.[57] It is unclear whether such techniques could or would have been utilised on a large scale during periods of particular strain in the worst of early modern plague epidemics. It was, however, part of medical diagnosis within these hospitals at other times.

During periods of observation, doctors would have looked out for a number of symptoms for the plague, as described in the introduction.[58] It is possible to compare general observations of symptoms with those made by doctors serving in the plague hospitals, including a brief statement by Nicolò Colochi and many brief comments in the Cucino letterbook. Writings survive from doctors to the *lazaretti* in other European cities but these tend to be more general pieces written as summaries after outbreaks rather than a daily record of events. Cucino and Colochi both refer to symptoms in those still alive, signs in corpses and Cucino's account has the added bonus of descriptions regarding the progression of the disease within particular individual cases in Venice, such as the account with which this section began.

In describing the living, who were suspected of having contracted the disease, Nicolò Colochi identified a number of the common symptoms. Colochi wrote that the plague often manifested itself at the beginning with fever, pain in the back and painful headaches. The second day was when *giandusse* might appear – on the ear, hip or thigh (*coscia*) under the skin or other locations. These could be treated with an unguent to reduce the pain. For those whose disease came on without a fever, they were said to be certain of cure. For Cucino, one of the most telling and common signs of the disease was the distinctive *carbone*. He refers to these signs a number of times in his letterbook, mentioning them particularly on arms and on thighs. References are also made to the rage and madness associated with the disease – a feature which was discussed in detail in the previous chapter.[59] Thebaldi's account of 1630 refers to blisters (*vessicatorii*), tumours and black *petecchie*. Thebaldi describes the latter, the black and blue blemishes (*il concorso di macchie..livide et nere*) as one of the most common signs of the disease. None of the Venetian *lazaretto* doctors mention nausea and vomiting in their accounts of the plague sick, although this was a common element in seventeenth-century descriptions elsewhere – and Father Antero described it as one of the worst

---

[57]   Cucino 100v (2 October 1557).

[58]   See introduction, pp. 29–30.

[59]   Cucino 37r (26 May 1555).

features of the disease. In a description unlike anything else I have found, Colochi also provided a method for testing for infection before any swellings had appeared – crucially this was something which could be done easily, in the home: the patient should hold their head still, roll the eyes as many times as possible up to the sky and then right and then left. If this brought on tears, severe pain and bloodshot eyes then it was necessary to act to treat the disease.

Since dead bodies were believed to be a potential conduit of the disease, it was also important that signs of the plague could be identified in corpses so that people could be safely buried. The description provided by Colochi may help us to understand why individuals were thought to be frightened to death at the sight of plague corpses. He wrote that dead bodies with signs of the disease would remain with their eyes still open, open mouthed with frothing or saliva from the mouth (*la spiuma fuori*), a black tongue, bruising to the back, visible *carboni* of varying sizes and bruised, sweaty testicles (*li testicoli et li vedrai pavonazi et sudati et cosi sarai certo d'il male*). What a sight! It is interesting to note that Colochi felt that *giandusse* withdrew into the body when individuals died of the plague and so would not be visible to the naked eye when inspecting a corpse.[60]

Medical Treatments and Secrets

Father Antero Maria, writing of Genoa, recorded the low esteem in which some people held the *lazaretti* and their treatments. He wrote that the ignorant population referred to costly cordials as poisonous potions and to medicines as drinks of death. He described many jars of compound cordials, almost all from distilled waters, *confettioni di Alchermes* and *Diagiacinto*, and many with syrup of pearl, of bezoar and other precious ingredients. Of one hundred patients, he wrote, only ten would accept the remedies. The rest said that they would rather die as quickly as possible from plague, a disease sent by God, than of man-made poisons. It was a miracle to see, he wrote, that those things were provided in abundance for the poor and yet they refused them with disdain; these same items could not be bought by the rich in the city for love nor money. Who would have believed, he asked, that this *lazaretto* which had been thought so abhorrent could become so longed for that people brought letters of recommendation and were eager to enter because of the problems in the city beyond. This fascinating insight indicates that patients may have refused the treatments on offer, as well as giving a sense of problems of supply within the city.

The purposes of medicine for the plague were numerous and included preventing and curing disease. Advice on how to prevent the disease was given to individuals by Health Offices and in the form of printed physicians' treatises. Instructions included eating good food in moderation, fresh air, the airing of clothes, the avoidance of excessive exercise, thinking pleasant thoughts, attending

---

60   BMC, Dona delle Rose 181/I 1–16.

Mass, temperance in the emotions (particularly avoiding anger), plenty of sleep, spraying the face with rose water and clean living accommodation.[61] For the sick, medicines were designed to minimise pain, cleanse the humours, strengthen the body and neutralise poisons. Medical treatment was informed by the principles of ancient medicine. As outlined in the introduction, the humoural theory lay at the heart of early modern medical knowledge and underpinned treatments including purging and bloodletting. In addition to concern for the *regimen sanitatis* and the spiritual health of the sick or suspected, which have been considered in previous chapters, medical treatments were drawn primarily from elements of the natural world. This fits with the general approach to early modern medicine which suggested that the cause and cure of a disease could originate in the same place. In general terms, those substances with the characteristics dry and cold were thought most appropriate to counter the plague.

Theriac was often recommended as a cure-all.[62] *Mithridatium* and *theriac* were the two most famous panaceas of the early modern period and were considered to be antidotes to poisons.[63] Both were composite treatments, notoriously difficult to manufacture to a high standard. Venice was renowned as a centre for the production of highest quality *theriac*. Venetian *theriac* developed its reputation on the basis of the high quality, exotic ingredients imported into the city from the East. Great worth was placed on both items and a belief in their ability to prevent and cure the plague was by no means unique to Venice.[64] The wonderful qualities of *theriac* were also thought to include curing fevers, preventing internal swelling and blockages, alleviating heart problems, treating epilepsy, inducing sleep, improving digestion, strengthening limbs, healing wounds and protecting against poisons and animal bites.[65] Like *theriac* and *mithridatium*, *terra sigillata* was a traditional remedy for poisons and had been used as a cure for the plague since the time of the Black Death. A natural clay, it was advocated by Galen as an

---

[61]   These are outlined in the works detailed in note 128 on p. 29, particularly Bernardino Tomitano, *De le cause et origine*, 23r. See also the useful documents printed in Paolo Preto, *Peste e società a Venezia nel 1576* (Vicenza, 1978) and *Venezia e la peste*, p. 66.

[62]   See Gilbert Watson, *Theriac and mithridatium: a study in therapeutics* (London, 1966).

[63]   For detail on *theriac* production in Venice see Richard J. Palmer, 'Pharmacy in the Republic of Venice', pp. 108–9. For *theriac* elsewhere see Gilbert Watson, *Theriac and mithridatium*. The other universal cure was *mithridatium* which took its name from Mithridate V of Pontus (132–63BC) who was said to have protected himself against potential poisoning by taking small doses of poison until habituated. *Mithridatium* was said to combine all known antidotes. For a discussion see Vivian Nutton, *Ancient Medicine* (New York, 2004), p. 142. For the characteristics of antidotes and a discussion of another famous example, that of Orvietan, see David Gentilcore, *Healers and healing* pp. 100–103.

[64]   See Christiane Nockels Fabbri, 'Treating medieval plague: the wonderful virtues of theriac', *Early science and medicine*, 12 (2007), pp. 247–83.

[65]   Ibid., p. 254.

external treatment for use on wounds and later also taken as an internal treatment, said to be used as an antidiarrheal.[66] The physician Gratiolo recommended it along with *bolo armeno* and pearl as a good preservative against corruption.[67]

Other treatments included plasters, which could be applied to swellings on cloth or leather or, in the case of *cerotti* (wax plasters), on wax-based substances.[68] These, like items such as onions, were used to draw out poisons and corrupt material. Unguents and balms could be applied; distilled waters or electuaries could be ingested orally.[69] The physician Prospero Borgarucci, for example, lists a number of waters which he felt were appropriate for the treatment of the plague including rose, myrtle and cedar flowers.[70] Copious sweating and purges were common responses to sickness during the period, cleansing the body by removing excess and harmful humours in order to restore the body's equilibrium. Cordials were revitalising and strengthening. Antidotes were designed to remove or neutralise poisons in the body.

During the outbreak of 1556, the Health Office confirmed the prices of the particular medicines needed for the *lazaretti* and for the treatment of the sick. Distilled waters were sent – both the 'ordinary' waters and the exceptional which included *lentivo, sebastien*, rose, daffodil and plum. *Mithridatium*, rosewater, *bolo armeno,* an electuary (*diacatholico*), *terra sigillata*, pink and violet *violepo*, extracts of pearl, perfumes, rose balm and common plasters, ointments, oils and syrups were all listed. So too were pills: aura, shell, masticine and commune.[71] James Shaw and Evelyn Welch have illustrated that pills were some of the most standardised treatments distributed at the Giglio. They were thought to be potent and effective at getting unpleasant medicines into the body, since they could be coated in sugar or wax depending on the cost.[72] We cannot be sure of how the other medical materials were combined at the *lazaretti* but some general observations can be made about the substances which were sent. Historians have suggested that plants and herbal remedies were associated with the medicine of the poor, in contrast to the animal and mineral products, spices and powders of the wealthy.[73] The medicines sent to the *lazaretti*, however, combine substances and so shed

---

[66]   Ibid., p. 251.

[67]   Andrea Gratiolo, *Discorso di plague ... nel quale si contengono utilissime speculationi intorno alla natura, cagioni e curatione della plague, con un catalogo di tutte le pesti piu notabili de' tempi passati* (Venice, 1576), p. 48.

[68]   See David Gentilcore, *Medical charlatanism*, p. 221.

[69]   The difference between unguents and balms was one of consistency. For a discussion of these individual treatments see ibid., pp. 217–26.

[70]   Prospero Borgarucci, *Dove ciascuno potrà apprendere il vero modo di curar la peste et i carboni et di conservarsi sano in detto tempo* (Venice, 1565).

[71]   ASV, Sanità, 730 79r (13 October 1556).

[72]   On pills see James E. Shaw and Evelyn Welch, *Making and marketing medicine*, p. 250.

[73]   See the work of Katherine Park, Samuel Cohn and David Gentilcore all cited in Sheila Barker's essay 'The making of a plague saint', p. 122 note 94.

little light on the social status of patients in their own right. Some were common treatments. At the Giglio in Florence, for example, *diacatholicon* was the best selling drug and was often used in purges for its laxative effect.[74] On the other hand, pearl was an expensive addition to treatments. The medicines which made use of medical 'simples' in the *lazaretti* would have been selected on the basis of the qualities (hot, cold, wet or dry) associated with each.[75]

The natural essences listed by the Health Office were referred to by physicians as being of a cold nature or moderately warm. Endive, for example, was bitter, cold and dry and would have offset the natural characteristics of plague as a disease of heat and moisture. It often features in purges. Similar characteristics were associated with *piantazene* which was useful for drying ulcers. A number of other treatments were temperate in their nature, such as rose and camomile. Some, such as *lentivo*, were refreshing. Some were famed for a number of potential health benefits – rhubarb, rose and pearl, in particular. Rhubarb was thought to clarify blood and help with pain and stomach problems. Rose was thought to purify the blood, comfort the heart and act as a purgative. Pearl was said to be of a dry nature and to be very useful at treating weakness of the heart. Daffodil, the yellow treatment referred to in the introduction to this chapter, was also used because of its dry nature.

Sweets and sugar products commonly accompanied medical treatments – and, indeed, were believed to fulfil a medical function themselves. Sugar and sweets were thought to be warm and moist in their nature, increased blood in the body and were easily absorbed.[76] In the surviving statutes for the hospital, the only instruction regarding medical treatment states that sweets, confectionery and *theriac* should be given only to those who had need and not to anyone else. The *lazaretti* documentation does not specify what the function of these items was believed to be, although the phrasing of the instruction makes it clear that contemporaries thought that they could do more than cure. Since confectionery was given as gifts for special occasions, it may also have been that patients were trying to consume these things because they enjoyed them or that they felt that the sweets played a role in accompanying preventative treatments. Either way, the Health Office was keen to limit the distribution of these products, presumably on the basis of their cost.

External treatments were applied to swellings. The purpose of ointments and poultices was to draw out the poisons from the body, particularly away from the major organs. The distinctive growths which were symptoms of the plague were believed to be the body's way of removing poisons. The cauterisation or lancing of these swellings was one way of removing or destroying harmful matter. Other approaches were to try to neutralise the poison. There were two ways of drawing

---

[74] Ibid., p. 244.

[75] For a full explanation of the contemporary views of pharmacology and simples see James E. Shaw and Evelyn Welch, *Making and marketing medicine*, p. 233.

[76] On sweets as medicine see ibid., particularly pp. 210–11.

out poisons. The first was to apply a substance opposite to the characteristic of the poison. The second, and the more memorable, was to apply a poison, since substances were believed to be attracted by things of a similar as well as an opposite nature. Frogs, serpents, scorpions, chickens and even half of a live puppy could be recommended by doctors.[77] Specific examples of such animals being used to treat children are described below.

Beyond these general observations, it is difficult to access specific treatments used within the *lazaretti*. Many surviving reports from doctors at work within the city are similar in focus to that of the Paduan physicians who reported on the plague in Venice in 1576: they concentrated on the quality of the air, housing and diet rather than providing specific recipes for medicines. Similarly, specific details regarding the treatments used within the *lazaretti* rarely survive. Cucino, for example, was instructed to use his own methods to disinfect houses as well as treat the sick and the suspected. Even with the detailed Cucino letterbook, however, we still do not know the nature of Cucino's own treatments nor are we able to match up particular cases with particular treatments. However, there are some fragments with which to work.

Detail regarding treatments survives in the Health Office archive and in the copy of Nicolò Colochi's internal treatments for individuals and external treatments for their *giandusse* and *carboni*. Colochi offers different levels of preservative and treatment for those considered healthy or suspected of the disease alongside the sick. Finally, printed physicians' treatises provide points for comparison. A significant proportion of these latter publications was dedicated to the causes and nature of the plague and ways in which to regulate the environment, particularly the quality of the air. As previously mentioned, physicians would have traditionally treated the sick on an individual basis but in their printed treatises they included a number of recipes and cures in order to increase the appeal and boost circulation of the tracts.

A printed treatise by the physician Thebaldi provides information about treatments in the *lazaretti* during the outbreak of 1630.[78] Thebaldi wrote that the priorities of doctors treating in the hospitals should be, first, to evacuate excess humours, second to protect the heart and third to treat the external symptoms, particularly the swellings. He also stressed the specific needs of those treating within the *lazaretti*. He provided a checklist of three qualities which should distinguish medicines for the plague hospitals: encouragingly for the patients, his first criterion was that treatments should be appropriate to the illness, his second was that the medicines must be easily prepared and administered on a large scale, the third that the ingredients be easily available and plentiful. The recipes he provided catered for five hundred people at a time. His recipe, for internal consumption, made use

---

[77]   Andrew Wear, *Knowledge and practice in English medicine, 1550–1680* (Cambridge, 2000), p. 347. This reference is part of his useful chapter on 'Prevention and cure of plague', pp. 314–49.

[78]   BMC, Codice Cicogna 3261.

of senna leaves boiled with cinnamon and reduced. Half a cup was to be served to each patient three hours before eating. For blisters, Thebaldi wrote that a quick and easy recipe consisted of strong vinegar, mustard and euphorbia. The need for mass catering for the plague within the *lazaretti* did, therefore, necessarily affect the medicines which were used, making it particularly likely that the substances combined were common and readily and cheaply available in large quantity.

In his account of plague in early modern England, Paul Slack has written that 'no one could argue that the appeal of contemporary medical knowledge lay in its instrumental success'.[79] In many ways this is a convincing argument. In Benedetti's account of Venice in 1575–77, he denounced the owners of various recipes and cures which, instead of curing the plague, simply produced upset stomachs and disturbed the balance of the body's constitution. Prominent amongst these treatments was that of Antonio Gualtiero, a merchant from Flanders, whose preservative required an individual to drink a measure of his own urine at dawn, with the sick required to do the same every morning and evening.[80] *Giandusse,* wounds or sores were treated with hot faeces rather than balms, as generally recommended, and cleansed with urine if necessary. Benedetti recounted how Gualtiero went, in order to prove his secret, to the houses of the quarantined poor, where he contracted symptoms of the disease, treated himself according to his own recipe and within a short time was sick to his stomach and died.[81] The use of bodily excretions in medical treatment fits into wider understandings of disease, since these substances were thought to be characterised by the contraries, and so could offset characteristics of disease.[82] Nevertheless, the fate of the secret's owner would hardly have inspired confidence in the remedy. Bellintani wrote that many people

---

[79]   Paul Slack, *Impact of plague in Tudor and Stuart England* (Oxford, 1985), p. 35.

[80]   Stale urine or water in which dung had been steeped was used in washing as a source of ammonia according to Carole Rawcliffe in 'A marginal occupation? The Medieval Laundress and her work', *Gender and history* 21:1 (2009), pp. 147–69.

[81]   'Antonio Gualtiero mercante fiandrese che offerendosi di liberar la Città in otto giorni ricordò che i sani à digiuno su' l'alba bevessero tre sorsi della propria urina ... e gli infetti usassero medesime*nte* di bevar della sua, cosi la mattina come la sera, mettendo invece d'empiastro sù la giandussa del proprio sterco caldo con tener mandata la piaga con l'urina ... et che per giustificar il secreto andava alle case delle povere persone sequestrate à persuaderle che cosi facessero venne per mala sorte un giorno à cader per terra et ammocossi un braccio, su'l quale sendogli venuto un poco di tumore entrò in sospetto, che fosse principio de giandussa; onde per repararvi postovi sopra l'empiastro dello sterco e dandosi da tutte le hore à bever quanto più poteva dell'urina, come fosse vidoppo se gli alterò di modo il sangue e spiriti vitali che frà pochi giorni vomitando l'anima venne ad uccider se stesso co'l suo rimedio' Rocco Benedetti, *Relatione d'alcuni casi occorsi in Venetia al tempo della peste l'anno 1576 et 1577 con le provisioni, rimedii et orationi fatte à Dio Benedetti per la sua liberatione* (Bologna, 1630), p. 24.

[82]   See Margaret Pelling, 'Medicine and the environment in Shakespeare's England' in *The common lot: sickness, medicine and the urban poor in early modern England* (London, 1998), p. 19. See also the introduction, pp. 12–13.

came forward in times of plague with promises of true remedies of the plague and none were successful. However, from the Venetian records, one cure stands out from the rest as highly praised and valued, purchased at great expense by the Venetian Republic and used throughout the sixteenth and seventeenth centuries in Venice and beyond. This cure was owned by the Health Office doctors Nicolò Colochi and later his son-in-law Ascanio Olivieri. In this case a strong claim was made for successful, effective treatment, similar to the confident assertions of efficacy made of plague remedies until the mid-fifteenth century which have been considered by Samuel Cohn.[83] It is worth, therefore, examining the nature of this treatment in more detail and, in particular, to use the information it contains on the treatment of children.

In Colochi's account, recipes were provided to treat painful and non-painful *giandusse* and *carboni*. Medicines were applied to the *giandusse* in order to draw poisons to the surface and then the swelling was cut, squeezed well in order to push out the pus and rot (*la marcia et il cattivo*) and then a second ointment would be applied to the wound including rose oil. The whole thing was then covered with fabric (*stopa*) followed by a layer of egg white. For *carboni*, a similar process was used but because these swellings would generally be smaller, the process seems to have been less invasive: a remedy was applied which, it was said, made cutting unnecessary, but if it was necessary to cut the *carbone*, a cross-shaped incision would be made and a treatment, along with candied sugar, put inside the growth.

Colochi also provided treatments for those suspected of having contracted the sickness. A recipe was described for the first day of illness using extracts of daffodil, rhubarb and rose along with compound essences. A water of *bocolosa* or of endive was prescribed with a diet of soup and water and no wine.[84] The second day was treated with a water of myrtle (with the waters from the previous day), bloodletting if the patient was too hot and a poultice and ointment or balm for *giandusse* and *carboni* including various herbs such as *piantazene*, linseeds and saffron with rose water. A distinction was made by Colochi between patients on the basis of age. Children were often accommodated separately within the plague hospitals. There is little evidence, however, as to how they were treated once they were beyond the age at which they were breast fed. Colochi provided separate instructions for children aged ten to fifteen (who were given a smaller dose of the above medicine) as well as for those aged three to eight who were treated with gentle oils such as sweet almond with some added sugar and saffron to defend and purge the body.

In the context of Genoa, Father Antero Maria gives a sense of how difficult it must have been to administer medicine to children in the plague hospitals. He wrote that as soon as the children saw a surgeon, they began to shout and tried to run away because they already knew to fear pain. It was necessary for the wet nurse to hold them down by force and for the surgeon, with great skill and patience, to

---

[83]   Samuel K. Cohn Jr, *Cultures of plague*, pp. 11–13.

[84]   The diet was to consist of *panada* which was a soup made with bread.

administer any treatment. It seems that staff also practised the age-old technique of distraction – he recorded one child who would not be treated unless the surgeon let him hold forceps and a lancet.[85] Father Antero recorded a memorable treatment used on children in Genoa – this time to combat putrefaction on the scalp. There were said to be such disgusting and deep rooted scabs on the children's heads that it appeared as though part of the skull had become rotten. A Scottish surgeon suggested finding two black hens. These were cut in two and each child had one of these placed on his or her head and tied like a bonnet so that it would stay in place when the children moved their heads. The hen hats remained in place for two days and two nights. When they were removed, it was said that they had absorbed all of the corrupt material and scabs from the scalp. Thereafter the children were treated with ointment for ordinary sores and they recovered completely.[86] Samuel Cohn has recorded that similar remedies were recommended elsewhere: in Rome, a Bolognese doctor wrote that an *aposteme* could be cured using a plucked hen, whose sexual organ would be placed over the swelling; the physician Ingrassia from Palermo recorded the same; in Milan Archileo Carcano substituted the bird's anus.[87]

Colochi's treatment, as one might expect, was more conventional and more easily used for a large number of patients. The key feature of his remedy was the herb *smartella* (myrtle) and his instructions were very specific regarding the species of plant to be used. Colochi recorded that three varieties were to be found in the city. The first grew to the size of a man and had large leaves, which was not to be used for the recipe. The second was about *tre quarte* (which broadly equates to twenty-four inches) in height and that was also not to be used.[88] The third variety, which grew to a height of approximately two arms' length, was said to be perfect. It was also stressed that only the leaves should be used, not the fruit or seeds which were harmful.[89]

Colochi's medical secret was one of many in the context of early modern medicine; however, it was without doubt one of the most successful and was subsequently sold to the Health Office by Colochi's son-in-law, Ascanio Olivieri having come into his possession as his wife's dowry.[90] Such treatments were also used by other *lazaretto* doctors. In 1556, Cucino claimed to possess a secret which

---

[85] Father Antero Maria da San Bonaventura, *Li lazaretti della città e riviere di Genova*, pp. 477–8.

[86] Ibid., p. 479.

[87] Samuel K. Cohn Jr, *Cultures of plague*, p. 79.

[88] A *quarte* was approximately a quarter of an *ell* – a form of measurement which varied in length in Europe and ranged from 30–45 inches.

[89] BMC, MSS Dona delle Rose no 181, 10/32.

[90] On the story of this medical secret see my forthcoming article 'Family fortunes: gender, public health and selling secrets for the plague in early modern Venice' in the Special Issue edited by Sharon Strocchia entitled *Women and health care in early modern Europe*.

would be of great benefit to the health of the city.[91] The Venetian Senate requested that Cucino go to the *lazaretto vecchio* to prove the efficacy of the remedy despite his service of over a year in the hospitals. It may have been that Cucino was offering a new remedy to Venice on the basis of his already established role. However, it appears that this was a standard response from the Senate. Olivieri too had offered to illustrate the success of the cure on 'a number of sick' providing that they were sent for treatment on the first day of showing symptoms. If this condition was met, Olivieri guaranteed that 'most' would be cured.[92] No further documentation survives, however, for Cucino's secret leaving the nature and ultimate fate of the cure difficult to establish. In the surviving correspondence from the Health Office, however, Cucino is asked to take his preservatives and medicines for the people within the *lazaretti*, illustrations that he made use of these recipes in his service to the hospitals.[93]

On the basis of the available documentation for Nicolò Colochi, Ludovico Cucino and Ascanio Olivieri, who between them served the Health Office for forty years during the sixteenth century, it appears that a medical secret was a common tool of Health Office doctors to the *lazaretti*. Such secrets were not the preserve of these *lazaretto* doctors. The physicians appointed to other areas of the city, such as particular *sestieri*, could also sell their secrets.[94] In these cases, doctors submitted their cures accompanied by attestations by parish officials regarding the efficacy of the treatment.[95] These cures were important features of the medicine provided within the *lazaretti* and were valued for their contribution to the public health of the city. In 1690, over a century after the sale of the secret and in the context of significant changes in medical thought, the Venetian Protomedico was asked to investigate preservatives and cures for the plague. His response drew attention to the tried and tested cure first revealed by Olivieri back in 1576 and used during the outbreak of 1630. Health Office officials ordered that the secret be registered in the statutes of the Health Office in order to be of universal benefit to the public health (*comune salute*) of the city.[96]

Medical secrets during the early modern period have received a significant amount of historiographical attention; the works of William Eamon and David Gentilcore are most notable.[97] The former drew attention to the existence of printed 'books of secrets', which brought together 'formulae and recipes: techniques in

---

[91]   Cucino 80r (19 March 1556).

[92]   ASV, Sanità reg. 14 312r (3 September 1576).

[93]   Cucino 12r (12 April 1555).

[94]   See the anonymous recipe offered in 1576 by one of the officials from Castello, whose letter is recorded in ASV, Consiglio dei Dieci, parti comuni reg. 32 145v (21 July 1576).

[95]   ASV, Sanità reg. 3 22r (4 July 1576).

[96]   ASV, Sanità b. 86 345 (9 January 1690).

[97]   For a consideration of secrets and treatments in early modern Milan see Grazia Benvenuto, *La peste nell'Italia nella prima età moderna: contagio, rimedi, profilassi*

the manual arts, tricks of the trades, medical specifics and formulae employed to work strange effects'.[98] Eamon considered the increased production of these printed books during the sixteenth century as an indication of the development of the concepts of 'openness' and 'public knowledge' in science which he saw as marking the road to 'modern science'. A separate facet of the early modern secret was studied by David Gentilcore in the course of his work on charlatans. Gentilcore considered the spectacle of secret-selling by charlatans as one of the aspects of the system of medical pluralism. These 'tried and tested' secrets, sometimes published in booklet form, were marketed as working by hidden or artificial rather than natural means.[99] Gentilcore characterised this period as one of an increased 'commercialisation of the economy as a whole and of drugs in particular' in which 'charlatans became synonymous with the secrets they marketed'. They combined 'spectacle and treatment', capitalising on this developed market.[100]

Both Eamon and Gentilcore offer specific and fascinating insights into the nature of early modern medical secrets. The use of the *lazaretti* as sites for the testing of medicines and the selling of these remedies to the state by their owners provides a new facet to the historiography of early modern medical secrets. These sales could prove to be valuable both for the seller and for the cities involved. Some of the treatments are described in Paolo Preto's account of the plague of 1576 in Venice.[101] In the list of documents at the end of the book, the 'antidotes' and 'preservatives' are considered under the heading of 'pseudo-medicine' in contrast to those of the 'official medicine' of the section which precedes them. This is a confused and misleading distinction, however. The three 'official' contributions identified by Preto are by Gerolamo Mercuriale, Andrea Gratiolo and Leonardo Fioravanti [1518–88], an unlikely trio. Mercuriale could indeed be seen as setting the mould for the medical establishment figure of the sixteenth century. A prolific writer, he held the chair of practical medicine at Padua and served as physician in the service of both Maximilian II and Cosimo de' Medici. Andrea Gratiolo, in contrast, was a physician of a more modest condition from Salò who published

---

(Bologna, 1996) pp. 116–28 and Paola Borghi, *Antidoti contro la peste a Milano* (Milan, 1990) chapter three.

[98] William Eamon, 'Books of secrets in medieval and early modern science', *Sudhoffs Archiv: Zeitschrift fur Wissenschaftsgeschichte* 69 (1985), p. 30.

[99] David Gentilcore, 'Charlatans, the regulated marketplace and the treatment of venereal disease in Italy' in Kevin Siena (ed.), *Sins of the flesh: responding to sexual disease in early modern Europe* (Toronto, 2005), pp. 57–80 and *Healers and healing*, chapter four, 'Charlatan and his secret'.

[100] Ibid., pp. 112–18. Gentilcore's monograph on charlatans has developed our understanding of the remedies and selling techniques of these figures. See *Medical charlatanism*, section II, 'Goods and services', pp. 91–267 and III, 'Communication', pp. 267–370.

[101] Paolo Preto, *Peste e società*. For a study of a sixteenth-century Milanese recipe see Paola Borghi, *Antidoti contro la peste a Milano*.

works on the causes of the plague and served the Venetian Republic in the role of *perito* (or expert) to the *Provveditori sopra i beni inculti*.[102] Fioravanti in many ways defies classification according to traditional labels. A surgeon, natural philosopher, popular healer, inventor, entrepreneur and reformer according to the various studies by William Eamon, Fioravanti was a member of the 'community of experimenters' and one of the 'professors of secrets' of the period.[103]

Preto contrasts the writings of these 'official' figures with ten 'pseudo-medicinal' cures. These cures were written by four doctors, one barber surgeon, a priest, a merchant, a *nutrido*, one from the account by Rocco Benedetti and one anonymous recipe. His distinction in terms of authors is unhelpful, however, since both groupings contained a diverse mixture of individuals and cures offered. The emphasis should more fruitfully be placed not on the status of the author but rather on the medium which was used to communicate the remedy. No absolute distinction can be made between the secrets sold to the state and those which were published since some printed remedies were dedicated to Health Offices. However, what Preto's distinction obscured was that his 'official' treatments were circulated in the form of treatises whereas the 'pseudo medicinal' cures were offered for sale to the Venetian state. It is precisely this involvement with the state which opens up the issue of innovation, encouraged by the Health Office, in times of plague.

Elsewhere, in Padua, a medical secret was used in the *lazaretto* by Giacomo Coppa, a figure described by David Gentilcore as 'one of the most famous [charlatans] of his day'.[104] An attestation (*processo*) is preserved in the *Archivio di Stato* in Padua of the works of Coppa during the *plague* of 1555 and 1556 in the Paduan *lazaretto*.[105] The collection of documents included an entry by Coppa himself, which explained the purpose behind the attestation. The documents also recorded interviews held with patients who had been treated by Coppa during the outbreak within the city and the *lazaretto*. Finally, privileges obtained by Coppa from governments and Colleges of Physicians, including Mantua, Vicenza, Padua, Ferrara, Bologna, Naples and Venice were confirmed. Coppa's preface to the attestation stated that he had been working in Padua since 1541 but that the service which he was seeking to highlight was during the outbreak of 1555 and 1556 within Padua itself, its territory and its *lazaretto*.

Coppa claimed to have healed an enormous number of people during the epidemic in Padua through internal and external treatments both within the

---

[102]   Andrea Gratiolo, *Discorso di peste*. For examples of his reports made in his role as 'expert' see ASV, Beni inculti, b. 291 'Relazioni dei periti non pubblicati 1569-99'.

[103]   See William Eamon, '"With the rules of life and an enema": Leonardo Fioravanti's medical primitivism' in Judith V. Field and Frank A.J.L. James (eds), *Renaissance and revolution: humanists, scholars, craftsmen and natural philosophers in early modern Europe* (Cambridge, 1993), pp. 29–45.

[104]   David Gentilcore, *Medical charlatanism*, p. 69 note 23.

[105]   ASP, Sanità, b. 353, 'Processo per rilevare le operationi del S Giacomo Copa medico di Modena per la plague nel 1555 e 1556 nel luogo del lazaretto'.

lazaretto and the city itself. Twelve interviews are recorded describing the effects of the syrups and plasters administered by Coppa. In some, descriptions were made of treatments applied to external symptoms, including both *carboni* and *giandusse*. In others, patients described how they had been almost unable to move but almost immediately upon receiving the medicine felt their spirits recover.[106] One couple who were interviewed claimed to have been healed within the space of just eight days.[107] In each interview, the witness was asked to comment (and in each case affirmed) whether or not they considered Coppa to be practised and able in the art of medicine.

Coppa's experiences were different from those of Health Office doctors treating within the *lazaretti*. He seems to have moved between medical categories, travelling throughout Italy, receiving licences to sell remedies *in banco* and in public and coming up against the various licensing bodies of Venice but also working within hospitals. The use of his remedies and cures in Padua during the outbreak of plague is a further indication of the approach of medical pluralism used by cities as well as by individuals in times of crisis. After his move to Venice, Coppa struggled to have his remedies accepted by the authorities for sale in the marketplace but had been given the freedom to treat in the time of crisis within the *lazaretto* and other hospitals. The example of Coppa underscores potential complications of categorisation of healers and opens up the spectrum of medical responses made to the plague in the course of public health measures.

The *lazaretti* provided a variety of medical treatments as part of a genuine attempt to cure the sick. Doctors, surgeons, barbers and female practitioners were all employed to serve the hospital. The medicine administered to patients included traditional approaches to the sick but also involved the development of new remedies for the plague, encouraged by the offer of sales to the state. Medical personnel made use of their experience within the hospitals, as well as accepted wisdom, to shape treatments. Working within the plague hospitals brought with it the opportunity to capitalise on experience gained, through the sale of secrets. There was, therefore, a degree of innovation and commitment to medical treatments, which has been underestimated in the historiography of the *lazaretti*. This does not mean, however, that contemporaries unanimously viewed these institutions as beneficial to health. The *lazaretti* were not only criticised for the poor conditions provided under the strains of epidemics. The nature and purpose of the institutions was also debated by physicians and governments alike.

---

[106] 'tuti doi che no se potevimo quasi mover retornassimo in noi et ritorno il vigor', ibid., 9r.

[107] Ibid., 10r.

Medical Views of the *Lazaretti*

It was said by some that 'to enter the *lazzaretto* without getting infected would be like jumping into water without getting wet or into fire without getting burnt'.[108] This is a powerful view of the nature of these hospitals. Contemporary views of the Venetian *lazaretti* were considered in Chapter 1, using two very different accounts – one of which emphasised a highly critical, contemporary perspective. The institution of the plague hospital was controversial amongst medical figures as well as those who were treated there, and their families. We have seen that the unpopular nature of the *lazaretti* in Florence led to the temporary closure of the structures after the outbreak of 1630–31. However, it was quickly discovered that it was more expensive and less efficient to attempt to minister to the sick in their homes throughout the city and the plague hospital was reopened – much to the disgust of contemporaries. Governments sometimes had to threaten individuals to go to the plague hospitals. Criminals were made to serve within the structures. The morality of using these institutions was debated but so too was their medical purpose. This debate centred around two issues: the quality of the air within the hospitals and the issue of contact within the institutions. Both of these points open up questions as to whether or not the institutions were more likely to exacerbate or to ease the problems of infection and mortality during epidemics.

The *lazaretti* played a high-profile role in public responses to disease and feature in the writings and reports of physicians within cities. During the outbreak of 1575–77, the Venetian Health Office requested reports on ways in which the city could be cured.[109] Four Venetian reports survive, each of which assesses the causes of and responses to the disease. Each too passed comment on the uses of the *lazaretti*. The first report assessed the plague as a disease caused by contagion in which goods had a large role to play and emphasised the importance of careful airing for thirty days and boiling in water. It lauded the use of the *lazaretti* but recommended that caution be used when allowing people and their goods back since either the individuals or the houses to which they were returning might not be clean. The use of monasteries near to or within the city was recommended for additional quarantine for twenty-five to thirty days. The report expressed a

---

[108] 'A entrar in un Lazzaretto, e non infettarsi, stimo sia poco meno che cascara nell'acqua senza bagnarsi, o nel fuoco senza abbruciarsi', cited in Father Antero Maria da San Bonaventura, *Li lazaretti della città e riviere di Genova*, p. 27.

[109] These are by Tiberio Superchio, Victorio Negroni, Alvise Venier and Zuane Ailano. Negroni was in the service of the Health Office as the physician appointed for Dorsoduro and part of San Polo. Ailano was one of the physicians appointed to the *contrade* to visit the sick at their doorways and had also served with the Paduan doctors. See the list of physicians appointed to the contrade in ASV, Secreta, MMN 95 10v (10 March 1576) and the three doctors appointed to help the Paduan doctors in ASV, Senato Terra reg. 51 85r (26 June 1576). Bibliographical information can be found in Richard J. Palmer, *The studio of Venice.*

fear of the reintegration of people and goods after quarantine rather than of the *lazaretti* themselves. This emphasised the important role of the *lazaretti* whilst also issuing a note of caution regarding potential flaws in the system, which was already cumbersome. The second and third reports underscored many of these same points. They pointed out the role played by the *lazaretti* in preserving the city through the disinfection of goods. The report stated that care should be taken with the goods and people returning from the *lazaretti*. It also emphasised the effective cleaning of houses and public areas within the city more generally. The final report consisted of a list of nine points, discussed almost as grievances against the existing system. It is certainly the most critical of the four regarding the use of the *lazaretti*. Its author, Zuanne Ailano emphasised the potential damage caused by lengthy periods of quarantine, the widespread destruction of personal possessions without compensation and the benefits of treating some of the sick within the city. His most pressing concern related to those who returned from the *lazaretti* destitute and dying of hunger, cold and thirst.

The *lazaretti* and policies of quarantine were also discussed by the visiting Paduan physicians in 1576. In their original supplication the physicians had set down a series of conditions, some of which expressed the Paduans' concerns to limit the number of people being sent to the *lazaretti* and being put under household quarantine.[110] They also requested that neither they, nor their confessors, other doctors, surgeons, barbers or other ministers would be quarantined or held within any restrictions on their movements. By 30 June, however, the two Jesuit priests who attended the houses with them had died and their barber and one of their servants were sick. The Paduan doctors, much to their disgust, were placed in quarantine for eight days. The *lazaretti* and the policy of quarantine and isolation that they represented again featured in their assessments of the disease although it is important to remember that these particular physicians famously felt that the disease affecting the city was not the plague and so would obviously have been against mobilising the public health structures to combat the disease.

A third report, presented to the Venetian Health Office in October 1576 by the doctors of the city, specifically addressed the issue of quarantine in the *lazaretto nuovo* for those returning to Venice. A discussion of the issue was said to have been motivated by a concern at the large sums of money being spent on the hospitals.[111] The group of physicians were asked to consider two issues, one of which was whether it was safe for individuals to return directly to their homes from the *lazaretto vecchio* or San Lazaro if they were given clean clothes and were then sent to carry out a period of household quarantine. The physicians advised that individuals could safely avoid a period of quarantine in the *lazaretto nuovo* as long as household quarantine was enforced and emphasised the threat posed by beds and materials which were not safely disinfected.[112] The report was

---

[110]   ASV, Secreta MMN 95 19r (20 June 1576).
[111]   ASV, Secreta MMN 95 108r–109v (3 November 1576).
[112]   ASV, Senato Terra reg. 51 130v (3 November 1576).

motivated not by a concern regarding the institution of the *lazaretto* in theory but by the considerable financial strain which the institutions placed on the city during outbreaks. It was a controversial decision to by-pass use of the *lazaretto nuovo* for those individuals returning from the *lazaretto vecchio*; just six days later a proposal was put to the Senate to suspend the decision. This was voted on twice and eventually passed, although without a significant majority.[113] The balance at work in assessing the high cost of the *lazaretti* versus the protection that they were seen to offer was a difficult one to maintain. The closing of the *lazaretti* for a period of disinfection at the perceived end of outbreaks provoked similar concern and fear. In December 1556, the Senate had refused the motion that the *lazaretto vecchio* should be closed despite there being only fifty-four people left there, two-thirds of whom were described as being out of danger. Not until 1558 was the hospital closed for disinfection, following a petition from the Health Office doctor still on site, Ludovico Cucino.[114]

Debates about the efficacy of *lazaretti* were published within plague treatises, particularly those of Leonardo Fioravanti [1518–88] and Hieronimo Donzellini. Fioravanti recorded five principles to be put into practice during epidemics. The first of these stipulated that people' should not be sent to frightening places, as is often done in our time'. The practice, he said, was enough to kill people.[115] Instead, Fioravanti recommends leaving people in their own homes and ensuring that they are visited regularly and treated by doctors. Donzellini recommends trying to clean rather than burn goods and trying to keep the sick within the city in clean houses rather than send to the *lazaretti*. Donzellini recognises, though, that there are some who would be left without the ability to procure necessary supplies and many of whom were disorderly and living without reason and wisdom and so it is necessary to distinguish between this group and those who live comfortably and who can be well-governed. For the former group, the *lazaretti* can be used and should be divided into four parts: for the sick; those suspected of infection; those who have been cured and those finishing their quarantine. There was no consensus regarding the ideal form for quarantine and the use of the *lazaretti*. Controversy abounded, not least because of the high cost of administering these structures, in print and in practice.

During the seventeenth century, the Health Office officials acknowledged that various problems could arise from an infection within the *lazaretti* because the islands were small spaces within which infection could spread quickly. Nevertheless officials reiterated a commitment to using the *lazaretti*, claiming that it was still better that people be there than within the city.[116] Elsewhere in Italy, and

---

[113]   ASV, Senato Terra reg. 51 131v (9 November 1576).

[114]   ASV, Senato Terra reg. 40 149r (12 December 1556).

[115]   'é il non mettere a loco spavento, over paura, come in questa notra etàtutti fanno' in Leonardo Fioravanti, *Il reggimento della peste* (Venice, 1594), book one, chapter thirty.

[116]   I am grateful to Alex Bamji for this reference to ASV, Sanità b. 17 189r–191r (6 December 1630).

in Europe more broadly, the *lazaretti* continued to be used in response to plague but were increasingly associated with the poor in cities. In Venice, the institutions altered in the course of the century in the main because of circumstances rather than a change of policy: after the outbreak of 1630–31, Venice was not again affected by an epidemic of the disease and as a result the institutions were reshaped to provide quarantine for merchants.

The *lazaretti* illustrate the considerable investment put into the treatment of the plague. The medicine provided was not without its critics but there was some optimism regarding potential success. Despite the criticism made of the hospitals, the *lazaretti* continued to provide a cornerstone of Venice's public health policies for the plague and were invested in as the best response to the disease. A number of individuals, from a variety of backgrounds, were involved in medical care. Despite the best efforts of these staff, the medicine which was provided and the successes which were had in providing cures, mortality rates within the hospitals during epidemics were distressingly high. How this issue of death on a vast scale was dealt with is the subject of the next chapter.

Chapter 5
Dying in the *Lazaretti*

For I was hungry and you gave me something to eat,
I was thirsty and you gave me something to drink,
I was a stranger and you invited me in,
I needed clothes and you clothed me,
I was sick and you looked after me,
I was in prison and you came to visit me.[1]

These acts of mercy were officially-endorsed approaches to charity, which were designed to shape the priorities of good Christians. The six acts were also widely acknowledged as principles which informed the aims of hospitals throughout the medieval and early modern period. This text from Matthew's gospel was not left to stand alone as a guide to charity. It was supplemented, by St Cyprian [*c*.258], St Ambrose [*c*.337–397] and later St Thomas Aquinas [1225–74], with words from the book of Tobit regarding the charitable and compassionate job of burying the dead. Centuries before the establishment of the Venetian *lazaretti*, the six acts of mercy became seven and burial was praised and prioritised within charitable institutions.[2] The memorable message of the acts, that the hungry and homeless were embodiments of Christ on earth and that caring for the dead was divinely commissioned work, can be contrasted with memorable accounts of burial in times of plague. Federico Borromeo, describing a plague epidemic in Milan, wrote of one body being moved by a *pizzigamorto* (body clearer). The worker went to pick up the corpse by its arm, which promptly came off in his hand because the body was so putrefied.[3] Taken together, statements about the ideal treatment of the dead and vivid pictures of experiences during epidemics draw attention to the tensions inherent in dealing with widespread mortality. This chapter will contrast the attempts made to ensure patients died 'a good death' within the hospitals with the contemporary accounts of the problems of dealing with death in the context of plague.

---

[1]   NT, Matthew chapter 25 verses 35–40.

[2]   For the significance of the acts in shaping medieval hospital structures see the work of Carole Rawcliffe. On the specific issue of the seventh act of mercy, see Carole Rawcliffe, 'The seventh comfortable work: charity and mortality in the Medieval hospital', *Medicina e storia*, 3 (2003), pp. 11–35. These ideas endure, as attested to by William Schupbach, *Acts of mercy: the Middlesex hospital paintings by Frederick Caley Robinson (1862–1927)* (London, 2009), p. 8.

[3]   Armando Torno, *La peste di Milano del 1630: la cronaca e le testimonianze del tempo del cardinal Federico Borromeo* (Milan, 1998), p. 73.

Burial was a charged and significant issue in early modern Europe and it was one firmly rooted in the parish and in the community. It was a process which was associated with honour and had both social and religious implications and functions. Across the social spectrum, individuals were encouraged to plan ahead and make provision for their death. The contemporary image of the seven ages of man was often reproduced in art and literature. Shakespeare in *As you like it*, described the seven ages, in the famous speech which begins, 'All the world's a stage' and ends, 'Last scene of all, /That ends this strange, eventful history, /Is second childishness and mere oblivion; /Sans teeth, sans eyes, sans taste, sans everything'.[4] This picture of life and its progressive stages was mirrored in paintings, such as Titian's 'Three Ages of Man' or the same trope by Hans Baldung Grien [1485–1545] [Plate 23]. In the image he shows three ages of women: an old woman warding off death; a young woman so occupied with her own reflection that she has not even noticed death standing over her shoulder; and, finally, an infant – the epitome of immature youth – viewing life through a veil.[5] Early modern Europeans were encouraged to plan for long life whilst receiving constant reminders about the fragility of life and the ever-present threat of death. Death and burial, regardless of social status, was something to be contemplated and prepared for.

In the course of distributing earthly wealth, spiritual wealth could be earned and testators were encouraged to think about not only loved ones but also those in need. Part of the preparation for death, therefore, was supposed to involve strengthening ties with the community through charitable giving. The reciprocal care required of the community towards the deceased was enshrined in law and in tradition; it included the fulfilment of bequests, funerary processions, burial and commemoration. These were affected by periods of infection when fulfilling communal duties could prove life threatening. Furthermore, one effect of the use of centralised hospitals during plague epidemics was that the space of death moved from the locality. In place of the death of the individual within the home and the family, death had to be dealt with on a much larger scale, which threatened to undermine local ties.[6]

This chapter will consider the effect of plague on the traditional structures surrounding death and the ways in which public health measures sought to facilitate ties between the individual and locality. It will explore mortality in the *lazaretti* – considering how likely death was for those who entered the hospitals. It will outline the process by which bodies were buried and sometimes burned. Finally, a rare insight will be gained into the patients from the plague hospital.

---

[4] William Shakespeare, *As you like it*, II vii 139–66.

[5] On these images see Lyndal Roper, *Witch craze: terror and fantasy in Baroque Germany* (London, 2004), p. 155 and note 74. Roper considers the borrowing of images between the Ages of Man images and Baldun Grien's erotic images of witches but also notes that the Ages of Man were often used in calendars.

[6] For insightful work on social ties maintained and made more visible in times of plague see Giulia Calvi, *Histories of a plague year: the social and the imaginary in Baroque Florence* (Oxford, 1989).

Amongst the various and notable studies of plague made in the past it is rare to find extensive discussion of the victims – the sources are difficult and often the terrifying statistics have been left to speak for themselves. The chapter will end by considering a series of wills made within the institutions, which are revealing about the patients themselves and their charitable bequests. Throughout the chapter, it will be clear that death and dying were contexts in which isolation would have been at its most dangerous and damaging, for individuals and communities alike. Public health measures, even during the most severe outbreaks, were attempts to counteract any sense of disconnection and ensure that these institutions responded to the acts of mercy and principles of charity with which the chapter began.

Within early modern Catholicism, salvation was tied to the ecclesiastical church. Dying a good death had genuine implications for the afterlife. The notion involved receiving visitation, extreme unction, viaticum and the commendation of the soul to God. After death, Catholics could go straight to Heaven (which was very rare), into limbo if they were unbaptised (particularly children), into Purgatory or straight to Hell (a fate reserved for the most ungodly). Movement between these realms was possible and could be facilitated by the intercessions of the living. As a result, Masses would be said for the dead – and were often requested in wills. Intercession for the dead was a key purpose of Catholic funerals. This tradition was attacked during the Reformation: the Protestant rejection of the doctrine of Purgatory meant that the destination of the dead was determined and fixed.[7] Nevertheless funerals continued to serve an important didactic purpose. The strain placed on traditional strategies for burial and commemoration, therefore, in the context of plague epidemics had wide implications because of the significance attached to rituals surrounding death. In times of plague, as the physician Ingrassia wrote, it remained essential that burials continued to be carried out in consecrated ground to avoid treating Christians as though they were 'Moors, Turks or other infidels'.[8] The way in which death and burial were handled formed part of defining the Christian community.

'Charnel Houses of Death'?

One criticism relayed by Father Antero in Genoa was that going into a *lazaretto* without becoming infected was as likely as falling into water without getting

---

[7]   This was one of the few areas of Protestant thought shared by Luther, Zwingli and Calvin. For an introduction to shades of Protestantism see Andrew Pettegree (ed.), *The Reformation World* (Abingdon, 2000). See Bruce Gordon and Peter Marshall (eds), *The place of the dead: death and remembrance in late medieval and early modern Europe* (Cambridge, 2000). On the effects of the Reformation on death and the afterlife see Craig Koslofsky, *The Reformation of the dead: death and ritual in early modern Germany, 1450–1700* (Basingstoke, 2000) and engaging chapters on burial and commemoration in David Gaimster and Roberta Gilchrist, *The archaeology of the Reformation 1480–1580* (Leeds, 2003).

[8]   Ingrassia, p. 267.

wet or into fire without getting burned. The view of the plague hospitals as sites which were saturated with infection was commonplace. Benedetti wrote that it would hardly be surprising, given the disgusting beds on which patients slept, if barely 10 per cent of people survived their stays within the hospitals and hundreds died every day.[9] In this section, two aspects of mortality within plague hospitals will be considered: first, the percentage of the total mortality within cities which took place in the *lazaretti* and second, the overall percentage of patients within the hospitals who died. Available contemporary statistics make the estimate of the former easier than the latter; a discussion of the available source material is provided below.

The records of those who died in plague epidemics (like those that registered the people who were sent to the hospitals in the first place) no longer survive in Venice as they do in Milan and Mantua. These may have been burned at the end of epidemics, like so many other documents, which was both a space-saving and public health measure.[10] There are a number of sources, however, which record information relating to mortality during plague. The bills of mortality for the city (*polizze*), issued by the Venetian Health Office and posted at Rialto and at St Marks every Sunday, provided varying amounts of information. They gave daily mortality figures and occasionally stated the gender or age of the deceased. They sometimes referred to the numbers sent to the *lazaretti*, although did not do so consistently.[11] Ambassadors made use of these official statistics in their lengthy reports regarding the state of the cities in which they were resident. Their reports were dispatched regularly, often every three or four days. The ambassadors' information expanded upon the official statistics in the *polizze* with details regarding the location of cases and the official

---

[9]   'Ne ci dobbiamo dar maraviglia, se apena dieci per cento ne campavano, e se ne morivano al giorno le centinaia sopra à quelli affumicati, e puzzolenti letti' in Rocco Benedetti, *Relatione d'alcuni casi occorsi in Venetia al tempo della peste l'anno 1576 et 1577 con le provisioni, rimedii et orationi fatte à Dio benedetto per la sua liberatione* (Bologna, 1630), p. 21.

[10]   The quantity of documentation generated during a plague was acknowledged to be extremely large. In 1522, the Health Office scribe was given a salary increase in recognition of the intolerable workload (*faticha intolerabile*) that he had during an epidemic. See ASV, Sanità 726 65r (31 July 1523). In 1559, the number of books from the *lazaretti* and confusion regarding record-keeping was acknowledged in ASV, Sanità 730 252r (12 December 1559).

[11]   The ambassadors' reports which have been looked at in detail pertain to the outbreak of 1555–58 and were written by ambassadors from Mantua, Florence and Modena. These are available on microfilm at the library of the *Istituto per la storia della società e dello stato veneziano* in the Fondazione Giorgio Cini in Venice. Some of these *polizze* were copied by ambassadors and sent back as part of their reports and are, therefore, available as parts of these sources. The Florentine ambassador, for example, records a set of these for three weeks between 7 June and 27 June 1556 in Cini, Florence, 2971, 562–83. In his report of 23 July 1556, the Mantuan ambassador wrote that every morning he saw on the *polizza* fifty-eight persons dead and more than 100 sick being sent to the *lazaretto* in Cini, Mantua b. 1489 (23 July 1556).

responses. Contemporary writers who attempted to summarise legislation and events at the end of epidemics also included mortality statistics of varying levels of detail and the records of the most serious plague epidemics provide estimates of the number of deaths which occurred within the *lazaretti* as well as the city.

The statistics that survive for Venice during the outbreak of 1575–77 have been widely reproduced from copies of the records of the Health Office scribe Cornelio Morello, which were used in Chapter 2 to assess the gender makeup of patients at the *lazaretti*.[12] Morello's statistics were listed in three sections, covering the periods from 1 August 1575 to the end of February 1576, 1 March 1576 until the end of February 1577 and from 1 March 1577 to the end of the outbreak. Morello wrote that for the final period he did not know how many people had died because the book containing the official figures had been lost, although he estimated the number to be 4,000. In total, Morello recorded a mortality figure of 50,721 people, which included 27,546 in the city and 19,175 in the *lazaretti*. The remaining 4,000 was not broken down by location.[13] This total mortality figure comprised just under one third of the total population of the city. The deaths that took place in the *lazaretti* during this epidemic, according to Morello, comprised 41 per cent of the total. This figure is comparable with that for earlier outbreaks. In 1478, for example, a total of 12,573 people were said to have died (estimated at 11 per cent of the population), although 1,946 were from diseases other than plague.[14] Of the total mortality 33 per cent of deaths happened in the *lazaretti*. Of the deaths from plague, 39 per cent were in the *lazaretti*. That over a third of the overall mortality of the city took place within the institutions is significant, considering the relative size of the *lazaretto* islands. It was also, of course, deliberate. One of the purposes of sending the sick to the *lazaretti* was to ensure that fewer corpses remained in the city, at the risk of decomposing without discovery and posing significant risk to public health. On the basis of available statistics, proportions of mortality in the *lazaretti* appear to have remained broadly consistent during the epidemics of the fifteenth and sixteenth centuries at around 40 per cent.

Statistics for the later outbreak of 1630–31 show a very different breakdown. Of 46,490 total deaths, just 6,743 people were said to have died in the *lazaretti*.[15] Mortality made up a substantial percentage of the population (about 33 per cent) but the percentage of people who died in the *lazaretti* decreased substantially, falling

---

[12]   See Chapter 2, pp. 102–4.

[13]   For Morello's statistics see ASV, Secreta, MMN 95 164r.

[14]   For the information on mortality see Richard J. Palmer, 'The control of plague in Venice and northern Italy 1348–1600' (unpublished PhD thesis, University of Kent, 1978), p. 60. Estimates of the population size of Venice before the sixteenth century are difficult to make. Sanudo writing in 1493 claimed that the city had a population of 150,000 but this is thought to be inflated. I have adopted an estimate of 110,000, using an alternative figure of 102,000 given by Sanudo for the size of population in 1509, excluding clergy and religious orders. See David S. Chambers and Brian Pullan (eds), *Venice: a documentary history*, p. 6.

[15]   These summary statistics are given in ASV, Sanità b.17 407r–408r (n.d.).

from 41 to 15 per cent.[16] This is a dramatic shift. In part, the change in mortality levels was affected by the way in which the statistics were recorded. Other islands were listed separately for this outbreak. When the figures from the other islands are included, the combined number of deaths on the islands made up 20 per cent of overall mortality. This is still half of that for the earlier outbreak. This shift must have been brought about either by fewer admissions to the hospitals or greater success in terms of cure. Contemporaries do not comment upon more effective hospitals during the later epidemic – a reduction of almost half of the number of deaths would seem worthy of note. The statistics given for this epidemic may be indicative of the overall capacity of the institutions. The seventeenth-century outbreak was concentrated within a single year. Even with the use of overflow islands, it may have been that the system was strained by the concentration of infection, which restricted the number of people who could be cared for within the hospitals. It is likely, however, given the significant reduction in number of deaths, that fewer people in the 'suspected' rather than 'infected' category were sent to the islands for treatment, because of concerns about the spread of the disease within the hospitals. During this epidemic the Health Office officials acknowledged, in a way that did not happen for the sixteenth-century epidemics, that problems could arise from an infection within the *lazaretti*. The islands were small and it was recognised that infection could spread quickly. Despite this, officials were committed to using the *lazaretti*, claiming that it was still better that people be there than within the city.[17] The Health Office continued to support the institutions rhetorically even if the officials did not send the numbers to the islands that they had done in earlier outbreaks.

During the outbreak of 1483–85 in Milan, 4,829 people died but only 262 (almost 5.5 per cent) of these died in the plague hospital of San Gregorio.[18] For Padua, the chronicler Canobbio recorded a total mortality during the outbreak of 1575–77 of 12,388 people with 2,977 (24 per cent) occurring in the *lazaretto*. A separate set of statistics has slightly different figures, with a higher proportion of deaths in the *lazaretto* (of 30 per cent).[19] These proportions indicate a less extensive use of the institution compared to Venice (no claim is made for higher cure rate by contemporaries) but it is also worth noting that these figures are comparable with information from elsewhere and with the statistics of seventeenth-century outbreaks. They are similar to the percentage of mortality recorded by Cipolla for the *lazaretto* in Prato in 1631 (27 per cent). Paul Slack's work on England, reflecting

---

[16]   For this figure see Paolo Preto, *Peste e società a Venezia nel 1576* (Vicenza, 1978) p. 112 notes 6 and 7.

[17]   I am grateful to Alex Bamji for this reference to ASV, Sanità b. 17 189r–191r (6 December 1630).

[18]   See Samuel K. Cohn Jr, *Cultures of plague: medical thought at the end of the Renaissance* (Oxford, 2010), p. 21.

[19]   4,201 people died in the city of Padua (49%), 1,810 in ninety-eight of the surrounding towns (21%) and 2,546 in the *lazaretto* (30%), giving a total of 8,557 in the summary statistics in ASP, Sanità reg. 49 25r (n.d.).

the different use of these institutions when compared with the Continent, records that 'just a fraction of the infected poor' was accommodated and died in the temporary structures of Newcastle, Windsor and Oxford. Slack highlights the case of Worcester during 1637, where a quarter of the deaths in the city were in the plague hospital, as having an unusually high number of deaths in the English context. He cites the case of Norwich in 1665–66, where the percentage of overall mortality within the pesthouse was less than ten, as more usual for the English case. In fifteenth- and sixteenth-century Venice, the *lazaretti* were used more extensively than elsewhere. In all likelihood this was because of the early foundation of permanent structures, which meant that they could be used immediately in times of infection.

In terms of accounting for change during the early modern period, it would seem that the shift in the percentage of overall mortality taking place in the *lazaretti* in Venice was caused by a reduction in the number of people being sent to the *lazaretti* during the seventeenth century, rather than an improvement in the effectiveness of medical care. The lack of source material relating to the numbers of people being sent to the *lazaretti* from the city makes this shift difficult to quantify precisely, however. The only source discovered to date which provides an insight into patient numbers at the *lazaretti* is a register which survives within the death registers of the Venetian archive. This source (register 810) details the number of people within each *sestiere* who died, were licensed or were sent to the *lazaretto vecchio* or *lazaretto nuovo* on a daily basis between 12 August 1576 and 16 July 1577.[20] This record is not complete, showing blanks when the figures from particular *sestieri* did not arrive or were lost in transcription. Out of a total of 350 days, only 260 are recorded in this *busta;* in other words, fewer than 70 per cent of the days' records are included.[21] Despite the incomplete nature of the source, this is the most useful register for assessing the use of the *lazaretti* during outbreaks in Venice during the early modern period. The figures from the *busta* can be converted to something approximating a full year's information. In order to achieve this, I first calculated the number of suspicious deaths in the city between 1 March 1576 and 28 February 1577 by supplementing the aforementioned death register with one other.[22] This information was used to produce Plate 24, which shows clearly the seasonality of the disease, as well as the fragmentary nature of the data, over the course of a year.[23]

Register 810 not only details the number of suspicious deaths but also contains information on the number of patients being sent to the Venetian *lazaretti* and

---

[20]   ASV, Sanità, Necrologi 810.

[21]   The end of the plague epidemic was declared officially on 13 July 1577. This *busta* contains records of three individuals who were licensed in Santa Croce and Castello after this official end (on 15 and 16 July). In order to calculate the number of days, therefore, I have allowed for complete months between August 1576 and June 1577 and then added sixteen days for July.

[22]   ASV, Sanità, Necrologi 809 and 810.

[23]   See Samuel K. Cohn Jr, *Cultures of Plague*, for example pp. 65–6.

has been used to produce Plate 25. This illustrates that, for the period 12 August to 29 December (after which date no suspected plague deaths are recorded in the registers, although the sources continue until 16 July 1577, two days after the end of the epidemic was declared), the number of people who were sent to the Venetian *lazaretto vecchio* followed a broadly similar trend to that of the number of suspected plague deaths in the city. I have used this broad correlation as the basis for my estimates of the number of people sent to the *lazaretti* for the five and a half months which are missing from register 810 (March, April, May, June, July and 1–11 August 1576), using comparable periods.[24] These calculations are shown in Plate 26. I have also adjusted the estimated figures, both for suspected plague deaths and numbers sent to the *lazaretti* using daily averages to account for days which were not recorded.

The estimated total number of people sent to the Venetian *lazaretti* during this year is 25,970. Morello provides a statistic for the number of people who died within the *lazaretti* in 1576 (m.v.), which provides the underlying level of mortality. Morello records the death of 10,213 men and 8,647 women between 1 March 1576 and February 1577. This gives a total mortality figure of 18,860.[25] This is 73 per cent of the estimated total number of people sent to the *lazaretti* during this period. The number of people being sent to the *lazaretto nuovo* may be conservative, given contemporary observations that more people were accommodated in the *lazaretto nuovo* than in the *lazaretto vecchio*, at least before the change in policy discussed in Chapter 2.[26] Were more accurate information available, this percentage might decrease although it remains a useful guideline. The statistic is broadly supported by contemporary observations. In 1559, in an account of the progression of a less severe plague outbreak, two-thirds of the people in the *lazaretto vecchio* were said to have died, which was said to be standard.[27] The 1575–77 epidemic hit on a scale unprecedented since the Black Death and so an increase in mortality within the institutions would not be surprising. It is important to note, however, that the statistics available also record that 81 per cent of those being sent to the *lazaretti* during this year went directly to the *lazaretto vecchio*: in other words, they had been diagnosed as sick. The mortality statistic of 73 per cent confirms the observation that will be explored in more detail in the following chapter that a number of those diagnosed with the plague did return from the plague hospitals and were thought to be cured.

Comparative material regarding mortality does survive for *lazaretti* elsewhere in Italy. In considering how likely death was within the *lazaretti* it is necessary to distinguish between cities and periods. A far lower mortality was recorded by

---

[24]   Comparable periods have been chosen on the basis of the number of suspicious deaths in the city.

[25]   These summary statistics are given in ASV, Secreta, MMN 95 164r (n.d.).

[26]   Discussed on pp. 83–4.

[27]   ASV, Sanità 730 258v (n.d. December 1559) 'A lazareto vechio verame[n]te p[er] l'ordinario, come esta sempre ne morinano poi li doi terzi in circa'.

Samuel Cohn for Milan in 1485: two-thirds of the people sent were said to survive the disease; however, this was during a far less deadly epidemic.[28] For the later outbreak of 1575–77 in Padua, Canobbio records that half of the people at the *lazaretti* returned and he estimates the number at more than 4,000 people.[29] For Florence in 1630–31, Henderson has calculated the number of deaths at sixty-nine per one hundred sick.[30] Cipolla's work on the Pistoian *lazaretto* recorded 51 per cent mortality and for Prato, 49 per cent mortality. In Genoa, Fra Antero Maria da San Bonaventura insisted that a stay in the plague hospital did not make death inevitable. He cited examples from December 1656 when 120 people and then 199 people arrived at the hospitals and were successfully cured. Later he records that about 70 per cent of the people in the plague hospitals died.[31]

In terms of comparison with general hospitals of the period, the *lazaretti* had high mortality levels, although their statistics survive only for periods of crisis. John Henderson's work has established mortality of 10 to 15 per cent for Santa Maria Nuova. Although the effects of plague on mortality in other hospitals cannot be generalised, some epidemics did increase the deaths within these hospitals significantly.[32] The information regarding mortality in the *lazaretti* remains fragmentary and can only be taken as broadly indicative of reality within these hospitals. On the basis of current information, it appears that, even during the worst of early modern outbreaks, approximately a quarter of the patients who were sent to the hospitals survived. More plentiful than statistics for mortality are the details regarding the practices which dealt with death during plague time, to which this chapter now turns.

A 'Good Death': Burial

During severe epidemics, much of what was recorded about the burial of corpses stressed the scale on which it was performed and the perceived lack of respect with which it was conducted – with one memorable simile, as we will see, comparing burial in mass graves to the layering of lasagna. In this section, archive records will be used which nuance our understanding of burial practices and relate them to contemporary sensibilities about death and burial. Archaeological and archival records show that the locations of burial were more varied than previously

---

[28]   See Samuel K. Cohn Jr and Guido Alfani, 'Households and plague in early modern Italy', *Journal of interdisciplinary history*, 38:2 (2007), p. 197.

[29]   Alessandro Canobbio, *Il successo della peste occorsa in Padova l'anno MDLXXVI* (Padua, 1576), 13r and 23v–24r.

[30]   John Henderson, '"La schifezza, madre della corruzione". Peste e società nella Firenze della prima età moderna: 1630–1631', *Medicina e storia* 1:2 (2001), p. 49.

[31]   He actually says that 30% died on p. 10.

[32]   See John Henderson, *The Renaissance Hospital: healing the body and healing the soul* (London, 2006), pp. 256–61.

understood. After considering the place of burial, the chapter will go on to explore the criticisms made by contemporaries of the way in which the dead were buried and the behaviour of the infamous body clearers (*pizzigamorti*) who, as I have explored elsewhere, captured the contemporary imagination and were described in vicious terms in contemporary writing.[33] Finally, will-making and charitable donations by patients will be considered.

Even more than visitors and cats or dogs, the way in which corpses were dealt with challenged the maintenance of health within the *lazaretti*.[34] Plague corpses were recognised to be dangerous if left to rot. Bodies were buried or burned in order to stop them releasing a stench (*fettor*), which was not only disgusting but believed to carry disease.[35] During recent archaeological work, the ground at the Venetian *lazaretto vecchio* was found to be saturated with human remains, not simply in areas of consecrated ground but across a number of open spaces. The nature of the graves varied.[36] For some, bodies had been carefully arranged, either in individual sites or in small groups. For the majority, however, corpses were arranged in pits, consisting of various layers – up to four deep. Here the optimal use of space was the priority and adults were laid out in the centre with children's bodies packed around the side. It is impossible to know how many bodies were buried in the *lazaretti* but it is clear that the authorities used all available space. That the public health authorities' intention was to bury as many bodies as possible is supported by material from Florence during the outbreak of 1630–31. John Henderson has shown that burial in the *lazaretti* on a month-by-month basis accounted for 43 per cent of the total at the beginning of the outbreak but that this percentage increased so that, by June 1631, 92 per cent of total mortality took place in the plague hospitals. Overall, the Florentine authorities buried 67.5 per cent of plague victims in the *lazaretti*.[37] Although similar statistical evidence does not survive for Venice, archaeological evidence indicates a similar intention.

The scale of burial in the *lazaretti* and city cemeteries elsewhere was vast. In Padua, Canobbio noted that the pits should be at least ten feet deep.[38] In Giovanni Boccaccio's description of burials in Tuscany during the Black Death, bodies were said to be stowed 'tier upon tier like ships' cargo, each layer of corpses being

---

[33]   See Jane L. Stevens Crawshaw, 'The beasts of burial: *pizzigamorti* and public health for the plague in early modern Venice' *Social history of medicine*, 24:3 (2011), 570–87.

[34]   For visitors, cats and dogs, see Chapter 3, pp. 147–9.

[35]   ASV, Sanità 730 140v–145r (1 May 1555) [25].

[36]   For comparative work on burial see Vanessa Harding, 'Burial of the plague dead in early modern London', in Justin A. I. Champion (ed.), *Epidemic disease in London* (London, 1993), pp. 53–64. Following archaeological work on the island of the *lazaretto vecchio* a catalogue of the findings should be forthcoming. Once this is available, information on burial on the islands is likely to be far more extensive than at present.

[37]   John Henderson, '"La schifezza, madre della corruzione"', p. 45.

[38]   Alessandro Canobbio, *Il successo della peste*, 11v.

covered over with a thin layer of soil til the trench was filled to the top'.[39] Regarding burial, Benedetti described the creation of a cemetery on the Cavanella near the Lido where enormous troughs were dug. Graves were described as consisting of corpses, chalk and soil, likened by a fourteenth-century Florentine chronicler to the layers in lasagne.[40] Emphasis on rotten flesh was developed by a Jesuit writer who described dead bodies 'packed like sardines' bringing 'a great stench and stink, even from the *lazaretto* as a result of the multitude of bodies and the burning of infected goods'.[41] It is interesting to note that archaeological work on the *lazaretto vecchio* has not found traces of chalk being used between the layers of the graves, despite the recommendation that chalk be used to minimise dangerous odours.[42] The stench of rotting flesh, therefore, may well have pervaded the island.

The development of mass graves required space and, in Venice, other lagoon islands were adopted as cemetery islands. Archive records and Benedetti's account state that heightened concern regarding the potential for bodies to infect the air meant that they were no longer to be buried within the city.[43] Sant'Ariano was adopted for the burial of corpses from 1565 when the island was enclosed by a perimeter wall. The island would become known as the *ossario* of the lagoon because of its frequent use for the disposal of dead bodies. This was the island visited by Frederick Rolfe [1860–1913] during the nineteenth century, whose arresting description of the place opens by asking whether the reader has ever seen a snake glide out from the eye socket of a skull.[44] Equally chilling sights were recorded in 1664 when Health Office officials inspected the site and found what they described as 'various pieces of human corpses' exposed and a distinct lack of sacred objects. As a result, a large, wooden cross was erected on the island and a pedestal was sculpted with the arms of St Mark and the family crests of the Procurators of the Health Office.[45] During epidemics, however, the concern was for quantity rather than quality in relation to burial. Sant'Ariano was used extensively until October 1576 when the Health Office officials decided that bodies should be sent to the graves on the Lido. An entry from 1577 estimated that 30,000 bodies

---

[39] Giovanni Boccaccio, *The Decameron*, (trans.) G.H. McWilliam (London, 1995), p. 12.

[40] 'e poi veniano gli altri sopr'essi e poi la terra addosso a suolo, a suolo, con poca terra, come si minestrasse lasagne a fornire di formaggio' reproduced in N. Rodolico (ed.), 'Cronaca fiorentina di Marchionne di Coppo Stefani', *Rerum italicarum scriptores* vol. 30 (Castello, 1903), p. 231.

[41] Cited in A. Lynn Martin, *Plague? Jesuit accounts of epidemic disease in the sixteenth century* (Kirksville MO, 1996), p. 51.

[42] On chalk to minimise odours see Ingrassia, p. 221.

[43] 'facilmente infetar l'aere il sepelir tanti corpi de rispetto nelli cimeteri della cita'. ASV, Sanità, 733 1v (13 July 1576).

[44] Fr Rolfe (Baron Corvo), *Tre racconti su Venezia* (Venice, 2002).

[45] ASV, Sanità 742 7v (12 August 1664).

had been buried on the Lido by the end of the outbreak.[46] This seems an extremely high figure, particularly since the period from October 1576 to July 1577 was one in which the effects of the disease waned. It may well be that this cemetery had been used in the earlier part of the outbreak for deaths on the Lido itself.

The regulations governing burial were specific and shaped by concerns regarding the transmission of infection. The Prior at the *lazaretto vecchio* was instructed, for example, that he should not allow the bodies to be stripped of clothing nor to have their hair cut before being buried, presumably because of the fear of infection on those materials although the authorities are not specific.[47] Sant'Ariano was used to bury bodies classed as *di rispetto* from the city in 1576 and specific boats were appointed for this task.[48] The boats were allocated to particular *sestieri*, with some serving San Marco, Castello and Cannaregio and the others San Polo, Dorsoduro and Santa Croce. The boats made two trips daily (one in the morning and the other after nine o'clock) and more often if necessary.[49] In the same instruction, the Health Office officials appointed two people to dig graves on the island, as deep as possible. Initially, instructions stipulated that the burial of corpses *di rispetto* could be done in coffins, but without any clothing, in deep graves in the ground but not in tombs.[50] The concern about tombs related to the issue of corrupted air. Official exceptions were made, for example, for the Prior and Prioress who were given the option of being buried in the tomb of the church at the *lazaretto* or in the ground.[51] In general, however, interment was preferred since the soil was thought to act like a protective layer around the bodies. Only ten days after issuing this proclamation, however, the officials instructed that burial of corpses *di rispetto* should be done without coffins and that those who chose to send bodies in coffins could do so at their own expense.[52] Here the motivation was financial rather than medical. The quantity of corpses led to the adoption of a policy of burning the bodies but this did little to alleviate conditions. This treatment of the dead, beyond plague time, was associated with heretics and witches. The religious implications of this Health Office policy were not fully engaged with. More attention was paid to the effects on the living than on the dead. Benedetti wrote of the hellish quality of the stench which disseminated from every side of the *lazaretto vecchio* and of the constant cloud of smoke from the burning bodies. He says that the smell became so unbearable that the Health Office was forced to return to burying bodies and ordered deep graves to be dug at Cavanella into which corpses could be placed.[53]

---

[46]   ASV, Sanità 733 192v (14 August 1577).

[47]   ASV, Sanità 730 142r (1 May 1557).

[48]   On this distinction see Chapter 2, p. 82.

[49]   ASV, Sanità 733 1v (13 July 1576).

[50]   ASV, Secreta MMN 95 35r (3 July 1576).

[51]   Cucino 29r (9 May 1555) and 89v (18 May 1557).

[52]   ASV, Sanità 733 44r (23 October 1576).

[53]   Rocco Benedetti, *Relatione d'alcuni casi*, p. 21.

It is clear, despite attempts by the Health Office to remove corpses from the city, burial also continued to take place, with or without the approval of the Health Office, in homes and parishes within the city from the fifteenth through to the seventeenth century. In 1490, Alexio Ruffian was said to be sick at the plague hospital, having buried a nine-year-old girl who had died of the plague in the cemetery of Santi Giovanni e Paolo. Alexio had been denounced to the Health Office and was said to have acted without respect for the office's authority.[54] In the early sixteenth century, the Health Office officials noted the case of five bodies in the parish of Sant'Aponal which had been buried in secret within a home. For obvious reasons the actions of the inhabitants were described as very dangerous and the case prompted officials to issue legislation regarding burials in secret: anyone caught would be banned *in perpetuum* from Venice and their estates would be used for the benefit of the *lazaretti*.[55]

In the mid-seventeenth century, two doctors compiled a report, which had been commissioned by the Health Office regarding the burial of plague-infected corpses within the city. Twelve doctors, two for each *sestiere*, had been asked to report on burial sites; this report is from Santa Croce. The doctors noted that 'many' infected people were buried in the city during the plague. They recorded that these bodies had been interred (*sotterate*) and, therefore, had been buried in line with the instructions issued by the Health Office that graves should be used in place of tombs for those infected with the disease so that the ground might act as a protective shroud around the body. The doctors' general observations expressed concern that these graves needed to remain well covered and remain undisturbed for a period of time deemed sufficient by the Health Office for any putrid air to subside. Otherwise, the doctors noted, opening up the graves would be like the opening of the gold casket in the Temple of Apollo at the time of Avidius Cassius when the soldiers expected to find treasure but instead met their death because a pestilential vapour was released. A number of the doctors' notes relate to the specific placement of bodies within particular churches. At San Giacomo dell'Orio it was noted that eight tombs within the church needed to be strengthened with metal bolts (*inarpesare*). The cemetery needed to be re-covered with fresh soil and paved with brick outside the door, where a number of corpses were said to have been buried. Eight protrusions (*eminenze*) had been discovered, beneath which there were said to be a number of corpses. At Santa Croce, it was noted that three infected members of the family had been buried in the burial place of Ca'Priuli, illustrating that even during epidemics there were opportunities for patricians to retain control over the bodies of members of their family.[56] Burial within the parish in times of plague was not unique to Venice. In England, Paul Slack illustrated that plague victims were interred within parish cemeteries, despite some reluctance on behalf of contemporaries to 'contaminate their churchyards with plague corpses'. Slack also recognised that a number

---

[54]   ASV, Sanità 725 4r–v (15 and 23 March 1490).

[55]   ASV, Sanità b. 2 8r (24 September 1506).

[56]   ASV, Sanità 740 42r (April 1645).

of plague victims were buried illicitly in gardens and fields.[57] The regulations governing burial in plague time were some of those contested most fiercely by the populace because of concerns about indignity and isolation after death.

Attempts made on behalf of the state to direct burial in plague times proved to be unpopular. The same was true of the methods used by those employed to move corpses to burial – known as the *pizzigamorti* (body clearers). Contemporaries expressed their shock at the behaviour of these workers, particularly in the light of the important ideas about charity and burial outlined in the introduction. Burial was a ritual firmly centred around key elements of individual identity, relating to place of residence and occupation. From artisans to Doges, the role which individuals had played in the life of the Venetian Republic was marked in the manner of their burial. For members of confraternities and guilds, fellow brothers would participate in processions and the route would depend upon the charitable geography of the city. For the city's Doges, funerals would follow a route including key sites within the city – including Rialto and St Mark's Square. In contrast to the collective participation of organisations based upon the identity of the individual, experiences of transportation to burial in plague time was markedly different. Benedetti wrote that patients in the *lazaretti* could be found in agony, or unable to speak or move; the body clearers would remove these poor souls to a mound of bodies and if any of them managed to move a hand, or foot, or call for help, it was a stroke of luck if any of the body clearers were compassionate enough to return them to the hospitals.[58] In place of Christian care, individuals were seen to be treated without respect or recognition.

Despite their notoriety during plague epidemics, body clearers for the plague had been permanent employees of the Venetian Republic since 1432.[59] The earliest responsibility of these men was to bury corpses; by 1484, their responsibilities included assisting with medical care for male patients in the *lazaretti*. Initially these men were paid in times of health and disease – and their salaries were doubled in the case of the latter.[60] Eventually the Health Office made use of the city's waterways to occupy their permanent body clearers beyond epidemics. The workers were given posts within Venice's *traghetti* stations, which lined the Grand Canal and served the city's population on short journeys. This work kept the body clearers fit and employed, ready to serve the Health Office by rowing corpses (as well as patients) between the city and the lagoon islands when there was need. Across Europe, temporary body clearers were also hired during

---

[57]   Paul Slack, *The impact of plague in Tudor and Stuart England* (London, 1985), p. 55.

[58]   Rocco Benedetti, *Relatione d'alcuni casi*, p. 21.

[59]   For a detailed discussion of these workers see Jane L. Stevens Crawshaw, 'The beasts of burial'.

[60]   In 1432 the *pizzigamorti* were paid more than other male servants and boatmen. In 1436 it is noted that the *pizzigamorti* should be given double pay in plague time. ASV Sal b. 6 reg. 3 78v (16 June 1436).

plague epidemics. These workers were often drawn from the poor and artisan classes. The role, therefore, was one which individuals could move in and out of.[61] Temporary body clearers were often foreigners, or at least were drawn from the Venetian state rather than the city itself. For example, eight body clearers were sent from Salò to assist during the outbreak of 1576, in response to a request from the Venetian authorities.[62] *Pizzigamorti* were also sent out from Venice to other areas of Venetian territory during periods of need.[63] Very little information survives regarding the temporary workers. Often only their names and salaries at the time of their appointment can be gleaned from surviving archival material.[64] The incentive to work as a temporary body clearer was said to be financial; Benedetti remarked that these men received both good salaries (*buona stipendio*) and benefits (*buona provisione*).[65] This perception, however, may have been shaped by resentment. Archival records show that during the outbreak of 1576, the *pizzigamorti* received salaries higher than some of the serving men and women but on a par with the boatmen and the guards, with whom their roles became interchangeable and overlapping.[66]

By 1630, Health Office officials recognised the need to improve the way in which *pizzigamorti* were moving corpses and ordered the Arsenal to begin constructing carts on which the bodies could be piled and transported to the boats to be taken for burial. In part this was introduced to speed up the process of body clearing but it was also done to protect the *pizzigamorti* from excessive contact with the bodies and from exposure to infection.[67] By the seventeenth century, occupational clothing had also been introduced for the *pizzigamorti*: they were instructed to wear tarred cloaks and advised to carry aromatics. Despite the introduction of the carts as a form of protection, the indignity of being taken to burial in such a way by public health workers, presumably, exacerbated the problem of the lack of proper burial.

---

[61] During the outbreak of 1575–77, there were 120 *pizzigamorti* based within the city, almost two per parish. In the later outbreak of 1630–31, 300 individuals were said to be have served in this role until the number was capped at 100. Additional *pizzigamorti* were based on islands of the lagoon. See ASV, MMN 95 66v (9 August 1576) and ASV, Sanità, reg. 17, 223r (19 December 1630).

[62] ASV, Sanità reg. 14 282v (18 August 1576) and ASV, Sanità 730 24r (6 September 1555).

[63] Two *pizzigamorti*, for example, were sent to Cattaro in 1572 in ASV, Sanità reg. 13 118r (7 July 1572).

[64] This information can be found in the *notatorio* series of the Venetian Sanità.

[65] Rocco Benedetti, *Relatione d'alcuni casi*, p. 22.

[66] The *pizzigamorti* received five ducats per month, the guards nine and the boatmen six in ASV, Secreta MMN 95 9v (11 March 1576).

[67] 'Per facilitar transporto cadaveri alle peate e preservar pizzigamorti, Reggimento Arsenale faccia construire numero di carretti ...', Nelli-Elena Vanzan Marchini, *Le leggi di sanità della Repubblica di Venezia* (Canova, 2000) vol. 3, 'Pestilenzie' (15 November 1630).

Ample description of the notorious *pizzigamorti* contrasts with the lack of documentation for those who died within the hospitals. It is only in the eighteenth century that some of the patients, who continued to be buried on the islands, can be identified by the inscriptions from the churches in the *lazaretti*.[68] A large number of deaths occurred within the *lazaretti* and of these few leave a trace in the archives. The following section will consider the exceptions to this rule in order to explore some individual cases in more detail: those whose wills survive in the Venetian Health Office archives.

A 'Good Death': Charitable Giving

Early modern wills often started by stating that 'nothing was more certain than death'.[69] The uncertainty of living a long life during the early modern period was pertinent to periods of plague, when the certainty of sudden death may have seemed particularly assured. A gruesome wax model of death during plague time, produced in 1657, illustrates this with the inscription 'It's my lot today, yours tomorrow' [Plate 27]. The scene shows plague skeletons in an environment of decay and ruin. A number of contemporaries made their wills during epidemics.[70] It is for this reason that Rocco Benedetti claims to have had such extensive knowledge of the city during plague time; as a notary he was called to take down the wills of the sick. In the files of his wills, moving examples like that of Anzola Brunacini survive. She was described as being in quarantine and affected by the plague in body although healthy of mind. Cornelia her niece had already been taken to the *lazaretto*. Anzola wrote that if Cornelia returned from the *lazaretto* alive she was to receive a number of items. Included with the will is a loose slip which records that Anzola was taken to the *lazaretto vecchio* on 5 August 1576 and died the following day.[71] The nature of the Venetian notarial archive means that a search for similar wills was beyond the scope of the present study, although it could make for a fascinating and revealing research project in itself. A series of seventy-four wills, made in the Venetian *lazaretti*, do survive in the records of the Venetian Health Office. The selection is spread throughout the notarial volumes and the reasons for

---

[68]   BMC, Codice Cicogna, 2018 (Iscrizione veneziane inedite), isole, b. 509:2 (Lazzaretto nuovo) and b. 509:3 (Lazzaretto vecchio).

[69]   Samuel Cohn pointed out to me that this is not a formula specific to the early modern period and is common in medieval wills. See his discussion of the preambles and formulas of wills in Samuel K. Cohn Jr, *Death and property in Siena, 1205–1800: strategies for the afterlife* (London, 1988), pp. 58–60.

[70]   It would be fascinating to know more about levels of preparation for death during the early modern period and how many individuals during epidemics made 'death bed wills' or had already made a will in good health. In Siena in 1500 Samuel Cohn has estimated that 44% of the wills surviving were of the former type. See ibid., p. 15.

[71]   ASV, Archivi Notarile, Testamenti, Atti Benedetti, b. 89, 9:3 (4 August 1576).

their inclusion in these volumes vary. For some, the Health Office was called upon to resolve conflicts with heirs or particular bequests. Of the tens of thousands of people who died within these hospitals across the period, this group offers a tiny proportion. The available wills do, however, offer an opportunity to glean more information about the elusive patients within the *lazaretti*.

Wills are not without their problems but have been widely recognised as rich sources. They have been used for purposes as varied as illustrating social networks, demonstrating change over time in relation to popular religious attitudes, highlighting characteristics of dialects and assessing female literacy levels in the early modern period.[72] They have also been used to assess the economic worth of individuals across the social spectrum.[73] Here, they will be used to facilitate a discussion of the process of will-making within the *lazaretti* and charitable bequests made within the hospitals in times of plague. The majority of these surviving wills were made in the *lazaretti*: fifty-four in the *lazaretto vecchio*, thirteen in the *lazaretto nuovo*, six within the city itself and one on a galley ship stationed at the *lazaretto vecchio*. The limited nature of the series makes it impossible to assess large-scale shifts in charitable giving. Overall, what the wills establish, though, is that the *lazaretti* were perceived as charitable institutions and were recognised in wills alongside more traditional charitable enterprises.

The seasonality of will-making from this selection follows a similar pattern to that of deaths within the hospital, with peaks in the summer months and in October. Some of those from the *lazaretto nuovo* were made because of different circumstances – such as the wedding referred to in Chapter 3 – but these were exceptional. The wills were an essential part of the preparation offered by the institutions for dying a good death, which seems to have been available to all patients. Testators range from the wife of a body clearer to wealthy widows. The gender breakdown of those making wills shows a predominance of men; of the sixty-seven individuals who made wills within the hospitals, thirty-nine were men and twenty-eight were women.[74] Although some wills were made concurrently by couples, the majority were made by individuals.

---

[72] See for social networks and servants and masters Dennis Romano, 'Aspects of patronage in fifteenth- and sixteenth-century Venice', *Renaissance Quarterly*, 46:4 (1993), pp. 712–33; on wills and changing religious belief see Ronnie Po-chia Hsia, 'Civic wills as sources for the study of piety in Muenster, 1530–1618', *Sixteenth century Journal*, 14:3 (1983), pp. 321–48; for will-writing as indicative of female literacy and education levels see Federica Ambrosini, '"De mia man propia" Donna, scrittura e praesi testamentaria nella Venezia del Cinquecento' in Mario de Biasi (ed.), *Non uno itinere. Studi storici offerti dagli allievi a Federico Seneca* (Padua, 1993), pp. 33–54. The variety of purposes to which historians have put wills is discussed in Samuel K. Cohn Jr, 'Last wills and testaments' in Margaret King (ed.), *Oxford Bibliographies Online: Renaissance and Reformation* (Oxford, 2010).

[73] Alison A. Smith, 'Gender, ownership and domestic space: inventories and family archives in Renaissance Verona', *Renaissance studies*, 12:3 (1998), pp. 375–91.

[74] For the gender make-up of patients see pp. 102–4.

In addition to the social and religious mores, the Health Office recognised the importance of will-making to avoid confusion and ambiguity after death. They laid down specific instructions for such a process in the *capitolari* of the *lazaretti*. Most of the surviving wills were recorded by the chaplains on the island and were witnessed by other workers. Of the fifty-five which record the name of the scribe, forty-five were written by a chaplain, three by a Prior, two by a Health Office scribe, two by other workers, two by other priests and one by a doctor. The introductory sections are sometimes revealing as to the process by which the will was made, particularly in wills written by Fra Marco Carmelitano, the chaplain to the *lazaretto vecchio* during the outbreak of 1575–77. Some of these simply note that an individual felt inspired by God (*Iddio Benedetti gli ha inspirato*) and called the Chaplain to them.[75] A standard case is that of Donna Madalena from Vicenza. Fra Marco recorded that she was in bed because of illness; he was called and informed the Prior, who instructed him to find four men of good standing and reason in whose presence he should write the will.[76] These witnesses included other people within the hospitals as well as those who worked there, ranging from members of the clergy and the medical profession to body clearers.

The format of the surviving Venetian wills is fairly standardised, with introductory sections dedicating the will to Creator God and the Virgin Mary. The testator then confirmed that they were healthy of mind and intellect although often sick of body and offered their soul to God and their body to the ground. Other studies of wills during this period have considered these introductory sections as indicative of religious belief more generally. R. Po-chia Hsia has made this assertion in the context of Münster wills where, he claims, 'there is no consistent pattern of invocation or commendation imposed on the testator by the clergy'.[77] In the context of the Venetian wills, however, the opposite can be observed. Of a series of fourteen wills made by Fra Andrea, the Chaplain to the *lazaretto vecchio* during the outbreak of 1528–29, for example, all of them record almost identical introductory sections.[78] Only one change can be found in the series and that is in a will of a Jewish man, where he was said to leave his soul to God (*il primo motore*) and his body to the composting earth and the Jewish burial.[79]

---

[75]   Will of Madonna Eufemia, ASV, Sanità 732 57r–59r (9 November 1575).

[76]   Will of Donna Madalena from Vicenza, ASV, Sanità 732 150r–151v (8 April 1576).

[77]   Ronnie Po-chia Hsia, 'Civic wills as sources for the study of piety', p. 327.

[78]   These read 'In the name of God the Creator and defender of all created things and of the glorious Virgin Mother Mary and of the divine Mark protector of our city of Venice and of all the saints of the heavenly court ... healthy of mind but sick in my fragile body and knowing that this life is fallible and transitory I leave in this my last Will my soul created in the likeness of God creator and uncreated to all the saints of the supreme court and the body, which is made up of four elements, I leave to the composting ground and to the ecclesiastical burial' in, for example, ASV Sanità 726 145v (27 June 1528).

[79]   Will of Ventura hebreo, ASV, Sanità 726 162v (6 July 1528).

Some of the wills give details of the particular times and places in which the will was made, such as for Donna Lucia on 6 March 1576 at 8pm in the female hospital in the *lazaretto vecchio*.[80] Others describe how long people had been in the *lazaretti*, such as Donna Justina, a widow from Santa Fosca, who had been taken to the *lazaretto nuovo* on 10 March. Two days later, the Chaplain recorded at the start of her will that he did not have time to gather together other people to witness it but immediately took up pen and paper and began to write. The will is just a few lines long. It ends with a confirmation by Fra Marco that it had been said in an intelligible voice, before noting that he had administered holy oil and recommended her soul to God before she died.[81] In the will of Zuan Maria de Altadona, a Venetian who was in the male hospital at the *lazaretto vecchio*, Fra Marco noted that, at midnight, the guard of the hospital had called him and told him that Zuan Maria wanted to write his will. Because of issues of contagion, it had to be confirmed by a reading at the doorway of the hospital. The testator called out from his sickbed that the details were right so that it could be confirmed by the guard from the Prior's house.[82]

In addition to providing an insight into the process of will-making, the selection can be used to illustrate some of the ways in which testators made charitable bequests in the period. Of the forty-two wills which detail such bequests, eighteen left money for Masses to be said, generally to the Virgin Mary and/or St Gregory but with one mention of St Roch.[83] The prominence of Marian and Gregorian Masses is unsurprising but the mention of St Roch is interesting. Existing histories of plague in Venice often emphasise the city's devotion to the saint in plague times. Crucially, however, the two plague saints were invoked in order to prevent the plague as well as offer consolation to the sick and the hope of cure.[84] Sheila Barker's careful essay on the cult of St Sebastian has emphasised his initial role, in line with that of other martyrs, of preventing disease. Later St Sebastian became associated with healing the sick. His image was used to inspire hope in the possibility of recovery as well as a reminder of the importance of preparing for death but did not tend to be used for intercession after death.[85]

---

[80]   Will of Donna Lucia wife of Battista di Ranzoli from San Pantalon, ASV, Sanità 732 128v–129v (6 March 1576).

[81]   Will of Donna Justina from Santa Fosca, ASV, Sanità 732 142r–143r (12 March 1576).

[82]   Will of Zuan Maria de Altadona, ASV, Sanità 732 101v–103r (29 November 1575).

[83]   For comparative examples see Grazia Benvenuto, *La peste nell'Italia nella prima età moderna*, chapter two, part three, pp. 129–42.

[84]   I am grateful to Professor Carole Rawcliffe for her comments on the roles of these saints in popular piety for the plague.

[85]   Sheila Barker, 'The making of a plague saint: Saint Sebastian's imagery and cult before the Counter-Reformation' in Franco Mormando and Thomas Worcester (eds), *Piety and plague from Byzantium to the Baroque* (Kirksville MI, 2007), pp. 90–132.

These funeral Masses were not always given a location but seven specifically asked for the Masses to be said within the chapels in the *lazaretti* and four asked for these to be said in parish churches. The sample size is too small to enable anything but observations to be drawn from the evidence. The significance of the parish church endured alongside the chapels at the *lazaretti* meaning that local and centralised foci for charity were compatible for contemporaries and that individuals attempted to preserve links with their communities from the public hospitals. The will of Vicenzo from Chioggia, for example, stipulated that money should be given to his parish church in Chioggia for a Mass to be said and that if he, his wife and all heirs were to die in the epidemic, that all of his estate should go to the Cathedral Church of Santa Maria on the island.[86] During the same outbreak, a widow from Malamocco left money for a chapel in a church there.[87] In 1575, Madonna Eufamia from Castello left money to sites in the *sestiere*.[88] There is clear evidence of the locality shaping charitable bequests. In other cases, membership of *scuole* dictated bequests. Zuan Antonio from San Basso left money to the church and *scuola* of Sant'Ambrogio.[89] In 1576, Agustin Bocchaler from San Barnaba left money to the *scuola* of San Michiel (Michele), requesting that he be buried there too.[90] Samuel Cohn has suggested that the concern about mass burial during the Black Death stimulated the desire of testators to specify a place of burial.[91] Only in seven of the surviving wills for the *lazaretti*, however, is place of burial specified: it is far less common that the instruction for intercessory masses in particular churches.

It is not always clear what determined the choice of institutions to which Venetians made pious bequests. Donna Justina from Santa Fosca left money to the convent of Santa Maria Maggiore and the Madonna del Anconetta (which was in San Marcuola) but her choice of sites was not explained.[92] In some cases,

---

[86] Will of Vicenzo from Chioggia, ASV, Sanità 726 154r–156r (2 July 1528).

[87] Will of Archilea a widow from Malamocco, ASV, Sanità 726 179v (21 September 1528).

[88] Will of Madonna Eufamia from Castello, ASV, Sanità 732 57r–59r (9 November 1575).

[89] Will of Zuan Antonio from San Basso, ASV, Sanità 730 113r–115r (11 February 1556).

[90] Will of Agustin Bocchaler from San Barnaba, ASV, Sanità 732 152v–153r (4 June 1576).

[91] Samuel K. Cohn Jr, 'The place of the dead in Flanders and Tuscany: towards a comparative history of the Black Death' in Bruce Gordon and Peter Marshall (eds), *The place of the dead*, pp. 17–43.

[92] Will of Donna Justina from Santa Fosca in ASV, Sanità 732 142r–143r (12 March 1576). On the Madonna del Anconetta see Flaminio Corner, *Notizie storiche delle chiese e monastery di Venezia e di Torcello* (Padua, 1758), p. 260.

ties of family, friendship, work and neighbourhood informed the decisions.[93] At other times, it is clear that bequests were influenced by testators' connections with particular institutions, including the Venetian *lazaretti*. Six testators gave money to the *lazaretti*, whilst other payments were made to individuals who worked there. These could be made in response to treatment which had been received, such as in the case of the doctors and the serving women.[94] It is clear that staff were not supposed to inherit or benefit from wills in order to prevent manipulation or bullying of the vulnerable dying. Bellintani recorded the need to keep an eye on serving women because they tried to convince patients to leave them things in wills.[95] Regulations against asking testators for money were introduced into hospital statutes as well as being the subject of specific Health Office regulation. In 1510, it was stated that neither the Priors nor other employees could be beneficiaries of wills made in the hospitals, nevertheless such payments were recorded.[96] Money was also left for services that had not yet been received – as in the case of the Chaplain who was asked to pray for the individuals.[97]

In addition to the specific sums of money left to the *lazaretti* and their workers, individuals also bequeathed areas of land to the institutions, so that the rent on the land would contribute to the annual, regular income. In 1513, for example, in Padua, five fields were left to the *lazaretto* with the only condition being that the Mass of St Gregory was said annually for the testator.[98] A few years earlier a bequest had been made by a separate testator to the *lazaretto*, this time promising bread each year in which there was plague within the city, to be distributed to the poor who were within the hospital.[99] In 1527, a clock was bequeathed, along with a half barrel of oil and two barrels of Puglian wine, to the Venetian hospital.[100] In addition to direct bequests by individuals, Venetian money was also given through the Procurators of St Mark, as mentioned in the introduction.[101]

Bequests to the *lazaretti* stood alongside sums given to more traditional and commonplace recipients of charitable bequests. Other hospitals and churches were mentioned by testators. Money was given to widows and poor orphans or young

---

[93]   For a discussion of how Venetians chose to make pious bequests in the context of the city's nunneries see Mary Laven, *Virgins of Venice: broken vows and cloistered lives in the Renaissance convent* (Harmondsworth, 2003), pp. 72–3.

[94]   For example ASV, Sanità 726 162r–163v, 727 223r–224v and 730 103r–104r.

[95]   Paolo Bellintani, *Dialogo della peste,* Ermanno Paccagnini (ed.) (Milan, 2001), chapter twenty-five, pp. 136–7.

[96]   ASV, Sanità reg. 1 (15 December 1510).

[97]   For example ASV Sanità 726 177r–178v (15 December 1528) and 189r–v (12 February 1528).

[98]   ASP, Sanità b. 555 (25 August 1513).

[99]   ASP, Sanità b. 555 80r (24 September 1509).

[100]   ASV, Sanità 726 127v (7 December 1527).

[101]   See for example ASV, PSMc b. 362 48r and b. 376. See the Introduction, p. 35.

girls for their dowries; the latter was a particularly popular form of charity amongst testators in the city.[102] The poor, particularly women and children, were thought to be effective intercessors for the rich and powerful in the early modern period since their humility and poverty was seen to bring them closer to God. Dowries for young girls were a popular form of charity.[103] With poor young girls or with orphans, testators could choose to give to known individuals or to institutions. The wills illustrate a variety of bequests. What is clear is that the *lazaretti* feature alongside traditional charitable causes. Although the selection in question is small, the wills underscore the importance and contemporary recognition of the *lazaretti* as charitable institutions, especially, but not only, during times of crisis. This is particularly significant, given the nature of early modern Venetian charitable giving. Brian Pullan has written that a principle of medieval charity had been for giving to begin at home and radiate outwards, touching the parish before the larger, centralised institutions.[104] It is clear that the structures of the *lazaretti* were intended to encourage patients to give locally as well as centrally, participating fully in the city's networks of charitable giving.

In the existing historiography, the temporary nature of a stay in the plague hospitals and, in some places, of the institutions themselves, is often emphasised. The institutions have not been seen to have a purpose beyond epidemics and even during periods of sickness they have been seen to have had a function limited to the containment of the sick. Where there were permanent plague hospitals, however, the institutions need to be characterised differently. In Venice, the hospitals cared for rich and poor alike. Despite the potential indignity of death and burial within the plague hospitals, structures were in place to facilitate the distribution of charity for the good of recipients as well as testators – enabling both to live as good Christians – and to connect individuals with their communities. The hospitals' policies encouraged patients to give charitably in their wills and die a good death, to give practical relief to others and spiritual relief to themselves. Although these hospitals were located outside the city, contemporaries had a clear conception of their pious purpose – so much so that some individuals were willing to trust the institutions (over the many other options in the early modern city) with the intercession for their eternal soul – it is hard to think of a stronger endorsement for understanding the *lazaretti* as sites of charity than that.

---

[102] Brian Pullan, *Rich and poor in Renaissance Venice: the social institutions of a Catholic state, to 1620* (Oxford, 1971), pp. 163–9.

[103] Dennis Romano, 'Aspects of patronage in fifteenth- and sixteenth-century Venice', p. 721.

[104] Brian Pullan, *Rich and poor in Renaissance Venice*, pp. 159–60.

Chapter 6
Returning to the City

Many people did not return from the *lazaretti*. As was seen in the previous chapter, during the worst of the early modern plague epidemics, only about a quarter of the people sent out to the islands in Venice were discharged from quarantine. This final chapter will consider the experiences of those survivors. For finite periods, those infected or suspected of the plague were treated in ways that were common to responses to the social margins. The return to the city of those who survived the disease though brings an important perspective to the study of marginal social groups and cautions against overly rigid discussions of fixed social categories. The emphasis on changing circumstances is also important for a discussion of goods, which were sent for disinfection. Goods were disinfected on the *lazaretto* islands in large quantity and returned to the city as key parts in Venice's trade economy. These ranged from the cheap and ordinary to the valuable and extraordinary and innovative methods were developed to deal with this variety of materials. Using influences from the material turn, the importance of considering goods in context is emphasised. Although disinfection techniques were often organised according to the materials used in goods, contemporaries distinguished, for example, between the goods of the rich and poor because of the different ways in which goods were used. A final perspective on the subjectivity of categories of dangerous, infected, polluted goods is given in a discussion of theft. A number of items were branded as dangerous because they had not finished time in the cleaning processes laid down by the Health Office.

The chapter concludes with a look at what happened when an epidemic ended. Those who were released from the *lazaretti* often returned to the city without their possessions – with a number of people lacking even the clothes on their back. Outside epidemics, the process surrounding a departure from the *lazaretti* was embedded in the structures for trade. Merchants were responsible for paying their guards, collecting any belongings which had been entrusted for safekeeping to the Priors and gathering the correct paperwork to enable their merchandise to be taken into the city. Although quarantine was seen to be irritating in terms of the time and money wasted, it was a relatively straightforward system. This was not the case for the departure from quarantine during epidemics. The sheer number of patients made administration complex – even more so since patients, like the staff members, as seen in previous chapters, were liable to flee from the plague hospitals. Details such as these remind us that isolation was difficult to maintain, despite the best efforts of the authorities, and that issues of illness were affected by spheres beyond the medical, including the economic and social.

Departing from the *Lazaretto*

The Health Office authorities acknowledged their great fear of liberating patients prematurely, given the spread of the disease within the city.[1] In order to leave the *lazaretto*, patients had to be cleared by the *lazaretto* doctor as free of sickness and suspicion and the Health Office also requested that administrators record the number of individuals, their location within the *lazaretto*, their name and surname, their age and condition and place of residence in Venice. For Cividale del Friuli, there is more detail regarding the process of inspection. Patients – including men, women, youth, children, nobles, artisans, poor, rich and peasants – were inspected naked by a Health Office official and the doctor from Venice (Olivieri at the time). Women were seen naked to the waist (*fin alla cordella delle trezze*).[2] Ulcers, where *giandusse* and *carboni* had been, were pointed out by two *pizzigamorti*. Those who had been cured came out one by one. New, clean clothes were prepared and distributed to those in need. The patients were then taken in procession with priests to carry out their second quarantine before returning home.[3]

Charity and piety infused the funding and administration of the *lazaretti* in a number of different contexts. These ideas can also be identified in contemporary accounts of those returning from the hospitals. For Padua, the account by Canobbio describes the return of individuals from the *lazaretto*. Some, he writes, were blackened as though with soot (*cingani*), with ripped clothing. At other times they resembled the people of Israel, wandering in the desert. He describes their processions, expressing a mixture of pain, joy and fear, singing litanies and accompanied by the priests and other ministers of the *lazaretto* who carried a crucifix, images of St Roch and other saints, torches and candles. Canobbio estimates the numbers that returned from the Paduan *lazaretto* in this way at more than 4,000.[4] Although similar processions existed for other early modern institutions, as well as the return from *lazaretti* in other Italian cities such as Florence and Mantua, such practices do not appear to have taken place in Venice.[5]

---

[1]   Cucino 24r–v (2 May 1555).

[2]   *Cordella* refers to *usoliere* (*asoliere*).

[3]   Mario Brozzi, *Peste, fede e sanità in una cronaca cividalese del 1598* (Milan, 1982), p. 40.

[4]   Alessandro Canobbio, *Il successo della peste occorsa in Padova l'anno MDLXXVI* (Padua, 1576), 23v–24r.

[5]   John Henderson, 'Plague, putrefaction and the poor in early modern Florence' (unpublished seminar paper, Institute of Historical Research, 19 January 2006). See Guy Geltner, *The medieval prison*, p. 77 for the ritual release of prisoners and their processions back into society in white garbs. For information on Mantua see the forthcoming dissertation by Marie-Louise Leonard at the University of Glasgow, 'Plague epidemics and public health in Mantua, *c.*1463–1577'. I have not read this dissertation but am grateful to Marie-Louise for sharing with me that these processions took place.

Those individuals who had survived periods of quarantine in the *lazaretti*, particularly those from the *lazaretto vecchio*, were not always allowed to put the period of strain behind them and get on, as far as possible with daily life. Individuals were sent into household quarantine, which was thought to provide additional security to the city. Once released, former patients were often put to work. The assumption underpinning their employment was that they would be safe in service. Benedetti, following his fierce criticism of the Venetian *pizzigamorti*, wrote that many men and women who returned healthy from the *lazaretto vecchio* were put to work within the city treating the sick and disinfecting goods.[6] This was not done out of choice but out of necessity and was not a policy which Benedetti retold with any degree of joy or pride. This was a policy which was adopted during the sixteenth century and which remained in force during the seventeenth century. Thebaldi recorded that women who were cured were used as serving women.[7] In some ways, in the context of a plague epidemic when patterns of work had already been interrupted by quarantine and public health, this could have been an opportunity to make money in a time of severe strain. It is not clear, however, whether or not these individuals were paid or whether this was an obligation placed upon individuals who had their periods of care in the *lazaretti* paid for by the state.

We can only imagine the emotions felt by those who returned to Venice having undergone quarantine. We cannot know how the city and their homes had altered. For some, their families may have been devastated. In the aftermath of the outbreak of 1631, the Venetian Senate was forced to recognise the number of children who had been left orphaned by the plague. These orphans became the responsibility of the *Provveditori sopra gli Ospedali*, who were to send those still nursing to the *Pietà* and distribute others as they saw fit. It was common practice for the children at the *Pietà* to be sent out to foster parents and then returned to the hospitals between the ages of four and seven to be taught skills and given an education.[8]

Many people arrived back from the *lazaretti* without their goods. The Health Office officials noted the problems of people returning, particularly from the *lazaretto nuovo*, whilst their goods were still in quarantine, without the ability to clothe themselves and without bedding. The Health Office had to provide mattresses, sheets and clothing for these individuals as an expression of the piety of the Venetian government to its faithful population.[9] In December 1575, the poor returning from quarantine in the *lazaretto nuovo* were described as utterly

---

[6]   'Et molti cosi' huomini, come donne, ch'erano tornati sani dal Lazzaretto Vecchio s'introducevano, spinti dalla necessità, nelle case à curar gl' appestati, et à sborar robbe infette'. Rocco Benedetti, *Relatione d'alcuni casi occorsi in Venetia al tempo della peste l'anno 1576 et 1577 con le provisioni, rimedii et orationi fatte à Dio benedetto per la sua liberatione* (Bologna, 1630), p. 25.

[7]   BMC, Codice Cicogna 3261.

[8]   See Brian Pullan, 'Orphans and foundlings in early modern Europe', p. 13.

[9]   See ASV, Secreta MMN 95 99r (14 October 1576).

miserable, without anything to cover their bodies. In winter, the situation was thought to be particularly dangerous, running the risk that the sick might die of the cold.[10] Two hundred ducats were given to each *sestiere* for clothing for those returning for the *lazaretti*, which would have supplied approximately one hundred and twenty people in each of the six areas of the city.[11] They were said to be given the clothing out of charity.[12] In the same year, instructions were given to those whose parents or members of their families were at the *lazaretto vecchio* or San Lazaro to make provisions for clothes in which to dress these individuals and also to ensure that there were clean houses to which the individuals could return.[13] Those people still within infected houses in the city were to be provided with similar items before being taken to the *lazaretto nuovo*.[14] The cost of supplying clothes to the poor was significant and, in 1576, it was noted that this was an unreasonable cost for the Health Office to cover. Although it was said to be important that the poor were given clothing with which to return to the city and that the items were to be bought at the best possible price, a number of conditions were introduced regarding payment. Those individuals whose possessions had been burned and who had less than twenty-five ducats worth of credit with the Health Office were to be given the clothes without charge, in a manner appropriate to their poverty. Those who had a credit of twenty-five ducats or more, whether their possessions had been burned or not, were to cover the cost themselves.[15] The scale of the need to supply the healthy with clothes reached such levels that during the outbreak of 1630 other government magistracies were called upon to assist, being asked to provide the Health Office with clothes or the fabric to make clothes.

The distribution of such goods was motivated by piety, concern for public health and civic order. It was thought that the Republic had a duty of care for the sick. This did not develop from a fully-fledged notion of the accountable state. Instead, those in authority were thought to have certain responsibilities placed on them by God. Those who returned to the city without blankets, mattresses and clothes were given these things, paid for by the Republic, because of the importance of comfort in sleeping and adequate clothing. Clothing the needy was one of the acts of mercy considered in Chapters 3 and 5. In addition, the reduction of many inhabitants of

---

[10]   ASV, Secreta MMN 95 116v (16 November 1576).

[11]   This has been calculated using the prices provided by the Health Office for the seven items of clothing referred to in Chapter 3 (overcoats, hats, shoes, socks, shirts, trousers and vests). One of each of these items would have cost in total 209 soldi (10 lire 9 soldi), meaning that 118 sets could have been purchased with the 200 ducats. The prices for the items are given in ASV, Sanità 732 128r (9 April 1576) and the distribution of clothing is discussed in Chapter 2, p. 136.

[12]   ASV, Secreta MMN 95 7r (14 December 1575).

[13]   Ibid. 106v (30 October 1576). For instructions on cleaning houses in Palermo see Ingrassia, p. 243.

[14]   Ibid. 99r (14 October 1576).

[15]   Ibid. 12v (9 April 1576).

the city to a state of utter depravity was one which threatened to affect the health, order and reputation of Venice.

It is important to note that this process of return based upon medical inspection and charitable giving was the intention but not always the rule. It is clear that patients attempted to flee from plague hospitals and some succeeded. In 1555, the Venetian Health Office wrote to the Paduan authorities regarding those who had fled from the *lazaretto* and advised that anyone who was caught should be banished so that others would not follow suit.[16] In previous chapters, it was shown that some individuals arrived at the *lazaretti* surreptitiously and it is clear that others attempted to leave in the same way. Similarly, individuals attempted to hide their possessions from the Health Office authorities and some items were stolen and returned to the city beyond the system of control imposed on the circulation of goods.[17]

Dealing with Goods

Contemporaries such as Benedetti recorded the effect of plague upon the economy of the city, particularly trades associated with dangerous materials; he described the silk and wool merchants, who sustained two-thirds of the city, and who ceased to work during epidemics; commerce between merchants disappeared from squares across Venice.[18] The *lazaretti* played an important part in enabling trade to continue during and beyond periods of plague.[19] It was noted as being essential that adequate provision was made for merchants and their goods, otherwise the valuable income generated by the sale of such goods and the income received from customs' duty (*datii*) would be threatened.[20]

The system which governed movement between the *lazaretto vecchio* and *lazaretto nuovo* was a complex one, which became particularly convoluted during periods of infection. The movement of goods was difficult to track but important because these items were potentially dangerous. Some groups were particularly associated with dangerous goods: Jews were warned by the Health Office officials in the early sixteenth century against the dangers of transporting goods from all over the city because of the enormous risk that posed to public health.[21] This was one of the reasons that the Health Office clamped down on the important

---

[16]   ASV, Sanità reg. 12 174v (3 September 1555).

[17]   For the issue of hiding goods in Palermo see Ingrassia, p. 145.

[18]   Rocco Benedetti, *Relatione d'alcuni casi*, p. 19.

[19]   For recognition of the need to introduce systems to facilitate trade in the fifteenth century for Milan see Ann G. Carmichael, 'Contagion theory and contagion practice in fifteenth-century Milan', *Renaissance quarterly* 44 (1991) p. 227.

[20]   ASV, Sanità reg. 16 13r (10 September 1588) regarding trade coming via Corfu and Zante.

[21]   ASV, Sanità 726 2v (14 April 1516).

second-hand goods trade in Venice during times of plague.[22] In October 1575, for example, the purchase of rags, old cloaks, bed covers and used goods of any sort was forbidden, with the penalty of eighteen months' service on the Venetian galley ships.[23] The connections between the movement of goods and the importation of disease had underpinned the foundation of the *lazaretti*. Throughout the early modern period, the institutions were used to disinfect goods coming into the city through trading networks as well as goods thought to pose a public health risk from the city itself.

In 1540, the Prior at the *lazaretto nuovo* described the island as being more like a customs house than a hospital.[24] The emphasis placed on the disinfection of goods alongside the care of individuals was reflected in the building structures of the hospitals. The construction of the large-scale *tezon grande* (the largest warehouse in the *lazaretto nuovo*) took place in 1561.[25] Not all of the goods were stored in the warehouse. Particular rooms were used for the disinfection and storage of individual items, valuables or those belonging to workers. These rooms were locked and sealed by the Health Office.[26] Despite the increased capacity of the *lazaretti* to deal with the disinfection of merchandise, these structures were often insufficient for the size of the task. During epidemics in Venice, outlying islands were used both for people and for the disinfection of their goods. Outside epidemics, other islands were used solely for goods when a number of trading partners were infected. In 1601, for example, Cyprus, Alexandria, Constantinople and many other countries were said to be infected with plague and it was necessary to use San Clemente as an overflow island.[27] In 1601 the Health Office officials estimated that 50,000 *colli* (bundles of merchandise) were passing through the hands of the Prior at the *lazaretti* every year.[28] At that time the Prior at the *lazaretto*

---

[22]   See Patricia Allerston, 'The market in secondhand clothes and furnishings in Venice c.1500–c.1650' (unpublished PhD. thesis, European University Institute, 1996), chapter five for the impact of plague.

[23]   ASV, Secreta, MMN 95 1v (3 October 1575).

[24]   ASV, Sanità 728 46r–49r (3 January 1540).

[25]   See Chapter 1, pp. 68–9.

[26]   Cucino 90r (18 May 1557).

[27]   ASV, Sanità 737 113r (8 October 1601).

[28]   It is difficult to know the equivalent volume of these bundles or the number of galley ships involved in transporting this cargo. Frederic Lane has illustrated that the weight of a *collo* varied depending on the port of origin. For example, a *collo* from Alexandria weighted approximately 1120 lb whereas one from Beirut weighed approximately 290 lb. Capacities of ships tend to be given in tons. In 1501, Marin Sanudo estimated that the capacity of a galley ship was between 400 and 440 *colli*. This should only be taken as a rough guide, since the statistic for the quantity of merchandise at the *lazaretto* is given a century later. See Frederic C. Lane, *Venice and history: the collected papers of Frederic C. Lane* (Baltimore MD, 1966), p. 13 and p. 368 note 67.

nuovo was in prison and it was said to be virtually impossible to keep track of the quantity of goods coming in and out of the plague hospitals.

At the beginning of the seventeenth century, an auditor was elected for the *lazaretti* with the task of maintaining on a weekly basis (and more often when needed) a book of the names of merchants and the quantity of merchandise being brought into the hospitals.[29] In 1617 when the Republic introduced the *Sopraintendente sopra i lazaretti* one of the principal responsibilities of these magistrates was the supervision of goods moving on and off the islands. They were instructed to keep a book for each *lazaretto* in which the merchandise could be itemised.[30] The merchandise was recorded either as that arriving by sea (from east or west) or over land. The date, quantity and quality of goods, the number and name of any servants, the place of origin and name of the vessel were all recorded. The magistrates were obliged to visit the hospitals every fifteen days at least and to keep track of the men disinfecting the goods.

These records do not survive in the Health Office archive. Instead, there are fragments which refer to particular ships and sometimes describe their cargo. In the supplication and review of his career which Cristoforo de' Bartolis wrote to the Health Office he described some of the most notable cargos which were disinfected in the *lazaretto nuovo* during his time as Prior. He mentioned a ship from Turkey with wool, fleece and hides in 1522. In 1523, a galley from Constantinople arrived with things which were of value and had belonged to Andrea di Priuli, former Ambassador (*Bailo*) in Constantinople and who had died of plague. The galley also carried bundles of silk. From Rome, items belonging to a monsignore, amongst them vestments *alla gardenalescha* from an archbishop in Vicenza, arrived in the city. These goods were described as very beautiful. From Alexandria, sacks of linen, hides of different kinds and sacks of thread were sent.

The disinfection of goods in the *lazaretti* – both from incoming merchants and the contents of homes within the city – was a time consuming, burdensome, complicated and expensive task, which involved three steps: '*sborrar, nettar e profumar*' (air, clean and perfume). Individual disinfectors were allocated to clean particular cargoes. In 1609, the Health Office officials complained that too many individuals were trying to cash in on the disinfection of merchants' goods. The magistrates set down minimum limits of forty bundles of silk, wool and similar items to be disinfected by each worker. If the merchandise was made up of copper, wax, drugs and other substances not thought to pose a serious risk of transporting contagion then the minimum quantity per person was eighty bundles.[31] From the *lazaretti*, the goods would be taken to the customs house following a sufficient period of quarantine.[32]

---

[29] ASV, Sanità 737 114v (5 November 1601).

[30] ASV, Sanità reg. 3 102r (11 September 1617).

[31] ASV, Sanità 738 10v (10 July 1609).

[32] ASV, Sanità 729 20v (3 December 1542).

The process of disinfection was often physical. Bundles were placed in large piles into which workers had to thrust their hands twice every day, in order to remove any pockets of bad air. Fabrics were moved every week during the forty-day quarantine. A similar technique was used for wool, linen, silk and other similar items but it was stressed that these fabrics must be cleaned in an area where, both day and night, there was a prevailing wind.[33] This technique for airing goods remained part of the public health treatment for goods until the end of the seventeenth century and beyond. In 1693, for example, the College of Physicians reported back on methods for the disinfection of wool for forty days, which included the disinfectors thrusting their arms into the bundles. This method of handling and cleansing the goods was to be carried out in the precise form described by the College, on pain of death. The disinfectors were to ensure that they inserted their arms into the fabrics in such a way that their hands met in the middle with the hand of the disinfector working opposite them.[34] There were to be no half measures in carrying out this work, although considering the vast quantity of merchandise and the potential for infection gained through the work a lack of enthusiasm by workers for the technique is understandable. The importance and expense of disinfecting goods was clear and this made the role of the disinfector a vital one during epidemics. Servants, washer women, *pizzigamorti* and disinfectors were all employed in this role. In 1555 it was said that more than a hundred people were tasked with cleaning goods.[35]

There was hierarchy of goods which caused particular concern for the Health Office.[36] Certain items were thought to be more dangerous than others and, therefore, feature more prominently in surviving material, either because the goods arrived in great quantity, were of great worth or because the item was particularly susceptible to carrying infection.[37] At the top of the pestilential pyramid were fabrics and furs. In the account by Jacopo Strazzolini, he wrote that all of the items in a house needed disinfecting, except iron, copper and other metals, wooden items, clay jars and glass because these things were not subject to infection.[38] In 1671 the Venetian Senate reiterated the designated periods of quarantine for particular items – partly for the benefit for those involved in quarantine in Spalato. Medicines, drugs, *cremeti*, grain and other combustibles, which were not subject to infection, were exempted. Spices had, for a long while, been exempted from quarantine. In 1542, for example, the goods arriving on a galley ship from Aleppo were all to be retained at the *lazaretto* except for spices. Animals too were taken to

---

[33]   ASV, Sanità reg. 3 1r (1574) and Sanità 740 75v–76r (18 May 1647).

[34]   ASV, Sanità b. 86 489 (12 January 1693).

[35]   ASV, Sanità 730 260r (December 1559).

[36]   For the disinfection of different materials in Palermo see Ingrassia, pp. 246–51.

[37]   For the specificity of disinfection techniques according to the imports of particular locations see Ingrassia, p. 386.

[38]   Mario Brozzi, *Peste, fede e sanità*, pp. 44–5.

the islands: those with hides were exempted from quarantine but others, whether quadrupeds or winged, were subject to forty days' quarantine.[39]

Disinfection methods were extremely specific, with seemingly endless lists of the different techniques used for varying materials.[40] Elements of the natural environment were utilised, including running water, boiling water, sand and aromatics.[41] For the disinfection of goods in Padua, instructions had been given during the outbreak of 1555 that cloth should be washed in hot water and then thrown into the Brenta and left there for two hours, offering another example of the purifying potential of water.[42] Paintings and books were purged in the open air.[43] Disinfection of goods was also carried out within the city. In 1575, there were seven *chiovere* and four more were added because of the scale of the need. These sites were places for wool to be dried in the sunshine and the same sites were often used to supplement space at the *lazaretti* in times of need, for example for the cleaning of goods from houses where someone had died of the plague.[44] As with their handling of patients, Health Office officials tried to distinguish between categories of goods on the grounds of perceived risk: the least dangerous were allowed to remain in the city whilst the rest were taken to the *lazaretti*. Like the treatments given to individuals, the disinfection of merchandise did not simply involve making use of elements of the natural world – wind, water, land and fire – but also attempted to harness the characteristics of medical preparations. From a document described as 'extremely secret' from 1576 we learn that different processes were used for linen, bed covers, silk and fur. Goods were disinfected in tubs of water and then washed with ashes and the addition of strong vinegar and arsenic crystals, amongst other things.[45]

In 1576, a method of disinfecting goods in water which had been tested in Murano was adopted by the Health Office, which is interesting from the point of view of public health techniques within Venice and the islands. The technique, which was described in a letter sent by the *Sopraprovveditori di Murano*, illustrates the reciprocal assistance and advice which passed between Venice and the larger

---

[39]   ASV, Sanità 743 2v–4r (22 April 1671). For disinfecting animals (including horses) in Palermo see Ingrassia, p. 243.

[40]   For examples of subdivisions see ASVer, Sanità reg. 33 165r (undated) and for methods see ASV, Sanità, reg. 3 1r (1574). For information on disinfection techniques see Patricia Allerston, 'L'abito usato' in Carlo M. Belfanti and Fabio Giusberti, *Storia d'Italia 19: La Moda* (Turin, 2003), p. 578.

[41]   ASV Senato Terra reg. 49 148r (15 January 1576).

[42]   Cucino 55v (16 October 1555).

[43]   Mario Brozzi, *Peste, fede e sanità*, pp. 44–5.

[44]   ASV, Secreta MMN 95 72r (15 August 1576). These were used to dry wool – see Andrea Mozzato, *La Mariegola dell'Arte della Lana di Venezia 1244–1594* (Venice, 2002), p. 744 «tiratoio, speciale telaio dotato di chiodi dove veniva steso il panno per farlo asciugare o tirare (B)». ASV, Sanità 733 13v (15 August 1576).

[45]   ASV, Secreta MMN 55bis ('Secret of Zorzi dalla Valle').

lagoon islands. The Murano technique used salt water to clean goods and the Health Office officials adapted it for use in Venice and stipulated which canals should be used in each *sestiere*.[46] The letter from Murano stressed that no one who had handled the goods after they had been immersed in the flowing salt water had been infected. Items were placed in baskets or containers with a large weave in order to allow the water to access the goods easily. These containers were sealed in order to ensure that no thefts took place – a lead weight was placed on the lid of the container. Once the items had remained in the water for between three and five days, they were washed and then dried. This method was thought to be suitable for all fabrics except for feather mattresses and any sort of hide. In illustrating the effectiveness of the method, the authorities in Murano emphasised that no sign of contagion had been seen since the technique had been adopted and that those individuals whose goods had been disinfected in this way had worn the clothes and handled the items for a period of forty days and more and no sign of infection had been seen. These 'natural' methods were recognised to be safe and, crucially, cheap. The Health Office officials stressed that using these methods was saving a great deal of public money, with reference to a technique which boiled items in salt water and used sand to clean them.[47]

In Chapter 4 medical secrets were considered which were sold to the Health Office for the treatment of individuals during plague. In addition to secret techniques to treat the sick and preserve against the plague, individual remedies were used in the treatment of both goods and houses. The instructions of Marc'Antonio Lancia Quadrio di Valtolina were published regarding the disinfection of houses using fumigation, the cleaning of goods through boiling in water, the use of sand on 'important' goods and finally the use of salt water.[48] His method also incorporated particular aromatics. His technique required men to be paired up. One of the men was termed 'suspected' and would handle goods and administer treatments; the other (termed 'clean') would then take the disinfected goods and ensure they were dried and handled in the appropriate way.[49] It is clear which of these roles would have been preferable. Recipes and secret techniques for the disinfection of goods were offered for sale and readily accepted by the city, although these were fewer in number than those concerned with the cure of individuals. Two examples survive from the outbreak of 1576.

Benedetti wrote about the best known of the disinfectors in Venice during the outbreak of 1575-7. The Grisoni were a company of disinfectors who were appointed to clean goods within the city. Depending on the quantity of merchandise, the process took up to three days. The disinfection made use of a thick smoke, so

---

[46]   ASV, Secreta MMN 95 102 r–v (24 October 1576) and 105r (23 October 1576).

[47]   ASV, Secreta MMN 95 108r (3 November 1576).

[48]   BMC, Donà della rosa, 181 10/22 (9 November 1576).

[49]   ASV, Secreta MMN 95 111v–113r (8 November 1576). It is not clear whether those suspected of the plague were used in this work or whether the terms were used simply to distinguish the roles of these two workers.

dense that it was said if you lit a candle you would not be able to make out things that were just an arm length's away. Benedetti described seeing the Grisoni leaving an infected house looking like the Cyclopes thunder and lightning coming out of the forge of Vulcan (*tanti Tronti e tanti Steropi*).[50] Benedetti noted the Grisoni's miraculous achievements – working in many infected houses and handling infected goods without being affected. Benedetti also recorded the work of Felice Brunello. In place of smoke and air, Brunello made use of running water and was hired to serve the Republic by disinfecting goods in purpose-built fishermen's huts in the *canal di Marani* close to Vignole and Sant'Erasmo.[51] He cleaned the goods in salt water and considered himself expert in the disinfection of silk, linen and wool.[52] In November 1576, he wrote to the Health Office regretful that his technique had brought him considerable praise but no financial reward and left him in a state of poverty.[53] In return for his work in the service of the state, he was granted exclusive right to disinfect goods in huts or similar structures, recognition of successful marketing of his technique to the state. From 1577 he was given the wood necessary for his technique by the State.[54] Both remedies illustrate that in its responses to the plague, the Health Office officials recognised the need to clean goods and homes as well as cure the sick and protect the healthy; as with Olivieri's treatment for individuals considered in Chapter 4, the Health Office published instructions regarding disinfection in line with both the Grisoni and Brunello's methods.

Health Office doctors were asked to provide advice for the disinfection of goods and homes and the treatment of individuals.[55] In 1583, for example, the doctor Alvise Venier assured the Health Office that feathers which were left in freshwater and cleaned for ten days would be free of infection.[56] In 1576 the Venetian College of Physicians was asked to report on two questions – one of which has already been considered.[57] First, the physicians were asked whether or not the quarantine

---

[50] *Sterope* is the name given to lightning and *tuoni* to thunder in Classical mythology, although the former is the Greek name and the latter is Roman – it is not clear why the two have been mixed in Benedetti's reference. In the Wellcome copy, the reference is simply to *tanti seropi* found in Rocco Benedetti, *Relatione d'alcuni casi*, p. 25.

[51] ASV, Secreta MMN 95 109v (11 November 1576).

[52] ASV, Secreta, MMN 95 106v (30 October 1576), 110v (6 November 1576) and 150v (24 September 1577).

[53] ASV, Secreta MMN 95 110v (6 November 1576).

[54] ASV, Consiglio dei Dieci, parti comuni reg. 33 26v (22 May 1577).

[55] See Mario Brozzi, *Plague, fede e sanità*, pp. 80–82 for Olivieri's method for disinfecting goods.

[56] ASV, Sanità reg. 3 44v (31 October 1583). Venier had served the Health Office during the plague of 1575–77. By 1583 he was also physician to the *Derelitti* hospital (from 1576 until his death in 1587) but obviously continued to advise the Health Office on matters related to public health for the plague. For information on Venier see Richard J. Palmer, *The studio of Venice and its graduates in the sixteenth century* (Padua, 1983), p. 124.

[57] See Chapter 4, pp. 179–80.

in the *lazaretto nuovo* for those who had been cured in the *lazaretto vecchio* or San Lazaro was superfluous. Second, they were asked whether or not those who had been cured at the *lazaretto vecchio* and carried out a period of quarantine at the *lazaretto nuovo* with the same clothing that they had brought from their first period of quarantine could return to the city safely with these same clothes. This second issue, acknowledged the physicians, was complicated and less easily answered than the first. The issue at the heart of the problem was whether or not clothing could continue to carry infection after a period of quarantine which was sufficient for the body to be cured. It was said that neither the heat of the human body nor exposure to the air could guarantee that the clothes had been cleansed. The only certain methods were boiling and purifying the fabric.[58]

Given the methods that were employed to disinfect objects, it is hardly surprising that a number of contemporaries complained about their goods being ruined by disinfection. This was true during times of plague and beyond. Leon Modena lamented the loss of goods from the Ghetto on a large scale in his account of the epidemic of 1630–31. He wrote of 'seven hundred and fifty bales worth much money [which] were sent to the Lazzaretto, and almost all of them were destroyed or lost'.[59] Similar observations were recorded in the merchants' supplications regarding the dangerous, damaging, open nature of the hospitals which left goods at the mercy of the elements and of thieves.[60] Even worse for the owners, however, was the shift in Health Office policy towards burning goods as a more expedient option than disinfection, as the quantity of goods increased. Whilst this was effective in dealing with the mountains of goods, the policy produced problems of its own. The owners of the goods had to be compensated for the loss of such objects. In 1557, set prices were determined by the Health Office as compensation for burned goods.[61] A covering letter to a series of inventories from the Prior at the *lazaretto nuovo* survives from 1575. This refers to the contents of the inventories as being, in general, items of low value which would take unjustifiable expense and a long period of time to disinfect and states, therefore, that they were to be burned.[62] Thirty-three individuals are mentioned in the list, although many shared the same houses.[63] In 1577 the Health Office was given 5,304 ducats to compensate the owners of burned beds, bolsters, pillows, mattresses, blankets and furs.[64] All of these items were acknowledged as being difficult to clean and required long

---

[58]   ASV, Secreta MMN 95 109r (3 November 1576).

[59]   Mark R. Cohen, *The autobiography of a seventeenth-century Venetian rabbi: Leon of Modena's Life of Judah* (Princeton NJ, 1988), p. 135.

[60]   See Chapter 2, pp. 96–7 and a selection of supplications dating from the 1590s and copied in ASV, Sanità reg. 16 between 16v and 19r.

[61]   ASV, Sanità 730 153r (18 June 1557).

[62]   ASV, Sanità 732 49r (29 September 1575).

[63]   ASV, Sanità 732 49r (29 September 1575).

[64]   ASV, Senato Terra reg. 41 20r (9 May 1577).

periods of disinfection during earlier outbreaks.[65] These items, along with clothing, were thought to be bad for the stench they gave off because of rotting.[66] The policy of burning goods was incredibly expensive for the Republic.[67] In 1528, policies of burning difficult goods had led to individuals being made creditors of the Health Office.[68] A decade later, however, it was noted that many of these creditors were still owed for these goods by the Health Office.[69] In his account of the epidemic of 1575–77, Benedetti described an extraordinary amount of money being spent by the state for this purpose.[70]

The bureaucracy surrounding the removal of goods from houses, the transportation of items to the *lazaretti*, the disinfection within the warehouses and the subsequent return of items to their owners was extraordinary. In most cases when individuals were transported to the islands their possessions were taken from their homes. Some individuals were granted permission to carry out the disinfection of goods within their own homes, if they were considered to be suitably sized and located. Assessments of the suitability of the home were made by those appointed by the Health Office at parish level, who were instructed to record the number of those who had died or become infected within the house, its capacity and site, the rent paid and whether disinfection within the house would place neighbours at risk. Items could be disinfected on balconies but would only be licensed if this was done for forty days and if those who handled the goods remained healthy.[71] The disinfection of goods in a home was reserved for those with houses considered to be airy and spacious (*commoda et capace*).[72] The removal of goods from properties was done, for the majority, so that the individual items and the house itself could be disinfected. The *pizzigamorti* were commanded to ensure that not even a rag remained in the homes – fabric, of course, was one of the worst culprits in contemporary eyes for spreading disease. Sometimes complaints were made by the Health Office via officials (particularly the doctors) to those carrying out the cleaning. Ludovico Cucino, for example, was given notice of an unsatisfactory clean of a house: benches, desks and similar items had been left, even though a woman had died there. Pieces of clothing including shoes and socks were also left,

---

[65] ASV, Sanità b. 2 15v (12 December 1528) and Senato Terra reg. 40 148v (12 December 1556).

[66] ASV, Sanità 732 116r (18 March 1576).

[67] For examples of payments see ASV, Senato Terra reg. 41 20r (14 May 1557) and for overall costs see ibid., 82v (5 March 1558).

[68] ASV, Sanità b. 2 15v (12 December 1528).

[69] ASV, Sanità 727 321r (24 July 1536).

[70] Rocco Benedetti, *Relatione d'alcuni casi*, p. 18. Financial records revealing government debtors and creditors during plague would be revealing regarding the scale and distribution of spending but these were not found.

[71] ASV, Secreta MMN 95 107v (2 November 1576).

[72] ASV, Senato Terra reg. 51 91v (18 July 1556). For a description of the qualities of spacious houses in Palermo see Ingrassia, p. 360.

posing considerable danger.[73] As was seen in Chapter 2, disinfection of homes was made more difficult by the problem of people hiding their goods in order to preserve and protect these possessions. This was an act which became associated particularly with the poor.[74] Lack of care and attention by Health Office employees and deliberate strategies by inhabitants made the effective clearing of household contents to the plague hospital islands very difficult to achieve.

Once on the islands, the goods were divided into three groups: goods to be burned, goods to be retained for the benefit of the *lazaretti* and goods to be returned to their owners. The goods retained for the hospitals were those belonging to patients who had died and which would prove useful: beds, blankets, bed covers and furs.[75] The goods were then subdivided according to the *sestiere* from which they derived.[76] Each group was inventoried separately. These inventories were used alongside the inventories drawn up when goods were shipped to the *lazaretti*, which recorded in detail clothing and household furnishings. Inventories also accompanied individuals as they were sent to and between the *lazaretti*. At times, inventories were made of an entire *lazaretto*, which must have been a major logistical challenge.[77] The inventories, along with records of people at the *lazaretti* and the wills made on the island, were sent to the Health Office. Just a few slipped through the cracks and still survive. One, from 1691, lists a variety of pieces of clothing along with protective clothing, a sword, a razor, money and tobacco.[78] Others included paintings and metal goods.[79]

Elsewhere, a number of these inventories survive, for example in Padua and Verona. The Veronese archive contains a series of seventy-three inventories of disinfected goods from the outbreak of 1576. This series includes some joint inventories made by married couples or sisters and some multiple entries for the same people, containing different items. The majority of these were made by men – forty-three of the total. Of the thirty made by women, ten are noted to have been widows. The entries vary as to the level of detail and length of entry – some consist of just a few lines and others cover a number of pages. Each of the entries was recorded by *lazaretto* workers. Valuables, particularly jewellery and money, were witnessed by more than one worker and the inventories as a whole were signed off by the Rector (the equivalent of the Prior) of the hospital. The jewellery often included rings and other items made from gold and silver. Rosary beads are listed separately, including those made from amber (*ambro*) and silk (*seda*). These inventories detail household items – including clothing, linen, beds and some

[73]   Cucino 44v (19 July 1555).

[74]   Elisabetta Girardi, 'La peste del 1630–1 nell'altopiano dei Sette Comuni', *Archivio Veneto*, 205 (2008), p. 82.

[75]   ASV, Sanità 730 144r (1 May 1557).

[76]   ASV, Senato Terra reg. 49 148r (15 January 1576).

[77]   Cucino 80r (27 March 1557).

[78]   ASV, Sanità b. 86 354 (recorded on 28 March 1691 for a death on 29 January 1691).

[79]   ASV, Sanità 736 101v–102r (15 December 1592).

basic kitchen equipment. Some of the most common items include aprons, collars, caps, bodices, handkerchiefs and woollen stockings made of a variety of fabrics. Weapons were also included in the lists, often swords or daggers. A surviving example for a *pizzigamorto* includes a high quantity of kitchen items and a large variety of clothing, although there tends to be just a few examples of each item. The quality of the items is difficult to assess because of the lack of detail which only needed to be sufficient to allow identification of the goods. These inventories, as opposed to probate inventories, were practical, working documents designed to record goods which were to be taken for disinfection rather than determining a person's wealth. As a result, descriptions tend only to mention the quantity and make brief reference to the materials from which the items were made.

For Padua, forty-two inventories survive which specifically mention the *lazaretto*. A number describe the process by which goods were taken to the plague hospital. Some goods were placed in chests and tied. Others were simply placed onto carts in bundles with names attached. In general, broken items or those of insignificant value were not noted. The surviving inventories vary: some list sums of money only; others include only bulky items, such as beds, and their accompanying linen; others are much more detailed. In these more detailed examples, clothing, household items and valuables are all itemised, including jewellery and paintings (often of religious subjects, particularly the Virgin Mary). Twenty-six record the owner: the majority were male with seven recorded for women. Some were joint entries and one survives for an institution, the Monastery of Santa Maria dei Servi. Very few of the entries record the occupation of the owner.

Despite the limited nature of the information, it is clear from wills and inventories alike that valuables were taken to the *lazaretti* by individuals. Testators would refer to money being held by the Prior (*in man' del Prior*) when making bequests. The process governing such valuables had been set down in the *capitolari*. In the earliest version, it was noted that when the sick arrived with silver or money in their possession these could only be removed for safe keeping in the presence of the Prior. They were then to be kept in a chest (*chassa*), locked with three different keys and were noted down, with details of amounts and ownership; presumably this was done without a period of disinfection because metals were not thought to be dangerous in the context of plague. In subsequent archival entries, it was noted that the sick were arriving at the *lazaretto vecchio* with silver, jewels and money. The money was only to be removed by the Prior in the presence of the doctor and Chaplain, it was to be carefully noted and, for silver, the identifying marks (*contrasegni*) were to be recorded. In the case of death of the owner, items were sent to the Health Office and then passed onto heirs. In the case of no heir being found, they were sold 'to the benefit of the *lazaretti*'. In 1556, money, gold, silver and jewels were sent from the *lazaretti* to the Health Office either because testators had left them in their wills to the hospitals or because individuals had died without heirs.[80] During the outbreak of 1575, the amount of gold, silver and money sent to

---

[80]   ASV, Sanità 730 74v (29 September 1556).

the Health Office reached such a level that officials began to send it instead to the heads of the *sestieri* for distribution.[81]

In 1560, the Health Office possessed a certain quantity of valuable goods, including silver, rings and rosaries, which had been sent for safe keeping from the *lazaretti* during the recent outbreak. Since these items had not been claimed in the two years since the end of the outbreak, they were to be sold, with the money being given to the Health Office to utilise as they saw fit.[82] The deaths of many of the owners meant that the end of epidemics often saw vast quantities of unclaimed items. In 1578, following the disinfection of the two *lazaretti* there was still said to be 16,880 ducats worth of goods in the *lazaretto nuovo*. The Health Office officials were anxious, having just declared the city to be free from infection, not to allow these goods to be reintroduced into the city, declaring that they ran the risk of reinfection, as had been seen in the past. The items were to be burned and 7,514 ducats worth of compensation was to be given.[83] Dealing with the goods left behind after epidemics was tackled in the interest of public health. In 1642, for example, old goods which had been on the island since 1637 were becoming increasingly rotten. The blankets, loose cloaks (*gabani*) and sacks which could be sold on were and the others were to be burned.[84]

Although the rhetoric surrounding the disinfection and quarantine of goods was one of separation and distance, the Health Office also sold goods from the *lazaretti* in order to raise money in times of particular financial strain. In the aftermath of the outbreak of 1528, for example, officials determined that all of the blankets from the *lazaretti*, which had been cleaned and disinfected and were free of all suspicion, should be sold to the public and the money given to the Health Office.[85] Similarly in 1533, it was noted that there were a large number of creditors to the Health Office with no funds to satisfy them. The number was said to be growing daily. It was determined that the beds at the *lazaretti*, thought to be superfluous owing to the lack of infection within the city, were to be cleaned and disinfected and then sold along with the blankets from the hospitals.[86] The beds were noted to be deteriorating in quality, although they were certified as being clean and free of all suspicion by the Prior. The following year, a similar process took place whereby the beds, blankets, bolsters, covers and mattresses which had been cleaned, and were said by the Priors to be free of suspicion, were sold. These items were valued by Andrea de Jacomo and Bartholamio de Todaro, both brokers in the Ghetto, and were sold to the Jewish buyer Mazo.[87]

---

81 ASV, Secreta MMN 95 125v (18 January 1575).
82 ASV, Sanità 730 292v (2 December 1560).
83 ASV, Senato Terra reg. 41 82v (5 March 1578).
84 ASV, Sanità reg. 3 136r (1 May 1642).
85 ASV, Sanità 727 201r (24 July 1532).
86 ASV, Sanità 727 237v (20 December 1533).
87 ASV, Sanità 727 257r (4 March 1534).

The value of beds (*letti*) as well as those complete with mattress, sheets, pillows and blankets (*letti completi*) was high within early modern society. These items could form part of dowries at the point of marriage and be passed on through wills.[88] Beds often feature on the inventories of goods sent to the *lazaretti* for disinfection. The purpose of the documents – to record the items sent and distinguish materials for the purposes of disinfection – means that the details given are often limited. In surviving inventories from Padua, sometimes the beds are described simply as new, old or used. In a few cases, only mattresses and covers are described. In most instances, however, the beds are described as *un letto di penna* (feather beds) and in one instance it was stated specifically that the bed was new and made of goose feathers (*penna d'occha*).[89] In one inventory, for the monastery of Santa Maria de Servi, the feather beds were described as *letti di piuma*, perhaps to distinguish the quality of the materials, and twelve large and small pillows made of feather and wool were also described. Beds were valued for their role in fighting the cold and did vary in type. The earliest and simplest forms consisted of either a mattress or straw on top of wooden boards or trestles. It was this sort of bed which was constructed in large number during the worst of plague epidemics and which can be seen in paintings showing the sick in the *lazaretti*, such as in Plate 2.[90] In Palermo, Ingrassia determined that the sick should be sent to the *lazaretto* with their goods and clothing but old or torn beds would be burned. He was specific, however, and distinguished between different parts of the bed. Beds were to be sent without the planks, trivet, mattress or accompanying undersheet which could be saved for the sake of the hospital.[91] He recognised the importance of beds within the hospital and how easily the institution could be left short of these essential items.[92]

Sales were also made after the outbreak of 1575–77 of mattresses, blankets and other goods.[93] These items had been used on the *lazaretto vecchio* and then disinfected on San Giacomo di Paludo. They were to be handled and disinfected for eight days before being sold. Similar action was taken in Padua and the money from the sales was given to the *monte di pietà*.[94] These were pragmatic acts designed to recuperate some of the high costs of operating the institutions during outbreaks. In 1644, the hundreds of blankets and mattresses which were still in the *lazaretto nuovo* and which were described by the Health Office notary as 'useless'

---

[88]   On beds as part of dowries see Raffaella Sarti, *Europe at home: family and material culture, 1500–1800* (London, 2002), pp. 45–7.

[89]   ASP, Sanità b. 54. Beds are mentioned in most of the inventories detailing goods sent to the *lazaretto*. For examples of feather beds see 15–19 (7 June 1576) and for the goose feather see 855–6 (15 February 1577). Inventories also survive in Verona, although less detail is provided about the beds, in ASVer, Sanità, Atti dei Registri, reg. 157.

[90]   On different sorts of beds see Raffaella Sarti, *Europe at home*, pp. 119–23.

[91]   Ingrassia, p. 257.

[92]   Ibid., p. 258.

[93]   ASV, Secreta MMN 95 147r (24 September 1577).

[94]   ASP, ACA, Atti del consiglio, b. 18 318r (28 April 1578).

were to be distributed to the hospitals within the city, particularly the *Incurabili* and *Mendicanti* before they deteriorated further. The straw mats, which were said to be 'completely useless', were to be sold. A note in the margin records that 218 items were distributed: 120 to the *Mendicanti* and 98 to the *Incurabili* and many others were burned because they were 'good for nothing'.[95]

A variety of considerations affected the treatment of goods during epidemics. Contemporaries, particularly during epidemics, did not consider all goods of the same 'type' in the same way. Despite this, broad regulations were set down by the Health Office which made clear that particular substances were more prone to the transmission of infection than others – particular the furs and fabrics which were of concern not only in the context of the disinfection of goods but which also affected wider public health policies such as the slaughter of cats and dogs. Despite the detailed regulation and significant investment put into dealing with goods in the *lazaretti*, a number of problems continued to thwart the Health Office's attempts to impose a strict and carefully managed system. Foremost amongst these was the problem of theft.

The Problem of Theft

Goods returned in a variety of ways from the *lazaretti*. Those of merchants went via the customs house. If they were lucky, individuals would have their own returned to them in almost the same condition as when they sent them for disinfection. There were two alternative possibilities for the return of goods to the city: via the sale of objects and theft from the plague hospital. The former method, as just considered, was Health Office directed whereas the latter was of genuine concern to the authorities. In 1517, the Health Office officials described how, on 26 January, several unknown persons had scaled the walls of the *lazaretto vecchio*, broken down the doors and furtively stolen several items from the *lazaretto* and removed them from the islands.[96] Similarly in 1525, the Health Office published details of a crime on the *lazaretto nuovo* in the course of which a door of the *lazaretto* was broken and goods were stolen with the serious threat of infecting the site to which they were taken.[97] The issue of goods being stolen from the plague hospitals was in no way unique to Venice. Giulia Calvi has described hospitals, lazarets and clinics as 'magical theatres in which linens, clothes, blankets and mattresses disappeared'.[98] Thefts of such goods were not only illegal but the stolen goods held the potential to spread infection. In reference to one such theft in Verona in 1576, the Health Office officials stressed that the body clearer who had committed the crime had operated without fear of God, or respect for the

---

[95]   ASV, Sanità 740 22v (7 March 1644).

[96]   ASV, Sanità 726 12r (29 January 1517).

[97]   ASV, Sanità 726 95r (11 March 1525).

[98]   Giulia Calvi, *Histories of a plague year*, p. 197.

Health Office or concern for public health. The Health Office records also include sentences from other cities within Venetian territory.[99] In Brescia in 1631, for example, the Podestà (Venetian governor) recorded that soldiers had robbed all of the infected goods from the *lazaretto* and requested advice regarding the 'rigorous' proclamation that should be issued in response.[100]

The issue of theft was of enormous importance to the Health Office. Thefts were thought to pose a significant danger to the public health of the city.[101] The entire purpose of the *lazaretti* was to remove infected persons and their possessions from the urban environment until they had been safely treated. Thefts cut short the period of disinfection of goods and reintroduced these items back into the city, prematurely in the eyes of the authorities. An indication of the importance of this issue to the Health Office is the mention in 1635 of a reward given for careful and faithful service by Lodovico Capretta who, it was said, had spent a great deal of time compiling information on an important case against thieves from the *lazaretti*. Motivations for theft balanced the perceived threat of infection with the desire for money-making. The theft of coffee, for example, during a period when Venice was not infected by the plague was one thing.[102] The theft of beds on which the infected sick may have slept was quite another.[103]

The responsibility for investigating thefts in the *lazaretti* was in the hands of the hospital Priors. A letter is recorded in the Cucino letterbook addressed to the Prior Hieronimo Mauritio. In 1555, Mauritio was asked to announce that anyone who had stolen goods within the hospital could turn themselves in within two days, naming the nature of the goods which had been stolen and the place in which they had been hidden and these individuals would be absolved of their crime. If the thefts had been undertaken by a gang of thieves, it was said that if one of the thieves denounced the others, that individual would receive a reward as well as being cleared of the crime.[104] This is a strong indication of the danger attached to these thefts in the contemporary mind. In the short term it was felt to be much more important to find these goods and prevent the spread of plague than to punish those responsible. A reward was also promised to anyone who provided correct information regarding the theft of goods, particularly a silk vest which had belonged to the former Prior Jacomo Antonio Mauritio.[105]

---

[99] For example someone banished from Brescia in 1601 is recorded in ASV, Sanità 737 100r (6 April 1601).

[100] *Relazioni dei rettori veneti in terraferma vol. 11: Podestaria e capitanato di Brescia* (Milan, 1978), p. 344.

[101] For Palermo see Ingrassia, p. 355 and pp. 368–9.

[102] ASV, Sanità 758 84r (14 March 1765).

[103] ASV, Sanità 726 6v (30 July 1516). It is difficult to compare the resulting sentences, however, because of the lack of detail surviving in the archive.

[104] Cucino 21r (24 April 1555).

[105] Cucino 21r–v (24 April 1555).

Although it was the responsibility of *lazaretto* staff to investigate thefts, crimes were carried out by a cross section of staff as well as patients. Some crimes were specific to the roles involved. Cases against chaplains, for example, tended to involve fraud in recording wills on the island or similar administrative errors.[106] Crimes by the Priors have already been referred to and often involved allowing goods or individuals to bypass Health Office bureaucracy. Shortly after issuing the above proclamation on behalf of the Health Office, Hieronimo Mauritio was sentenced to a ten-year banishment from Venice and its dominions. He was said to have allowed people into the *lazaretto vecchio* without the permission of the Health Office. Even worse, he had allowed the same people to leave the *lazaretto* and return to Venice, exposing the city to the threat of infection. Hieronimo was said to have acted without respect for his own honour and without fear or reverence for God or for the city of Venice. The sentence stressed that small transgressions by employees of the Republic could cause enormous damage, at great expense for the city, and that, amongst these employees, the Prior of the *lazaretto* was foremost.[107]

In order to retain financial support for the family, Francesco, Hieronimo's brother, was given the position of Prior at the *lazaretto vecchio* in his place. By April of the following year, however, Francesco was accused with a doctor, captain, body clearers and others of having allowed unlicensed goods out of the *lazaretto*.[108] On 10 June 1557, he was banished permanently from Venice to Capo d'Istria. He was fined 600 *lire*, his goods in the *lazaretto* were confiscated and he lost any credit he had with the Health Office.[109] His sentence did not sit quietly. In 1567 he appeared again, this time in the records of the Council of Ten. His banishment was being challenged by a request for a permit for safe conduct (*salvoconducto*). Francesco Mauritio had found himself a powerful patron – Cardinal San Sisto (Hugo Boncampagno), the future Pope Gregory XIII – by becoming a servant (*camariero*) in his household. Francesco's own supplication claimed that he had become Prior at a tender age. He said that he had been falsely accused of allowing goods to be taken from the *lazaretto* and that he had been banished for life to Capo d'Istria. Having served ten years of banishment, he blamed his young age and inexperience of the ways of the world and stressed his personal ruin as a result of being removed from his home.[110] The *salvoconducto* was granted and the following year, Francesco submitted a supplication to the Health Office directly accusing the procurer of supplies for the *lazaretto* (*spenditore*) Gentil di Marchiori, whom Francesco described as his half-brother (*fratel uterino*), of fraudulent activities. Five years after the issuing of the first *salvoconducto*, Francesco reapplied for a

---

[106]   ASV, Sanità 725 113v (1 April 1506) and 730 61r (27 June 1556).

[107]   ASV, Sanità 730 35v (9 November 1555). Hieronimo's sentence was reduced a month later because three witnesses were found to have made false depositions.

[108]   In Cucino 77v (9 March 1557) the Prior is described as being in chains.

[109]   ASV, Consiglio dei Dieci, parti comuni, filza 71 155r (12 January 1557).

[110]   ASV, Consiglio dei Dieci, parti comuni, filza 100 (22 August 1567).

further five year extension.[111] He claimed that, on return to Venice, he had become the head of his household, following the death of his father and his two brothers in the service of the Republic. Again, his application was approved. Then in 1577, Francesco applied for a third time, with the support of the then Pope Gregory XIII and the Ambassador in Rome Antonio Tiepolo but this time for a ten-year extension.[112] No further applications survive for Francesco and the date of his death is unknown. His will is dated 1574, in which he describes himself as sick and confined to bed.[113] This unusually well-documented case of a *lazaretto* Prior illustrates the significance of the role for the Republic, the seriousness with which theft was viewed and confirms the observations made in Chapter 3 regarding the social status of the men who took on the role of Prior during the sixteenth century.

The merchandise in the *lazaretti* was supposed to be meticulously documented by those in charge. In 1608, however, the Health Office officials noted that a number of reports had reached them regarding pieces of merchandise which were going missing in the course of disinfection on the islands. It was felt that those carrying out the disinfection, the *bastazi*, had to be involved. The magistrates reiterated the punishments for thefts and failure to clean goods properly and also stressed the need for a license in order to go to the *lazaretti*.[114] The largest number of cases against Health Office and, more particularly, *lazaretto* workers involve thefts by the *pizzigamorti*, but thefts and misdemeanours were carried out by a variety of *lazaretto* employees.[115] In 1516, the gardener at the *lazaretto nuovo* was accused of stealing beds and bolsters and transporting them back to the city. Later in the century, accusations of theft were aimed at the guards of quarantined ships.[116] Cases often involved one or more workers complicit in a crime or fraud. In 1505, the doctor was accused alongside boatmen and a serving woman. In 1555 two *pizzigamorti* were in league with a serving woman.[117] More often than not, these individuals worked together in order to facilitate the movement of goods out of the *lazaretti*. These thefts are not surprising considering the time period which this study covers. The number of cases is not excessive and they tend to be clustered during outbreaks. What is particularly interesting about the records of these crimes is the method by which they were brought to the attention of the authorities within the Health Office.[118]

---

[111] ASV, Consiglio dei Dieci, parti comuni, filza 115 (29 July 1572).

[112] ASV, Consiglio dei Dieci, parti comuni, filza 130 (13 November 1577).

[113] ASV, Archivi Notarile, Testamenti, b. 12 (Atti Alcherio Antonio) (14 April 1574).

[114] ASV, Sanità 738 1v (1 April 1608).

[115] For a comparative case see Giulia Calvi, *Histories of a plague year: the social and the imaginary in Baroque Florence* (Oxford, 1989), pp. 146–7.

[116] ASV, Sanità 726 6v (5 July 1516) and 729 190v (11 March 1550).

[117] ASV, Sanità 725 108r (7 January 1505) and 730 37v (2 December 1555) and 45r (23 March 1556).

[118] This has been affected by the number of studies which have accessed periods of disease through criminal records. See in particular Alessandro Pastore, *Crimine e giustizia*

That some people would have taken advantage of the opportunities presented by outbreaks to make some extra money in addition to the Health Office salaries is neither new to studies of hospitals nor to a study of institutions. Having noted that these crimes existed and were followed up by the Health Office, the remainder of this section will focus upon the mechanism by which these crimes were reported. Whilst thefts offered an opportunity to supplement a Health Office employees' income, so too did denouncing fellow employees. This was a strategy which brought about many of the cases which have already been mentioned. Amongst the various cases and trials recorded by the Health Office, some include details of the origins of accusations. These were often made by denunciations. This was a method encouraged by the Republic. The 'lion's mouth' letterboxes into which individuals could slip anonymous reports against others were placed throughout the city, with each *sestiere* having multiple sites, often designated for accusations of particular crimes, such as those against health [Plate 28]. The *Palazzo Ducale* also contained a large number of these denunciation boxes, the majority of which have since been destroyed. Of the denunciations which survive in Health Office records, some describe individuals removing goods from quarantined houses or lodging beggars illegally.[119] A number of these include specific mention of Health Office employees, often those employed to work in the *lazaretti*, as perpetrators or accusers or both.

The rewards for correct denunciations were published by the Health Office at Rialto. In 1600, for example, the potential benefits of successfully bringing to light the perpetrators of the attempted theft of 15 March 1599, when the thieves were frightened off by the discovery of the guards, and the successful theft of 10 May, when a bundle (*fagotto*) was stolen from outside the *lazaretto vecchio*, were advertised.[120] Boatmen, disinfectors, chaplains, body clearers, doctors and others were all denounced during the outbreak of 1555–58. Their crimes and subsequent punishments varied. In 1557, a disinfector was found guilty of sending a chest back to his own home in San Nicolò which was perceived to have reinfected his house with plague. He was sentenced to serve on the Venetian galley ships for eight years. Other workers received similar sentences, either confined for life or for a specified period on the galley ships or within a prison. Others were fined.[121] These denunciations were sometimes drawn to the attention of the Council of Ten, an indication of the serious nature of the crime. In 1576, for example, several principal workers at the *lazaretto* were accused of smuggling covered baskets of goods from the hospitals into the city.[122] On the *polizza* from 14 June, it was noted

---

in tempo di peste dell'Europa Moderna (Rome, 1991) and Giulia Calvi, *Histories of a plague year*.

[119]   ASV, Consiglio dei Dieci, parti comuni, filza 69 67r (19 October 1556) and ASV, Sanità 730 2v (3 January 1554).

[120]   ASV, Sanità, reg. 3 74r (14 June 1600).

[121]   ASV, Consiglio dei Dieci, parti comuni, filza 71 155r (12 January 1557).

[122]   ASV, Consiglio dei Dieci, parti comuni, reg. 33 12v (10 April 1577).

that a doctor, a barber surgeon and three body clearers had been found guilty of selling cloth from the hospital within the city and had been hanged.

Of particular interest here is the role of Health Office officials in making accusations against fellow workers. Of nine surviving cases against *lazaretto* workers during the outbreak of 1555–58 and one from 1577, eight were brought following accusations by Health Office employees. Zuan Jacomo de Zuane, a *fante* of the Health Office made five accusations and the Prior at the *lazaretto nuovo* Zorzi Nassin made three. Zuan Jacomo's supplications refer to further denunciations the details of which have not survived.[123] He accused both a female worker and one of the disinfectors of the *lazaretti* who returned home after a period of work on the *lazaretto* with goods without a licence. His next target was the chaplain to the *lazaretto nuovo* who was accused of stealing three chests of disinfected goods and sending them back to a woman's house in San Moise in Venice. The chaplain was banished *in absentia* and was implicated alongside two body clearers. The following year he accused the scribe at the *lazaretto nuovo* and one body clearer of illicitly opening compartments within the warehouses.[124] As *fante*, Zuan Jacomo was well-placed to operate as the eyes and ears of the Health Office, moving throughout the city and between the city and the *lazaretti*. For him, contact with the *lazaretti* and the workers proved to be profitable.

It was not simply the *fante* who was in a position to make such denunciations. As Prior, Zorzi Nassin made three denunciations during the outbreak of 1555–58. The first, in 1555 was made against the doctor to the *lazaretti* along with three body-clearers.[125] The second two were higher profile. The first, recorded in January 1557, was against Francesco Mauritio, along with the chaplain and scribe at the *lazaretto vecchio* in conjunction with nine other workers in 1557.[126] Finally in 1558, he denounced Piero Rega the doctor to the *lazaretti*.[127] In his denunciations, Zorzi Nassin was fulfilling the role of the Prior as the representative of the Health Office. Denunciations were made against workers of differing status within the *lazaretti*. Such cases were actively encouraged by the Health Office. Whilst these two men were not the only Health Office officials to make denunciations, they feature most prominently in the records. In their denunciations they may have been motivated, as their supplications express, by a loyalty to the Republic and a piety for God. Other factors may also have played a part.

Within Health Office cases and the Venetian judicial system more generally it was fairly standard practice for fines to be issued and for a proportion of the money to be given to the accuser of the crime. Such a policy was also in place for the denunciations against the crimes mentioned above. Sums of 500 *lire* and more

---

[123] ASV, Consiglio dei Dieci, parti comuni, filza 71 95r (29 December 1557).

[124] ASV, Consiglio dei Dieci, parti comuni, filza 72 52r (24 March 1558).

[125] ASV, Sanità 730 38r (2 December 1555).

[126] ASV, Sanità 730 188v–189r (19 January 1557) and ASV, Consiglio dei Dieci, parti comuni, filza 71 155r (28 January 1557).

[127] ASV, Consiglio dei Dieci, parti comuni, filza 74 94r (11 January 1558).

were offered to both men in return for their information. In both cases, however, the men rejected the money offered in favour of a different compensation. These cases had been reported in association with the Council of Ten and the preferred payment of both men was to seek absolution for banishments issued by the Council of Ten. Zuan Jacomo chose to release Silvestro di Agassi who had been banned for a year from the city for murder (*homicidio puro*). Later the same year, Zuan Jacomo was offered 2,000 *lire* for the denunciation of the Chaplain of the *lazaretto nuovo*, scribe and body clearers or was offered the opportunity to clear a sentence which had less than three years remaining, as long as the banishment had not been sentenced for sedition, sodomy, homicide or counterfeit fraud (*monetarie*). For Zorzi Nassin's bumper denunciation of twelve individuals, his cut would have been 4,500 *lire* but instead he chose to release one guilty individual. Such a method of payment was obviously familiar to early modern Venetians. In one supplication of 1556 it was expressly requested in the original denunciation letter.[128] The process by which this took place is not clear but it operated as an incentive for denunciations. Although the Health Office employees who made the denunciations did not receive financial compensation, they certainly benefitted from the nature of their roles.

The location of the *lazaretti* and the significant quantity and sometimes quality of the goods sent for disinfection meant that the temptations for theft affected patients and staff alike. The Health Office and wider government of the Republic attempted to increase the benefits of denunciations to encourage fellow staff members to monitor and report on one another's behaviour, with some degree of success. The central role of goods in perceptions of disease transmission made this area of the *lazaretti* structures vital to the maintenance of health and prevention of epidemics, as well as the cure of the city when plague hit.

The End of the Epidemic

Contemporaries felt that a number of different factors contributed to bringing about the end of an epidemic – including both divine grace and the physical cleanliness of the city. In describing one of the religious services at St Mark's during the plague, Benedetti recorded the pleas that were made to God, citing two Bible stories. The first was the rescue of the people of God from slavery in Egypt, through the Red Sea, which submerged the powerful enemy. The second was the famine in the desert, when manna fell from the sky and when thirst was quenched by the flowing of fresh water from the stone. The place of water in each of these stories is significant, as a source of protection and provision, echoing the discussions of the Venetian lagoon with which this book opened. The Venetians were, Benedetti recorded, firm in their faith that God would not abandon the city

---

[128]   ASV, Consiglio dei Dieci, parti comuni, filza 69 69r (19 October 1556).

to the plague but, once sins had been accounted for, that the disease would cease as a result of changes in the environment.[129]

Declaring an end to an epidemic was not entirely straightforward: the levels of infection which determined the end of an epidemic were, like those which determined the start, qualitative. When, for example, in December 1556 there were said to be only 54 people left in the *lazaretto vecchio* and two-thirds of these were out of danger, the proposal was put to the Senate that the Health Office doctor Cucino, who had been overseeing activities in the *lazaretto vecchio* should be allowed to move to the *lazaretto nuovo* to tackle the vast quantity of goods requiring disinfection. The Senate, however, was obviously not as comforted by the number of sick in the hospital as the Health Office had been and the proposal was rejected.[130] By 1558 the city was described as 'entirely healthy' and both *lazaretti* were said to have been cleaned. The only traces of the epidemic which remained were the large quantity of goods in the *lazaretto nuovo*. In spite of the expense associated with reimbursing the owners of these items, the Health Office officials had no intention of letting these items return to the city. Too many people had died, too many families ruined and too much public money spent in the course of the plague to run the risk of reinfecting the city.[131] This statement obviously rang true for those in charge of making such decisions since it was directly quoted again in February 1575 when, in the course of the new epidemic, vast quantities of goods had again been accumulated in the *lazaretto vecchio*, *lazaretto nuovo* and San Giacomo di Paludo. Motivated by issues of cost and the risk of theft, the Senate had them burned.[132]

Once the epidemic was declared to be over, a number of processes were put into place, including some relating to the *lazaretti*.[133] Cleaning the hospitals included tackling the buildings as well as the items within the structures and the people who had run them. Ordinary disinfection processes were used on walls of buildings and on goods still in quarantine. For staff, during the fifteenth century, a period of two months outside Venice was thought to be necessary for disinfection after their service was finished.[134] Staff were sent into quarantine at various points during epidemics – particularly when it seemed that the worst of the epidemic was over. Unfortunately sometimes these decisions were made prematurely.[135] Individuals were also sent into quarantine mid-way through epidemics when they

[129]   Rocco Benedetti, *Relatione d'alcuni casi occorsi*, pp. 25–6.

[130]   ASV, Senato Terra reg. 40 149r (12 December 1556).

[131]   ASV, Senato Terra reg. 41 82v (5 March 1558).

[132]   ASV, Senato Terra reg. 51 45r (24 February 1575).

[133]   For a description of the process at the end of the epidemic of 1575–77 in Palermo see Ingrassia, pp. 391–5.

[134]   ASV, Sanità 725 132r–134r [26] (26 April 1486).

[135]   Cucino 43v (17 July 1555).

were no longer needed by the Health Office.[136] For most, however, quarantine was necessary when the end of an epidemic was declared.[137]

At the end of epidemics the impact of plague was visible not only in the depleted population, the friends and relatives who had died and the shops which were left empty but also in the damage caused to the physical fabric of the city. In 1577, for example, a small house in San Fantin which had been inhabited by the *pizzigamorti* during the outbreak was said to be ruined and stripped of many things.[138] The owner of this house was the nobleman Marco Bragadin, who left a record of the outbreak of 1575–77. Bragadin expressed his less than happy reaction to the state of the eight or so houses in San Fantin which were used by the Health Office for approximately ten months during the epidemic. *Pizzigamorti* and cleaners stayed in the houses as did those carrying out periods of quarantine. Goods had also been disinfected within the homes.[139] Buildings on the lagoon islands which had been used by the Health Office were also damaged. San Lazaro and San Clemente, for example, were said to have damaged floors, broken windows and were in need of general cleaning and repair.[140] San Giacomo di Paludo and other islands, including San Secondo, were said to have sustained significant damage to the gardens as well as in a number of other areas.[141] Even the building occupied by the Health Office at *terranova* was affected. In 1577, the Health Office notary recorded that the Procurators wished to return to that building but that some of the furnishings had been stolen and others had been taken to the *lazaretti* and burned during the epidemic, because of the sickness of some of the serving men and women. New pieces were commissioned and purchased in anticipation of the return to normal.[142] These physical effects would endure long beyond the official end of the epidemic, as would the economic effects on individuals and the state.[143]

As the cleaning and repair work began to hospitals, to outlying islands and their buildings and to homes in the aftermath of an epidemic, the traces of the plague were slowly cleansed from the fabric of the city. Two epidemics were sufficiently severe, however, for the Venetian Republic to feel that the effects should not be erased without a trace. The end of the plague was declared, after the outbreak of 1575–77, on the day of the Incarnation, which, by a happy coincidence, was also the date on which Venice was said to have been founded. In the years following

---

[136] Cucino 92r (28 May 1557).

[137] The quarantine of the Prioress, for example, is referred to in Cucino 99v (7 September 1557).

[138] ASV, Secreta MMN 95 134v (30 March 1577).

[139] BMC, MSS Dandolo Pr. Div. C. 941: carte di Ca Dandolo et suoi autori dal 1575 settembre al 1580, 106: 1577 ricordata Marco Bragadin (26 July 1577).

[140] ASV, Secreta MMN 95 140v and 141r (23 and 30 June 1577).

[141] ASV, Secreta MMN 95 148v (24 September 1577).

[142] ASV, Sanità 733 190r (14 August 1577).

[143] For a case of a widow petitioning for some release on her rent on Cavanella because of the effects of the plague see SEA b.78 78r (6 March 1581).

the outbreaks of 1575–77 and 1630–31, two votive churches were completed. The vow to build the church of the Redentore was taken by the Venetian Senate in 1576, the building work started in 1577, after the end of the epidemic, and the church was completed by 1593. It was designed by the architect Andrea Palladio [1508–80]. Santa Maria della Salute was also commissioned by a vow on behalf of the Venetian Senate, this time in 1630, and was started in 1631, at the end of the epidemic, by the architect Baldassare Longhena [1596/97–1682].

The churches were both prominent within the city: deliberately so since they would become important parts of the ritual geography of Venice, which remain sites of annual processions to this day [Plates 29 and 30]. On the third Sunday in July, for the Redentore, the doge visited the church of the Redentore in the morning before witnessing a grand procession in *Piazza San Marco*, involving members of religious and lay communities. These individuals would then process across a temporary bridge of boats to the Redentore itself.[144] Whereas the *lazaretti* were put to military use and eventually abandoned altogether, the churches of the Redentore and Santa Maria della Salute were adorned and adored.[145] The changing nature of the *lazaretti* was reflected in imagery produced of the islands. The sketch by Giacomo Guardi illustrates the later form of the hospitals [Plate 31] and emphasises the prosaic and accessible form of the islands during the eighteenth century, with the islands surrounded by boats and individuals. The *lazaretti* in Venice never became ceremonial sites as they did elsewhere and lacked a sense of ritual or grandeur. Instead it was the two votive churches that represented all that the Republic wanted to commemorate about the public responses to plague: the generosity, the piety and the end.

---

[144] For the Redentore celebrations see Edward Muir, *Civic ritual in Renaissance Venice* (Princeton NJ, 1981) p. 216.

[145] A Redentore church was also built in 1599 in Cividale del Friuli and completed in 1605. The main altar there shows the Redentore and Sts Roch and Sebastian, painted by Palma il Giovane.

Conclusion

Dealing with disease in early modern Venice involved addressing a broad range of social and medical issues and ideas: from the relationship between space and society to the interconnectedness of charity and cure. It also required rulers to hold in careful balance the protection of the city's trade economy, its reputation and the health of its populace. Public health for the plague drew upon and in turn influenced responses to other social and medical ills. These relationships of response can only be identified if early modern illness is considered from a contemporary perspective. Quarantine too can only be understood fully when it is viewed in context. Early modern isolation lacked the severity of its modern counterpart: it was believed that infectious disease could not be stopped through either social or religious separation. Instead, the ties of community and charity played vital roles in public health for the plague.

The connections between the Venetian *lazaretti* and the city took a number of forms. These ranged from the imagery applied to the hospitals in literary accounts of plague to the visits of the friends and family of patients to the sites. The purpose of these connections also varied. The ways in which the *lazaretti* were linked with other institutions in early modern Venice, through imagery, architecture and purpose, reveals more about the civic importance of the sites. The increased ability and desire of the government to regulate health and morality in early modern Venice sparked the establishment of charitable and welfare institutions in the context of the Renaissance and Catholic Reformation. From their foundation in the fifteenth century, the *lazaretti* became more closely interwoven with wider social, religious and physical forms of purification. The *lazaretti* were founded at the beginning of an intensive period of social and spatial shaping in early modern cities and developed alongside other key institutions. In their location and use of space, these latter institutions were influenced by the early public health measures in response to plague. In their administration and potential for reputation-building, these institutions influenced the *lazaretti*, as the plague hospitals developed a broader purpose in the course of the sixteenth and early seventeenth centuries.

During the fifteenth century, epidemics affected European cities on a smaller scale than they would in the following centuries. As a result, patient numbers were more easily accommodated and the hospitals' reputation for providing a reasonable quality of care was easier to maintain. Initially, it was not compulsory but voluntary for patients to go to the hospitals and so later vignettes of the sick being dragged from their homes were not yet upmost in people's minds. The purpose of the hospitals was also simpler: the protection of the city and the cure of the disease.

During the sixteenth and early seventeenth centuries, the new scale on which plague was experienced intensified the problems of providing care as well as its significance. Earlier Renaissance ideas regarding the significance of ordered cityscapes were supplemented by Catholic Reformation priorities, as the hospitals became part of an attempt at a system of defensive and protective architecture. By the seventeenth century, however, the idealistic attempts at all-embracing systems of social policy had ebbed away. Increasingly, the symbolic importance of the institution as a focus for religious purification declined and the medical and economic significance of the sites again became the primary purpose underpinning investment.

Personal connections between the island hospitals and the city included the movement of both visitors and staff. The presence of both groups at the *lazaretti* was intended to bring comfort to the patients and to minimise dark, dangerous emotions. The staff were also considered to be essential for monitoring the behaviour of patients and other colleagues; employees of the Health Office were tasked with reporting any misdemeanors. Bad behaviour threatened not only the reputation of the sites but also, particularly in the context of theft or sinful (often sexual) misconduct, the prolonging of outbreaks of plague. The Health Office, therefore, established structures which were intended to ease the widely recognised strain of plague epidemics for both individual patients and wider society.

The retention of family and friendship networks can also be seen in the sphere of charity. The ties which connected the *lazaretti* with the religious and charitable structures of the city were just as significant as the personal links. These ties ensured that the plague hospitals played the fullest possible role for the city, allowing plague, its victims and its institutions to be symbolically prominent whilst being physically separated. Charity enabled contact of the most positive and significant kind during epidemics. Such contact also played an important part in supporting the *lazaretti* financially, given the high cost of administering these institutions on a permanent basis.

The wealth, ambition and administrative ability of the Venetian Republic were critical factors which enabled the creation of *lazaretti* in the early fifteenth century. The scale of achievement in establishing and maintaining these institutions for centuries was immense. Systems within the hospitals, necessarily, evolved as contemporaries deepened their experiences of the disease and understood public health in new and varied ways. Nevertheless, the significance of the *lazaretti* as support structures for the Venetian trade economy endured. The Venetian authorities continued to consider trade as one of the most important (and potentially dangerous) elements of the economy, the avenues of which could open up the city to the wealth as well as problems of the wider world. The defences against the importation of dangerous substances, people and ideas were dealt with differently across Europe and the particular targets for attack changed over time. Nevertheless, regardless of time and place, *lazaretti* structures were important weapons in the arsenal of cities in the sphere of public health and were particularly powerful in places such as Venice, where the Republic's structures were capable of asserting significant acts of authority.

The *lazaretti* in Venice had distinctive features, shaped in response to the particular context of the city and its environment. Some of these distinctive features were practical measures necessary to deal with the problem of plague in a lagoon location (boatmen in place of cartmen, for example). More substantially, though, the Venetian hospitals were directed by the State rather than the Church; this does not downplay the significance of religious ideas within the structures but did affect the nature of the individuals serving and administering the sites. Notably, the Venetian institutions did not see the involvement of the religious orders in the way that most hospitals in Catholic Europe did elsewhere. Venetian effects to project a powerful, pious Republic beyond the subordination of Rome are well known. The state direction of a charitable and religious institution here is in keeping with the Venetian authorities' broader relationship with that of the Catholic Church and meant that the *lazaretti* were portrayed as sites shaped by religion rather than the Church.

The Venetian *lazaretti* were some of the earliest to be developed and were also distinctive in their location and architectural design. The original aim of the *lazaretti*, to provide a measure of protection for the Venetian trade economy, meant that the institutions were developed on available island sites; the locations chosen also reflected contemporary awareness of the significance of placing sites for the sick a distance from the main urban centre and the utility of using religious structures as hospitals. The location and administration of the hospitals is, however, also revealing regarding the city's relationship with the lagoon in Venice. It was not unusual for the city's authorities to make use of island sites, within or surrounding the city, for essential but potentially dangerous people – from the nuns whose sexual behaviour could threaten the morality of the city to the sick whose bodies posed a threat to its health. Island sites were well-placed to offer the access and security necessary for both care and control. The relationship between Venice and the communities on outlying islands continued to be one of close contact when that was considered, by either party, to be useful or necessary.

The early introduction of *lazaretti* in Venice is one of the reasons for the strong contrasts in architectural design between the Venetian hospitals and those developed elsewhere. In the latter institutions, the significant use of space in public health sometimes prompted the creation of purpose-built sites, the design of which reflected the function of the institutions far more effectively than it did in Venice. In these purpose-built sites, the ideas which would dominate the administration of the hospitals can be seen clearly: the need for observation and control of patients, which determined the ordered architecture, and the priority of providing medical and spiritual care, which required central wards and prominent chapel buildings. The nature of the architecture was as important as the location for ensuring a high quality, clean environment for patients, which would mean that patients could live as good Christians.

During the early modern history of the hospitals, attempts to ensure the high moral standards and behaviour of patients were not simply architectural. The original idea of administering the *lazaretti* using a Prior and Prioress, often a married couple, in line with other charitable and social institutions on the Italian peninsula and beyond, was affected by developing ideas about gender roles, authority and the patriarchal family. By the end of the sixteenth century, the role of Prioress had been altered significantly and the role of women in the administration of the hospitals had largely ceased. Gender continued to play a significant role in the treatment of patients, as men and women were separated in hospitals for the sick, and there is evidence too that the hospitals were gendered spaces, with a greater proportion of men being sent than women. Changing ideas about gender impacted on the administration of the hospitals, therefore, in relation to the experience of both staff and patients.

Just as both genders were treated in the hospitals but men may have been sent in higher numbers, so too were individuals sent from across the social spectrum, with the largest number being from the poor. The reasons for the predominance of the poor should not be overstated. Initially the reasons for sending higher numbers of the poor than the rich were pragmatic: the latter, for example, had homes within which they could be cared for, freeing up space in the city's institutions. Only during the seventeenth century did attitudes towards the poor solidify and a clear mould for the vilified poor, responsible for the outbreak or spread of the disease, was created. This change in attitude is easier to see beyond Venice, for example in Genoa, because the former city remained largely free of plague after 1631 but it is nevertheless visible in the emphasis on the lifestyle rather than the nature of the poor as a potential source of problems in earlier epidemics.

For rich and poor and men and women, one of the common features of experiences of quarantine was the significance attached to the treatment of the person, their goods and their homes. People and their environments (domestic, urban and natural) had to be addressed by public health measures. For merchants, this involved the disinfection of cargo and ships. For those living within the city of Venice, interventions were more extensive. The treatment of goods was not dealt with in a uniform manner – different materials were distinguished between, as were the way in which goods had been used and their recent histories (for example whether they had been stolen or disinfected). Plague hospital care, therefore, stretched far beyond the bodies of patients.

Public institutions are a product of the society in which they are created. The historiography of hospitals, over the past two decades, has illustrated that a study of such institutions cannot stop at the boundaries of the sites. Instead, hospitals provide a starting point or a window onto the history of a city and a society. In the case of the *lazaretti*, it is only when we recognise the complex, rich and interwoven discussions of an illness which was firmly rooted in the nature of the everyday that we can illuminate the ambitious hospital structures of the *lazaretti* and the genuine attempts made to clean up the physical, social and religious nature of patients and their wider cities. The plague sick and their institutions were not conceptualised as being permanently on the outskirts of society or the city. Instead, understandings of the place of these people and their spaces were richer and more varied. Perceptions of marginality of the plague sick were undermined not only by the temporary and cyclical nature of the plague but also by the role of charity within early modern healthcare systems.

In the second half of the seventeenth century and into the eighteenth century, the geographical spread of plague hospitals widened. A number of features which mark out the early modern Venetian *lazaretti* – the symbolic as well as practical use of space, the combination of charity and cure, the tempering of the influence of ecclesiastical ideas with the prioritisation of religious ones and the specific responses to perceptions of poverty – became less significant as *lazaretti* were subsumed into continent-wide and eventually global systems of public health. The simply defined idea, and complexly pursued policy, of public health for the city became a thing of the past.

Epilogue

Many of the ideas which have been explored in this study endured beyond 1650 and shaped public health structures beyond Venice.[1] In 1675, for example, the Venetian Health Officers recorded in archival material that they faced a problem. A commodity was being imported into the city on a large scale, but magistrates were uncertain of the risks it posed to the city's public health. An immediate investigation was ordered from Venice's College of Physicians.[2] The tricky merchandise in question was tobacco – which was being brought into city in bulk and also being carried by passengers arriving at the city's *lazaretti*. Although leaf and powdered tobacco were celebrated by contemporaries as preservatives against disease, particularly the plague, Venice's doctors determined that the merchandise required a period of quarantine. Tobacco and coffee were just two of the goods which were brought to the *lazaretti* of the seventeenth and eighteenth centuries and which required new responses from the Health Office and the structures for trade. The problem of tobacco endured, even forcing a smoking ban in parts of the islands that contained flammable materials by 1732, after a fire in the *lazaretto vecchio*.[3] There was significant variety in the commodities and foodstuffs brought into the city during the eighteenth century: from barrels of lemons in water to bovine animals.[4] Fabrics were of enduring concern and disinfection of wool continued to be a priority. In 1643, the demand for this service was so high that fifty disinfectors were said to be required.[5] New fabrics were also introduced: tiger pellets are recorded as having been left in the *lazaretto vecchio* in 1696; the Health Office officials were struggling to find the owners, after the pellets had been left by someone in quarantine two years previously.[6]

By 1675 in Venice, the two *lazaretti* had been adapted in line with new circumstances. Following the outbreak of 1630–31, the city remained free of plague epidemics and was virtually untouched by the outbreak of 1656–57 which caused very high levels of mortality in cities such as Genoa and Naples. As a result

---

[1] The best study to date of quarantine facilities after 1650 focuses on Britain, Malta and Marseilles and is John Booker, *Maritime quarantine: the British experience c.1650– 1900* (Aldershot, 2007).

[2] This is addressed in ASV, Sanità b. 86 331 (26 September 1690) and includes a copy of the report from the College of Physicians dated to 1675.

[3] ASV, Sanità 751 183r (13 December 1732).

[4] See, for example, ASV, Sanità b. 203 (letter dated 16 September 1720 'barille con li limoni in acqua') and references in ASV, Sanità 756 [1756–60].

[5] ASV, Sanità 740 10r (30 April 1643).

[6] ASV, Sanità 745 49r (9 April 1696).

of this change in the medical history of Venice, the hospitals lost the first of their two primary functions: to care for the inhabitants of the city when Venice was infected; nevertheless, the second purpose remained of paramount importance. The protection of the trade economy and the quarantining of incoming ships endured and was thought to be an important factor in ensuring that Venice remained free from infection. During the seventeenth century, a traveller from Baghdad to Europe wrote that he and his companions were put into a 'house of purification' for 41 days 'as is the custom. This *nazarīt* is outside of the city, and this is usual in Christian countries (*bilād al-Naṣārī*), because of their fear of the plague.' At the end of the quarantine period, the travellers were inspected by a doctor before being allowed into the city.[7] The administration of the hospitals was altered in line with the more limited function. Rather than keeping the *lazaretto vecchio* for the plague sick and the *lazaretto nuovo* for those suspected of infection, an instruction was issued in 1642 that incoming boats would be diverted alternately to each of the two islands; in essence, the islands became interchangeable.[8]

The surviving records of the city's *lazaretti* illustrate that these hospitals continued to play a vital role in protecting the city during the later part of the early modern period. These trusted structures received investment from the state and gifts from individuals. The chapels received bequests and were seen as charitable sites. In 1735, for example, a silver oil lamp was given for the main altar of the *lazaretto*, dedicated to the Virgin.[9] The make up of the patient base did, however, change. Quarantine was provided predominantly to travellers, merchants and foreigners.[10] In 1655, for example, the opera singer Anna Renzi underwent a period of quarantine in the Veronese *lazaretto*, as did a variety of other musicians.[11] Patients received their food from the sutlers (*vivandieri*), who were paid directly, using money which was left in salt water to disinfect it. For the early nineteenth century there are lists of the foodstuffs which were offered to passengers and the prices laid down by the Health Office for each. The diet was certainly more varied than in previous centuries with nearly fifty foodstuffs available, including a selection of meats and a variety of fish.[12] Although the concerns regarding foodstuffs and infection seem to have abated, instructions continued to be issued

---

[7]   I am very grateful to John-Paul Ghobrial for providing me with this description in translation of the Arabic account of a traveller named Elias who travelled from Baghdad to Europe in 1668.

[8]   ASV, Sanità 740 5v (24 July 1642).

[9]   ASV, Sanità 752 123v (18 January 1735).

[10]   For Dutch merchants in quarantine in the seventeenth century see Martje van Gelder, *Trading places: the Netherlandish merchants in early modern Venice* (Leiden, 2009), pp. 69–70 and p. 156.

[11]   Paolo Rigoli, 'Il virtuoso in gabbia. Musicisti in quarantena al lazzaretto di Verona (1655–1740)' in Francesco Passadore and Franco Rossi (eds), *Musica, scienza e idée nella Serenissima durante il Seicento* (Venice, 1996), pp. 139–50.

[12]   ASV, Sanità, b. 1009.

that a sensible distance should be maintained when supplying food to patients and that objects without rope or other materials should be utilised to pass food into the *lazaretti*, in order to prevent the spread of disease.

Just as the importance of quarantine and cleaning endured within the hospitals, so too did many of the old problems. Despite the development of bureaucracy, illustrated in surviving copies of the *capitolari* which continued to be issued to the Priors, who by the eighteenth century, remained in post for four years, the Health Office did not succeed in clamping down on illicit hiding and theft of goods. In 1704, for example, a *cassa* of silk and a sack of tobacco were pulled from the water – where they had been placed in an attempt to circumnavigate quarantine. The objects were burned and the guard banished.[13] The *lazaretto* also continued to be used as a prison.[14] This continued demand for the *lazaretti* took its toll on the building structures – now nearly three centuries old. In the sixteen inventories taken of the *lazaretto nuovo* between 1739 and 1800 it is easy to track the deterioration of the buildings. In particular, from 1750 the Church is noted as being in a poor state of repair and the rooms in which passengers were accommodated seem badly affected from 1764. No wonder then that in 1759, it was recognised that the degraded state of the *lazaretto nuovo* made it unsuitable for use. By 1777, it was again noted that the buildings were in a state of disrepair and the poor condition of the canals was making access difficult. The institution was still considered worth redeveloping. In 1808, a new site was built, the *lazaretto nuovissimo*, upon on the island of Poveglia.[15] Quarantine facilities were also developed in response to cholera during the nineteenth century on the island of Sacca Sessola. The nature of the structures is described, as Thomas Rütten has illustrated, in Thomas Mann's novella *Death in Venice*.[16]

In Venice, public health structures for the plague benefitted from direct state funding whereas, for other diseases, hospitals were established which straddled the public/private divide. The lack of dependence on private philanthropy meant that the Venetian plague hospitals continued to be funded, even during periods of crisis, and were retained as preventative measures even when the wider public had turned its attention and diverted its money to other causes. The *lazaretto nuovissimo* would never see the intensity of sickness of its predecessors. The important idea of holistic care, including bringing comfort to patients, receded into the background.

---

[13] ASV, Sanità b. 87, 921 (26 April 1704).

[14] ASV, Sanità, b. 200 (28 May 1691).

[15] Angelo A. Frari, *Cenni storici sull'isola di Poveglia e sulla sua importanza sotto l'aspetto sanitario* (Venice, 1837). For an account of the island's history from 1782 see ASV, Sanità b. 563 (6 February 1782).

[16] Thomas Rütten, 'Cholera in Thomas Mann's Death in Venice', *Gesnerus* 66:2 (2009), pp. 256–87. The quarantine structures are described on pp. 265–9. A number of examples could be given which hint at the enduring relationship of association between cholera and plague, for example Michael Durey, *The return of plague. British Society and the Cholera 1831–2* (Dublin, 1979).

The purpose of the institutions was cleansing and regulating. As a result, the structures were altered and the nature of isolation was simplified. Although contact was possible with friends and family through written correspondence, visiting from family and friends was minimal as was the attempt to care for the emotional state of patients. Spiritual care was still available, if decidedly less prominent. Even medical care was administered less frequently. For some, a period of quarantine became little more than a necessary inconvenience for the travelling merchants, philanthropists and wealthy tourists of Europe.

During the eighteenth century, new *lazaretti* were built across Europe and beyond.[17] Eighteenth-century accounts of plague, particularly in the aftermath of the outbreaks in Marseilles and Moscow, abound as do treatises on epidemic disease, such as those by Richard Mead and Patrick Russell.[18] Connections were often made by medical authors between plague and diseases such as small pox and yellow fever. A valuable source for the study of plague hospitals at the end of the eighteenth century is the publication by John Howard [1726–90], best known for his position at the forefront of the penal reform movement of the 1770s. His publication on 'The state of the prisons' of 1777 had established Howard's reputation on the domestic and international stage and has absorbed the attention of historians.[19] His 'Account of the principal lazarettos in Europe', first published in 1789, is an important and rarely considered work, with a broad geographical focus. His descriptions of the *lazaretti* of Spezia, Naples, Corfu, Dalmatia, Smyrna and Constantinople are brief. Those institutions which Howard described at length, included Marseilles, Genoa, Leghorn, Malta, Zante and Venice.

Howard had broad interests in matters of health in relation to a number of elements, which are prominent in his publications as well as in eighteenth-century medical thought more broadly: the environment, architecture, morality, poverty and the treatment of the individual. Howard's motivation for investigating *lazaretti* was not primarily economic. His interest in the potential economic advantages of *lazaretti* emerged, as he tells us in his preface, in the course of his research. Instead, his earlier study of prisons in Britain and Europe led him to speculate regarding the utility of a detailed study of plague hospitals. Howard designed an 'ideal *lazaretto*' [Plate 32] which is useful for exploring perceptions of the form and function of plague hospitals at the end of the eighteenth century. The design echoed his instructions in the text that plague hospitals should be of a 'cheerful aspect' and express visually the notions of order and harmony which he hoped

---

[17]   For the debate on quarantine and importance of the *lazaretto* in Malta see John Booker, *Maritime quarantine*.

[18]   Richard Mead, *A discourse on the plague* (London, 1744) and Patrick Russell, *A treatise of the plague* (London, 1791).

[19]   The best, however brief, discussion of John Howard remains Roy Porter, 'Howard's beginnings: prisons, disease, hygiene' in Richard Creese, William F. Bynum and Joe Bearn (eds), *The health of prisoners: historical essays* (Amsterdam, 1995), pp. 5–26. As yet, there has been little by way of in-depth study of Howard's interests in public health.

to see in their regulation and operation and which were central to contemporary medical thought. Howard complained that *lazaretti* often looked too much like prisons; the latter institutions, in his view, should express simplicity and plainness in their design. Howard's ideas regarding architecture and morality were related to understandings of contagion and corruption. Howard expressed concern, for example, regarding a lack of separation of individuals within prisons, young from old, men from women, experienced from novice offenders, which he perceived as a cause of moral corruption.

Throughout, Howard's concern with order in the design, regulation and site of institutions reflected a belief that such characteristics would feed through into their nature as well as the health of the individuals within them. This is true of his plan for the ideal *lazaretto*. Here, the use of space is clearly defined. The *lazaretto* is in a port and the ground closest to the sea is set aside for the burial of corpses as well as the disinfection and airing of foul goods, so that they could be transported directly from incoming ships without passing through the building structure. This area would also have been most fully exposed to the cleansing winds. The land entrance to the building complex is at the opposite side to this area for cleansing and adjacent to the governor's house and grounds, which were positioned so as to allow the individual in charge to supervise the land-based traffic. Inside the *lazaretto* complex, the importance of architectural symmetry is clear to see. The central bowling green is a new addition, presumably an element of eighteenth-century recreation but would also – as the area through which the pavements passed – have allowed for a beautiful garden at the centre of the building complex. A number of the elements emphasised by Howard within his plan had long been recognised as important features of *lazaretto* architecture, particularly the chapel and open spaces.

By the time of John Howard's publication, contemporary writings which make reference to *lazaretti* are no longer the vivid accounts of epidemics or effusive accounts of the histories of cities. The institutions did, however, continue to be used as emblems of diseased and infected states: John Aiken, for example, wrote that all hospitals run the risk of descending to the level of *lazaretti*, while a publication entitled the *The Walkers' Companion* deploys the *lazaretto* as an emblem for the world.[20] References to the sites are widespread in the writings of travellers and in works produced for maritime and seafarers. In particular, the sites at Leghorn, Marseilles, Venice and Malta take on a heightened strategic significance. Sites further afield are also referred to – including Cuba, Barbados and Kingston.

The accounts by travellers are often brief but can be used to shed light on the eighteenth-century *lazaretti*. Jean-Jacques Rousseau [1712–78] described his experiences of quarantine in his *Confessions*. He, unlike the rest of his fellow travellers, chose to carry out his quarantine within the *lazaretto* rather than on the ship he had been travelling on, despite the *lazaretto* being unfurnished. Once he had

---

[20]   John Aikin, *Thoughts on hospitals* (London, 1771), pp. 9–11 and *The Walkers' Companion* (London, 1787), p. 8.

been locked in, Rousseau recorded having much of the site at his disposal. He made use of a series of empty rooms, made his stay as comfortable as possible using his own goods and filled his time with work and reading.[21] In 1776, Richard Chandler recorded, in his *Travels in Greece* his experiences of quarantine in the *lazaretto* at Zante. He describes having had the opportunity to enjoy much that the region had to offer: from grapes to an earthquake characteristic of that area.[22] In 1797, the poet and diplomat Joel Barlow [1754–1812] stayed in the *lazaret* at Marseilles. The American Barlow had remained in Europe following the French Revolution and undertaken diplomatic commissions on behalf of the Republic. Simon Schama describes Barlow's stay and the writings he produced during his time in quarantine.[23] He writes of the room Barlow stayed in as a 'philosopher's cell'. Schama continued, 'His Purgatory was serene, the building cool and commodious with ample rooms.' Servants' quarters were provided. Patients ate Spanish oranges, olives and white cheeses. Much had changed in the two centuries between the descriptions of Mediterranean plague hospitals provided by Rousseau, Chandler and Barlow and the accounts by Sansovino and Benedetti of the Venetian *lazaretti*. By the time of Barlow's writing, the *lazaretti* had lost their dual nature as hospitals and quarantine centres and had become institutions more simply allied with the mechanisms of trade. Some things stayed the same. At Marseilles, the plague hospital was described as 'half sanitary, half military' with a double line of fifteen-foot high walls around the compound. It catered for merchants and traders, this time from Africa. Isolation, disinfection, defence and trade were all prominent in Barlow's account. Even Benedetti's image of Purgatory echoed in the later writings.

In these later writings, we also continue to see the importance of viewing these institutions, and their descriptions, in context. Many of the writings touch on wider contemporary debates. The treatment of slaves in the late eighteenth century, for example, raised discussions of the care provided by masters to slaves in times of sickness. In 1788, Hector Macneill wrote in his 'Observations on the treatment of the negros in the island of Jamaica' that these individuals were better treated than labourers in Britain because the latter were left to their own devices in periods of sickness whereas the former were sent, at the first sign of illness, to the '*lazaretto* or hot house'.[24] Discussions of quarantine and isolation also feature in writings on liberty. In 1787, the archdeacon of Carlisle, William Paley, specifically mentioned confinement in his discussion of civil liberty. He used the policy as an example of restriction of movement which was seen to be perfectly compatible with civil liberties as long as the policy was believed to be the effect of

---

[21]   Jean-Jacques Rousseau, *The confessions of J.J. Rousseau ... part the second* (London, 1790), pp. 44–6.

[22]   Richard Chandler, *Travels in Greece* (Oxford, 1776), p. 328 and p. 330.

[23]   Simon Schama, *Landscape and memory* (London, 1995), pp. 245–6.

[24]   Hector Macneill, *Observations on the treatment of negros, in the island of Jamaica* (London, 1788), p. 8.

a 'beneficial public law'.[25] This theme of freedom, liberty and the *lazaretto* is also evident in literary texts. In Charles Dickens' novel *Little Dorrit*, for example, the nature of confinement is explored. A prison and a *lazaretto* are meeting places for the protagonists of the novel.[26] A foundling hospital and debtors' prison seem to offer their inhabitants greater freedom than the outside world. The home and the mind are the most repressive, restrictive sites in the novel.

Debates regarding the purpose and impact of these institutions endured through the centuries, as did the institutions themselves. Originally designed for merchants and traders the institutions evolved into sites for those travelling within the increasingly-lucrative tourist trade. As the *lazaretti* came to serve those arriving from outside as opposed to those living inside cities, the prominence of the institutions diminished. Already physically located on the margins of the city, the sites were perceived far more simply as barriers against the introduction of disease. In addition, from the nineteenth century, these institutions ceased to be associated with European public health for the plague and were introduced more broadly, for example in the Ottoman Empire.[27] Plague was of continued concern in the eighteenth century and beyond but the disease was increasingly perceived as one which was caused predominantly through importation. It was no longer an omnipresent threat, firmly rooted in the nature of the everyday.

---

[25] William Paley, *The principles of moral and political philosophy* (London, 1787), p. 167.

[26] Charles Dickens, *Little Dorrit* (London, 1857).

[27] For the introduction of quarantine sites in the Ottoman empire during the nineteenth century and the concepts of disease causation which meant that such structures were not introduced in earlier centuries see Miri Shefer-Mossensohn, *Ottoman medicine: healing and medical institutions, 1500–1700* (New York, 2009), pp. 172–5.

Bibliography

MANUSCRIPT SOURCES

London

Wellcome Library for the History and Understanding of Medicine

Manuscripts ms. 223

Padua

Archivio di Stato

Archivio Civico Antico, Atti del Consiglio b. 14–18.
Ufficio di Sanità b. 5, b. 6, b. 7, b. 14, b. 27, b. 36, b. 46, reg. 49, b. 54, b. 186, b. 239, b. 240, b. 273, b. 295, b. 324, b. 325, b. 345, b. 353, b. 441, b. 452, b. 539, b. 543, b. 545, b. 570, b. 572, b. 575, b. 588, b. 589.

Venice

Archivio di Stato

Archivi notarile, testamenti b. 12, b. 193, b. 194.
Arsenale, Capitolare 9–13 and Terminazioni 133–6.
Cinque Savii all Mercanzia b. 56 and b. 60.
Collegio, Cerimoniali reg. 1, reg. 2.
Collegio, Relazioni di Ambasciatori, Rettori b. 32–3, 43 and 50.
Consiglio de Dieci, parti comuni reg. 1, 22, 32–3, 65–7, 69–74, 100, 115, 126, 128, 130, 132; filza 5–8, 24–6, 43–4.
Capi del Consiglio de Dieci, Lettere di Rettori e di altre cariche b. 81–2, 84, 92–5.
Inquisitori di Stato 925, 1256.
Miscellanea carte non appartenenti ad alcun archivio b. 16.
Procuratia di San Marco di Citra b. 85, b. 196, b. 223, b. 335, b. 360, b. 361, b. 362, b. 376.
Provveditori al Sal b. 6 reg. 3, b. 8 reg. 7, b. 9 reg. 8, b. 10 reg. 13, b. 11 reg. 15.
Provveditori alla Sanità reg. 1, b. 2, reg. 3, reg 4, reg. 12–18,b. 51, b. 85–7, b. 564, b. 566, reg. 809, reg. 810, b. 1009.

Provveditori di Comun b. 60.
    Notatorio 725–60.
Provveditori sopra i beni inculti b. 262, b. 291, b. 299, b. 300.
Savi ed Esecutori alle Acque 119, 231.
Scuola Grande di San Marco b. 101.
Secreta, Materia miste notabili b. 55 bis, b.95.
Senato, Terra reg. 2–3, 17–38, 40–46, 48–52 and filza 6, 67.

Archivio Storico del Patriarcato di Venezia

Parrochia di S Samuele, morti, libro II (1556–1602)
Parrochia di S Fantin, libro de battizati (1560–1629)

Fondazione Giorgio Cini, Istituto per la storia della società e dello stato veneziano

Archivio di Stato di Firenze, Arch Mediceo, Carteggi con Venezia filza 2971, 2974
    (bb. 28).
Archivio di Stato di Mantova, Carteggio esterno, carteggio ad inviati b. 1488 (bb. 61),
    b. 1489 (bb. 62).
Archivio di Stato di Modena, A.S.E. Cancelleria amb. a Venezia b. 44 (bb. 125–8).

Biblioteca del Museo Correr

MSS Donà delle Rose 181, 327, 466
Codice Gradenigo 43
MSS Dandolo Pr. div. C. 941
Codice Cicogna 2018, 2543

Biblioteca Marciana

MSS Italiani VII 2342 [=9695]

Verona

Archivio di Stato

Acta Ecclesiae Mediolanensis (Milan: Lugduni, 1682).
Archivio del Comune, Atti del Consiglio reg. 77, reg. 80–81, reg. 89.
Archivio del Comune, Collegio dei Medici reg. 610–11.
Ospedale di San Giacomo e Lazzaro alla Tomba 22–5, 26–8, 1464–85, 1587–98,
    1600–1618.
Ufficio di Sanità reg. 1, reg. 2, b. 3, b. 26, reg. 33, reg. 157.

PRINTED SOURCES

Aikin, J., *Thoughts on hospitals* (London, 1771).

Averlino, A. (known as Filarete), 'Sforzinda' in G.C. Sciolla (ed.), *La città ideale nel Rinascimento* (Turin, 1995) pp. 70–84.

Bacon, F., 'Of gardens' in *Essays* (London, 1992) pp. 137–43.

Baravalo, C., *L'historia della peste di Padoa* (Padua, 1555).

Bellintani, P., *Dialogo della peste,* E. Paccagnini (ed.) (Milan, 2001).

Benedetti, R., *Ragguaglio delle Allegrezze, Solennità, e feste, fatte in Venetia per la felice Vittoria* (Venice, 1571).

———, *Le feste et trionfi fatti dalla serenisima signoria di Venetia nella felice venuta di Henrico III. Christianissimo re di Francia et di Polonia* (Venice, 1574).

———, *Relatione d'alcuni casi occorsi in Venetia al tempo della peste l'anno 1576 et 1577 con le provisioni, rimedii et orationi fatte à Dio benedetto per la sua liberatione* (Bologna, 1630).

Bisciola, P., *Relatione verissima del progresso della peste di Milano ... dove si raccontano tutte le provisioni fatte da Monsignor Illustrissimo Cardinal Borromeo... dove si può imparare, il vero modo d'un perfetto Pastore amator del suo gregge e come in Principe deve governar una città nel tempo di peste* (Bologna, 1630).

Boccaccio, G., *The Decameron*, G.H. McWilliam (trans.) (London, 1995).

Borgarucci, P., *Dove ciascuno potrà apprendere il vero modo di curar la peste et i carboni et di conservarsi sano in detto tempo* (Venice, 1565).

Cantagalli, R. (ed.), *Diario di Firenze e di altre parti della cristianità (1574–9)* (Florence, 1970).

Canobbio, A., *Il successo della peste occorsa in Padova l'anno MDLXXVI* (Padua, 1576).

Cessi, R., Segarizzi, A. and Spada, N., *Antichi scrittori d'idraulica veneta* (Venice, 1987).

Chandler, R., *Travels in Greece* (Oxford, 1776).

Cherchi, P. and Collina, B. (eds), *Tommaso Garzoni, 'La piazza universale di tutte le professioni del mondo'* (Turin, 1996).

Contarini, G., *Della republica et magistrati di venetia libri V* (Venice, 1591).

da San Bonaventura, A. M., *Li lazaretti della città e riviere di Genova del MDCLVII ne quali oltre à successi particolari del contagio si narrano l'opere virtuose di quelli che sacrificorno se stessi alla salute del prossimo e si danno le regole di ben governare un popolo flagellato dalla peste* (Genoa, 1658).

de Ferrari, O., *Quorum duo priores de tuenda eorum sanitate posteriores de curandis morbis agunt* (Brescia, 1577).

de Pomis, D., *Brevi discorsi et efficacissimi ricordi per liberare ogni città oppressa dal mal contagioso* (Venice, 1577).

Dante, *The Divine Comedy* (Oxford, 2008).

Dickens, C., *Little Dorrit* (London, 1857).

Fioravanti, L., *Il reggimento della peste ... Nel quale si tratta che cosa sia la peste, et da che procede et quello che doveriano fare i Prencipi per conservar i suoi popoli da essa; et ultimamente si mostrano mirabili secreti da curarla, cosa non mai piu scritta da niuno in questo modo* (Venice, 1571).

Frigimelega, F., *Consiglio...sopra la peste in Padoa dell'anno MDLV* (Padua, 1555).

Gastaldi, G., *Tractatus de avertenda et profliganda peste politico = legalis. Eo lucubratus tempore, quo ipse Leomocomiorum primo, mox Sanitatis Commissarius Generalis fuit, peste urbem invadente Anno MDCLVI et LVII* (Bologna, 1684).

Glisente, A., *Trattato del regimento del vivere et delle altre cose che deveno usare gli huomini per preservarsi sani nel tempi pestilenti: continuando alla cognitione delle cause che producono la peste* (Venice, 1576).

Gratiolo, A., *Discorso di peste...nel quale si contengono utilissime speculationi intorno alla natura, cagioni e curatione della peste, con un catalogo di tutte le pesti piu notabili de' tempi passati* (Venice, 1576).

Howard, J., *An account of the principal lazarettos in Europe* (London, 1791).

Ingaliso, L. (ed.), *Giovan Filippo Ingrassia: Informatione del pestifero et contagioso morbo* (Milan, 2005).

Leoni, B., *Canzone fatta intorno allo stato calamitoso dell'inclita città di Vinetia nel colmo de' maggiori suoi passati travagli per la peste* (Padua, 1577).

Macneill, H., *Observations on the treatment of negros, in the island of Jamaica* (London, 1788).

Malespini, C., *Ducento novella di Signor Celio Malespini nelle quali si raccontano diversi avverimenti cosi lieti come merti e stravaganti con tanta copia di sentenze gravi, di odianzi e moti che non meno sono profittevoli nella practica del vivere humano che molto grati e piacevoli ad udire* (Venice, 1609).

Manzoni, A., *The Betrothed: and history of the column of infamy*, D. Forgacs and M. Reynolds (eds), (London, 1997).

Massa, N., *Ragionamento ... sopra le infermita che vengono dall'aere pestilentiale del presente anno MDLV* (Venice, 1556).

Mead, Richard, *A discourse on the plague* (London, 1744).

Milesio, G.B., *Beschreibung des deutschen Hauses in Venedig* (Munich, 1881).

More, T., 'Utopia' in S. Bruce (ed.), *Three early modern Utopias* (Oxford, 1996).

Moryson, F., *An Itinerary* (Amsterdam, 1971).

Odorici, F., 'I due Bellintani da Salò ed il dialogo della peste di Fra Paolo' in G. Mueller (ed.), *Raccolta di cronisiti e documenti storici lombardi inediti* (Milan, 1857), pp. 251–313.

Paley, W., *The principles of moral and political philosophy* (London, 1787).

Paré, A., *A treatise of the Plague* (London, 1630 [1568]).

Porcacchi, T., *L'isole piu famose del mondo* (Venice, 1572).

Portenari, A., *Della felicità di Padova* (Padua, 1623).

Raimondo, A., *Discorso nel quale chiaramente si conosce la viva et vera cagione che ha generato le fiere infermità che tanto hanno molestato l'anno 1575 et tanto il 76 acerbamente molestano il Popolo de l'invittissima Città di Vinetia* (Padua, 1576).

Rangoni, T., *Come i Venetiani possano vivere sempre sani* (Venice, 1565).

Ripa, C., *Iconologia* (Padua, 1611).

Rodolico, N. (ed.), *Cronaca fiorentina di Marchionne di Coppo Stefani* (Castello, 1903).

Rolfe, F., *Tre racconti su Venezia* (Venice, 2002).

Rousseau, J.-J., *The confessions of J.J. Rousseau ... part the second* (London, 1790).

Russell, P., *A treatise of the plague* (London, 1791).

Sabellico, M. A., *Le historie vinitiane* (Venice, 1543).

Sansovino, F., *Venetia città nobilissima et singolare, descritta in XIII libri* (Venice, 1663).

Sanudo, M., *De origine, situ et magistratibus urbis venetae ovvero la città di Venetia (1493–1530)* (Milan, 1980).

———, *I Diarii di Marino Sanuto*, R. Fulin (ed.) (58 vols, Venice, 1879–1903).

Scappi, B., *Opera* (1570).

Shakespeare, W., *All's well that ends well*.

Tomitano, B., *De le cause et origine de la peste vinitiana* (Venice, 1556).

Valerio, A., *Lettera consolatoria ... Nella quale essendo stata liberata essa città dal sospetto della peste, che l'ha per molti giorni travagliata, si consola col suo popolo, e l'essorta a ringratiarne la maestà di Dio, et a viver christianamente* (Venice, 1575).

Vasari, G., *Lives of the painters, sculptors and architects* (2 vols, London, 1996).

Vecellio, C., *Habiti antichi et moderni di tutto il mondo* (Venice, 1598).

The walkers' companion (London, 1787).

PRINTED SECONDARY SOURCES

Aikema, Bernard and Meijers, Dulcia (eds), *Nel regno dei poveri: arte e storia dei grandi ospedali veneziani in età moderna 1474–1797* (Venice: Arsenale Editrice, 1989).

Albala, Ken, *Eating right in the Renaissance* (London: University of California Press, 2002).

———, 'To your health: wine as food and medicine in mid sixteenth-century Italy' in Mack P. Holt (ed.), *Alcohol: a social and cultural history* (Oxford: Berg, 2006), pp. 11–25.

Albini, Giuliana, *Città e ospedali nella Lombardia medievale* (Bologna: CLUEB, 1993).

Alexander, John T., *Bubonic plague in early modern Russia: public health and urban disaster* (London: Johns Hopkins University Press, 1980).

Allerston, Patricia, 'Wedding finery in sixteenth-century Venice' in Trevor Dean and Kate J.P. Lowe (eds), *Marriage in Italy 1300–1650* (Cambridge: Cambridge University Press, 1998), pp. 26–31.

———, 'Clothing and early modern Venetian society', *Continuity and change*, 15:3 (2000), 367–90.

———, 'L'abito usato' in Carlo M. Belfanti and Fabio Giusberti, *Storia d'Italia 19: La Moda* (Turin: Giulio Einaudi, 2003), pp. 561–81.

Ambrosini, Federica, '"De mia man propia". Donna, scrittura e praesi testamentaria nella Venezia del Cinquecento' in Mario de Biasi (ed.), *Non uno itinere. Studi storici offerti dagli allievi a Federico Seneca* (Venezia: Stamperia di Venezia, 1993), pp. 33–54.

———, 'Toward a social history of women in Venice: from Renaissance to Enlightenment' in John Martin and Dennis Romano (eds), *Venice reconsidered. The history and civilisation of an Italian city–state 1297–1797* (London: Johns Hopkins University Press, 2000), pp. 420–54.

Appelby, Andrew B., 'The disappearance of plague: a continuing puzzle', *The Economic History Review*, 33 (1980), 161–73.

Appuhn, Karl, 'Inventing nature: forests, forestry and state power in Renaissance Venice', *The Journal of Modern History*, 72:4 (2000), 861–89.

———, 'Politics, perception and the meaning of landscape in late medieval Venice: Marco Cornaro's 1442 inspection of firewood supplies' in John Howe and Michael Wolfe (eds), *Inventing medieval landscapes: senses of place in Western Europe* (Gainesville FL, 2002), pp. 70–88.

———, 'Friend or flood? The dilemmas of water management in early modern Venice', in Andrew C. Isenberg (ed.), *The nature of cities: new approaches to urban environmental history* (Rochester NY: University of Rochester Press, 2005), pp. 79–102.

———, *A forest on the sea: environmental expertise in Renaissance Venice* (Baltimore MD: Johns Hopkins University Press, 2009).

Arbel, Benjamin, *Trading nations. Jews and Venetians in the early modern Eastern Mediterranean* (Leiden: Brill, 1995).

———, 'Colonie d'oltremare' in Alberto Tenenti and Ugo Tucci (eds), *Storia di Venezia: dalle origini alla caduta della Serenissima* (14 vols, Rome: Istituto della enciclopedia italiana, 1991–) vol. 5: 'Il Rinascimento: società ed economia', pp. 947–85.

Arbesmann, Ralph, 'The concept of "Christus medicus" in St Augustine', *Traditio*, 10 (1954), 1–28.

Armstrong, Lilian, 'Benedetto Bordon, "Miniator" and cartography in sixteenth-century Venice', *Imago mundi*, 48 (1996), 65–92.

Arnaldi, Girolamo, Giorgio Cracco and Alberto Tenenti et al. (eds), *Storia di Venezia: dalle origini alla caduta della Serenissima* (14 vols, Rome: Istituto della enciclopedia italiana, 1991–).

Arici, Graziano et al., *La galea ritrovata: origine delle cose di Venezia* (Venice: Consorzio Venezia Nuova, 2002).

Arrizabalaga, Jon, 'Facing the Black Death: perceptions and reactions of university medical practitioners' in Luis Garcia Ballester, Roger French, Jon Arrizabalaga and Andrew Cunningham (eds), *Practical medicine from Salerno to the Black Death* (Cambridge: Cambridge University Press, 1994), pp. 237–88.

Arrizabalaga, Jon, John Henderson and Roger French, *The Great Pox: the French disease in Renaissance Europe* (London: Yale University Press, 1997).

Avery, Harold, 'Plague churches, monuments and memorials', *Proceedings of the Royal Society of Medicine*, 59:1 (1966), 110–16.

Bagatta, Francesco, *Storia degli spedali e degli istituti di beneficenza in Verona dall'epoca cristiana a giorni nostri* (Verona: Stabilmento di Giuseppe Civelli, 1862).

Bailey, Gavin A., Pamela M. Jones, Franco Mormando and Thomas W. Worcester (eds), *Hope and healing: painting in Italy in a time of plague, 1500–1800* (Worcester MA: University of Chicago Press, 2005).

Ball, James G., 'Poverty, charity and the Greek community', *Studi veneziani*, n.s. 6 (1982), 129–45.

Ballon, Hilary, *The Paris of Henri IV: architecture and urbanism* (Cambridge MA: MIT Press, 1991).

Barker, Sheila, 'The making of a plague saint: Saint Sebastian's imagery and cult before the Counter-Reformation' in Franco Mormando and Thomas Worcester (eds), *Piety and plague from Byzantium to the Baroque* (Kirksville MI: Truman State University Press, 2007), pp. 90–132.

Barry, Jonathan and Colin Jones (eds), *Medicine and charity before the Welfare State* (London: Routledge, 1991).

Bartrum, Giulia (ed.), *Jost Amman* (Rotterdam: Sound and Vision Publishers, 2001).

Beier, Lucinda N., 'In sickness and in health: a seventeenth-century family's experience' in Roy Porter (ed.), *Patients and practitioners: lay perceptions of medicine in pre-industrial society* (Cambridge: Cambridge University Press, 1985), pp. 101–28.

Bellavitis, Giorgio, *L'Arsenale di Venezia: storia di una grande struttura urbana* (Venice: Marsilio, 1983).

Beloch, Giulio, 'La popolazione di Venezia nei secoli 16 e 17', *Nuovo archivio veneto*, n.s. 3 (1902), 5–49.

Beltrami, Daniele, *Storia della popolazione di Venezia dalla fine XVI alla caduta della Repubblica* (Padua: CEDAM, 1954).

———, *Forze di lavoro e proprietà fondiaria nella campagne venete dei sec XVIII e XVIII: la penetrazione economica dei Veneziani in Terraferma* (Venice: Istituto per la Collaborazione Culturale, 1961).

Beltrami, Luca, 'Il lazzaretto di Milano', *Archivio storico lombardo*, 9 (1882), 403–41.

Benvenuto, Grazia, *La peste nell'Italia nella prima età moderna: contagio, rimedi, profilassi* (Bologna: CLUEB, 1996).

Berengo, Marino, *La società veneta alla fine del Settecento: ricerche storiche* (Florence: G.C. Sansoni, 1956).

Bertelli, Sergio, Nicolai Rubinstein and Craig Hugh Smyth, *Florence and Venice, comparisons and relations* (Florence: La nuova Italia, 1979).

Bianchi, Francesco, *La Ca' di Dio di Padova nel Quattrocento: riforma e governo di un ospedale per l'infanzia abbandonata* (Venice: Istituto veneto di scienze, lettere ed arti, 2005).

Biancolini, Giambatista, *Notizie storiche delle chiese di Verona* (Verona: Dionigi Ramanzini, 1749–71).

Biow, Douglas, *The culture of cleanliness in Renaissance Italy* (London: Cornell University Press, 2006).

Biraben, Jean-Noël, *Les hommes et la peste en France et dans les pays européens et méditerranéens* (2 vols, Paris: Mouton, 1975–76).

Bisgaard, Lars and Leif Søndergaard (eds), *Living with the Black Death* (Lancaster: Gazelle, 2009).

Boccato, Carla, 'La mortalità nel Ghetto di Venezia durante la peste del 1630', *Archivio Veneto*, 5th series, 140 (1993), 111–46.

Boeckl, Christine M., 'Plague imagery as a metaphor for heresy in Rubens's "The miracles of Saint Francis Xavier"', *Sixteenth century journal*, 27:4 (1996), 979–95.

———, *Images of plague and pestilence: iconography and iconology* (Kirksville MO, Truman State University Press, 2000).

———, 'Giorgio Vasari's "San Rocco altarpiece": tradition and innovation in plague iconography', *Artibus et historiae*, 22 (2001), 29–40.

Boerio, Giuseppe, *Dizionario del dialetto veneziano* (Venice: Reale Tipografia di Giovanni Cecchini, 1867).

Booker, John, *Maritime quarantine: the British experience c.1650–1900* (Aldershot: Ashgate, 2007).

Borelli, Giorgio (ed.), *Mercanti e vita economica nella Repubblica Veneta sec XIII–XVIII* (2 vols, Verona: Banca popolare di Verona, 1985).

Borghi, Paola, *Antidoti contro la peste a Milano* (Milan: IPL, 1990).

Bound Alberti, Fay, 'Emotions in the Early Modern Medical Tradition' in Fay Bound Alberti (ed.), *Medicine, Emotion and Disease, 1700–1950* (Basingstoke: Palgrave Macmillan, 2006), pp.1–21.

Braddick, Michael J., *State formation in early modern England c.1550–1700* (Cambridge: Cambridge University Press, 2000).

Braudel, Fernand, *The Mediterranean and the Mediterranean world in the age of Philip II,* S. Reynolds (trans.) (2 vols, London: Fontana, 1975).

Bray, Xavier, *The sacred made real: Spanish painting and sculpture 1600–1700* (London: National Gallery Company, 2009).

Breda, A., 'Contributo alla storia dei lazzaretti (leprosari) medioevali in Europa', *Atti del reale istituto veneto di scienze, lettere ed arti*, 68 (1908–1909), 133–94.

Brockliss, Laurence and Colin Jones, *The medical world of early modern France* (Oxford: Clarendon Press, 1997).

Brown, Horatio F., *Life on the lagoons* (London, 1900).

Brown, Patricia Fortini, *Private lives in Renaissance Venice* (London: Yale University Press, 2004).

Brozzi, Mario, *Peste, fede e sanità in una cronaca Cividalese del 1598* (Milan: A. Giuffre, 1982).

Brunetti, Mario, 'Venezia durante la peste del 1348', *Ateneo veneto*, 32 (1909), 289–311.

Brusatin, Manlio, *Il muro della peste: spazio della pietà e governo del lazaretto* (Venice: CLUVA, 1981).

Burckhardt, Jacob, *The civilisation of the Renaissance in Italy* (London: Penguin, 1950).

Burke, Peter, 'Early modern Venice as a center of information and communication' in John Martin and Dennis Romano (eds), *Venice reconsidered. The history and civilisation of an Italian city-state 1297–1797* (London: Johns Hopkins University Press, 2000), pp. 389–419.

———, *Historical anthropology of early modern Italy: essays on perception and communication* (Cambridge: Cambridge University Press, 1987).

———, *Critical essays on Michel Foucault* (Aldershot: Ashgate, 1992).

———, *Popular culture in early modern Europe* (Aldershot: Ashgate, 1994).

———, *Varieties of cultural history* (Cambridge: Polity Press, 1997).

Burke, Peter, Brian Harrison and Paul Slack (eds), *Civil histories: essays presented to Sir Keith Thomas* (Oxford: Oxford University Press, 2000).

Bury, Michael, 'The fifteenth and early sixteenth-century *gonfaloni* of Perugia', *Renaissance studies,* 12 (1998), 67–87.

Bylebyl, Jerome, 'The school of Padua: humanistic medicine in the sixteenth century' in Charles Webster (ed.), *Health, medicine and mortality in the sixteenth century* (Cambridge: Cambridge University Press, 1979), pp. 335–71.

Calabi, Donatella and Paola Lanaro, *La città italiana e i luoghi degli stranieri XIV – XVIII sec* (Rome–Bari: Laterza, 1998).

Calvi, Giulia, 'A metaphor for social exchange: the Florentine plague of 1630', *Representations*, 13 (1986), 139–63.

———, *Histories of a plague year: the social and the imaginary in Baroque Florence* (Oxford: University of California Press, 1989).

Camerlengo, Lia, 'Il lazzaretto a San Pancrazio e l'ospedale della Misericordia in Bra: le forme dell'architettura' in Alessandro Pastore, Gian Maria Varanini, Paola Marini and Giorgio Marini (eds), *L'ospedale e la città: cinquecento anni d'arte a Verona* (Verona: Cierre, 1996), pp. 179–91.

Campbell, Donald, *Arabian medicine and its influence on the Middle Ages* (London: Routledge, 2000).

Campigotto, Luca, *L'Arsenale di Venezia* (Venice: Marsilio, 2000).

Caniato, Giovanni and Michele Zanetti (eds), *L'arcipelago dimenticato: isole minori della laguna di Venezia tra storia e natura* (Venice: Comune, 2005).

Carbone, Salvatore, *Provveditori e sopraprovveditori alla sanità della repubblica di Venezia: carteggio con i rappresentanti diplomatici e consolari veneti all'estero e con uffici di sanità esteri corrispondenti inventario* (Rome: [s.n.], 1962).

Carmichael, Ann G., 'Plague legislation in the Italian Renaissance', *Bulletin of the history of medicine*, 57 (1983), 508–25.

————, *Plague and the poor in Renaissance Florence* (Cambridge: Cambridge University Press, 1986).

————, 'Contagion theory and contagion practice in fifteenth-century Milan', *Renaissance quarterly,* 44 (1991), 213–56.

————, 'The last past plague: the uses of memory in Renaissance epidemics', *Journal of the history of medicine,* 53 (1998), 132–60.

Carter, Francis W., *Dubrovnik (Ragusa), a classic city-state* (London: Seminar Press, 1972).

Casini, Matteo, 'Fra città-stato e stato regionale: riflessioni politiche sulla Repubblica di Venezia nella età moderna', *Studi veneziani,* n. s. 99 (2002), 15–36.

Cassini, Giocondo, *Piante e vedute prospettiche di Venezia (1479–1855)* (Venice: Stamperia di Venezia, 1982).

Cattani, Manuel and Nicola Berlucchi (eds), *I magazzini del sale a Venezia: indagini storiche e diagnostiche per un intervento di restauro conservativo* (Venice: Marsilio, 2006).

Cavallo, Sandra, *Charity and power in early modern Italy: benefactors and their motives in Turin 1541–1789* (Cambridge: Cambridge University Press, 1995).

————, *Artisans of the body in early modern Italy: identities, families and masculinities* (Manchester: Manchester University Press, 2007).

Cavallo, Sandra and Silvia Evangelisti (eds), *Domestic Institutional Interiors in Early Modern Europe* (Aldershot: Ashgate, 2009).

Cecchi, Roberto (ed.), *Ritrovare restaurando: rinvenimenti e scoperte a Venezia e in laguna* (Venice: Soprintendenza per i Beni Ambientali e Architettonici di Venezia, 2000).

Chambers, David S., *The Imperial age of Venice 1380–1580* (London: Thames and Hudson, 1970).

Chambers, David S., Cecil H. Clough and Michael E. Mallett, *War, culture and society in Renaissance Venice* (London: Hambledon Press, 1993).

Chambers, David S. and Brian Pullan (eds) with Fletcher, Jennifer, *Venice: a documentary history, 1450–1630* (Oxford: Blackwell, 1992).

Chittolini, Giorgio, 'Cities, "city states" and regional states in north-central Italy' in Charles Tilly and Wim P. Blockmans (eds), *Cities and the rise of states in Europe AD 1000–1800* (Boulder CO: Westview Press, 1994), pp. 28–43.

————, *Città, comunità e feudi negli stati dell'Italia centro-settentrionale (XIV–XVI sec.)* (Milan: UNICOPLI, 1996).

Chojnacka, Monica, 'Women, charity and community in early modern Venice: the casa delle Zitelle', *Renaissance quarterly,* 51 (1998), 68–91.

————, *Working women of early modern Venice* (London: Johns Hopkins University Press, 2001).

Chojnacki, Stanley, 'Dowries and kinsmen in early Renaissance Venice', *Journal of Interdisciplinary history,* 5 (1975), 571–600.

————, 'Nobility, women and the state: marriage regulation in Venice 1420–1535' in Trevor Dean and Kate J. P. Lowe (eds), *Marriage in Italy, 1300–1650* (Cambridge: Cambridge University Press, 1998), pp. 128–51.

————, *Women and men in Renaissance Venice: twelve essays on Patrician society* (London: Johns Hopkins University Press, 2000).

Christensen, Peter, '"In these perilous times": plague and plague policies in early modern Denmark', *Medical history*, 47 (2003), 413–50.

Cicogna, Emmanuele A., *Corpus delle iscrizioni di Venezia e delle isole della laguna Veneta* (3 vols, Venice: Biblioteca Orafa di Sant'Antonio abate, 2001).

Cipolla, Carlo M., *Cristofano and the plague; a study in the history of public health in the age of Galileo* (London: Collins, 1973).

————, *Public health and the medical profession in the Renaissance* (Cambridge: Cambridge University Press, 1976).

————, *Faith, reason and the plague: a Tuscan story of the seventeenth century* (Ithaca NY: Cornell University Press, 1979).

————, *Fighting the plague in seventeenth-century Italy* (Madison WI: University of Wisconsin Press, 1981).

————, *Contro un nemico invisibile: epidemie e strutture sanitarie nell'Italia del Rinascimento* (Bologna: Il mulino, 1986).

————, 'Corfu: "chiave della cristianità" e la sua difesa contro la peste' in Carlo Cipolla (ed.), *Saggi di storia economica e sociale* (Bologna: Il mulino, 1988), pp. 327–43.

————, *Miasmi ed umori: ecologia e condizioni sanitarie in Toscana nel Seicento* (Bologna: Il mulino, 1989).

Ciriacono, Salvatore, *Building on water: Venice, Holland and the construction of the European landscape in early modern times* (Oxford: Berghahn Books, 2006).

Cockayne, Emily, *Hubbub: filth, noise and stench in England 1600–1770* (London: Yale University Press, 2007).

Cohen, Elizabeth. S., 'Seen and known: prostitutes in the cityscape of late sixteenth-century Rome', *Renaissance studies*, 12 (1998), 392–410.

Cohen, Mark R., *The autobiography of a seventeenth-century Venetian rabbi: Leon of Modena's Life of Judah* (Princeton NJ: Princeton University Press, 1988).

Cohn Jr, Samuel K., *Death and property in Siena, 1205–1800: strategies for the afterlife* (London: Johns Hopkins University Press, 1988).

————, *The cult of remembrance and the Black Death: six Renaissance cities in central Italy* (London: Johns Hopkins University Press, 1992).

————, *Women in the streets: essays on sex and power in Renaissance Italy* (London: Johns Hopkins University Press, 1996).

————, 'The place of the dead in Flanders and Tuscany: towards a comparative history of the Black Death' in Bruce Gordon and Peter Marshall (eds), *The place of the dead*, pp. 17–43.

————, *The Black Death transformed: disease and culture in early Renaissance Europe* (London: Harvard University Press, 2002).

————, *Cultures of plague: medical thought at the end of the Renaissance* (Oxford: Oxford University Press, 2010).

————, 'Plague and its consequences' in Margaret King (ed.), *Oxford Bibliographies Online: Renaissance and Reformation* (Oxford: Oxford University Press, 2010).

————, 'Changing pathology of plague' in Simonetta Cavaciocchi (ed.), *XLI Settimana di Studi: Le Interazioni fra Economia e Ambiente Biologico Nell'Europa Preindustriale, Secc. XIII–XVIII (Prato, 26–30 Aprile 2009)* (Florence, 2010), pp. 33–57.

Cohn Jr, Samuel K. and Guido Alfani, 'Households and plague in early modern Italy', *Journal of interdisciplinary history* 38:2 (2007), 177–205.

Cohn Jr, Samuel K. and Guido Alfani, 'Nonantola 1630. Anatomia di una pestilenza e meccanismi del contagio con riflessioni a partire dale epidemie milanesi della prima età moderna', *Popolazione e storia* 2 (2007), 99–138.

Concina, Ennio, *L'Arsenale della Repubblica di Venezia (*Milan: Electa, 1984).

————, 'Owners, houses, functions: new research on the origins of the Venetian Ghetto', *Mediterranean Historical Review*, 6 (1991), 180–89.

————, *Fondaci: architettura, arte e mercatura tra Levante, Venezia e Alemagna* (Venice: Marsilio, 1997).

Concina, Ennio, Ugo Camerino and Donatella Calabi, *La città degli Ebrei. Il Ghetto di Venezia: architettura e urbanistica* (Venice: Albrizzi, 1991).

Conrad, Lawrence I., Michael Neve, Vivian Nutton, Roy Porter and Andrew Wear, *The Western medical tradition 800 B.C –A.D. 1800* (Cambridge: Cambridge University Press, 1995).

Constable, Olivia R., *Housing the stranger in the Mediterranean world: lodging, trade and travel in late Antiquity and the Middle Ages* (Cambridge: Cambridge University Press, 2003).

Cook, Harold J., *The Decline of the Old Medical Regime in Stuart London* (Ithaca NY: Cornell University Press, 1986).

————, 'Good advice and little medicine: the professional authority of early modern English physicians', *The Journal of British Studies*, 33 (1994), 1–31.

Corbin, Alain, *The foul and the fragrant: odour and the French social imagination* (Leamington Spa: Picador, 1994).

Corner, Flaminio, *Notizie storiche delle chiese e monasteri di Venezia e di Torcello* (Bologna: Forni, 1990).

Cosgrove, Dennis, 'The myth and stones of Venice: an historical geography of a symbolic landscape', *Journal of historical geography*, 8 (1982), 145–69.

————, 'Power and place in the Venetian territories' in John A. Agnew and James S. Duncan (eds), *The power of place: bringing together geographical and social imaginations* (London: Unwin Hyman, 1989), pp. 105–24.

Costantini, Massimo, *L'acqua di Venezia: l'approvvigionamento idrico della Serenissima* (Venice: Arsenale Editrice, 1984).

Cozzi, Gaetano, 'Authority and the law in Renaissance Venice' in John R. Hale (ed.), *Renaissance Venice* (London: Faber and Faber, 1973), pp. 293–346.

———— (ed.), *Stato, società e giustizia nella Republica di Venezia (sec XV–XVIII)* (Rome: Jouvence, 1980–85).

———— (ed.), *Gli ebrei e Venezia secoli XIV–XVIII* (Milan: Edizioni Comunità, 1987).

————, *La politica culturale della Repubblica di Venezia e l'università di Padova* (Trieste: Lint, 1995).

Cozzi, Gaetano and Michael Knapton, *La Repubblica di Venezia nell'età moderna: dalla guerra di Chioggia al 1517* (Turin: UTET, 1986).

Cozzi, Gaetano, Michael Knapton and Giovanni Scarabello, *La Repubblica di Venezia nell'età moderna: dal 1517 alla fine della Repubblica* (Turin: UTET, 1992).

Crisciani, Chiara and Michela Pereira, 'Black Death and golden remedies: some remarks on alchemy and the plague' in Agostino Paravicini Bagliani and Francesco Santi (eds), *The regulation of evil: social and cultural attitudes to epidemics in the late Middle Ages* (Florence: Sismel, 1998), pp. 1–39.

Crislip, Andrew T., *From monastery to hospital: Christian monasticism and the transformation of health care in late Antiquity* (Ann Arbor MI: University of Michigan Press, 2005).

Crouzet-Pavan, Elizabeth, 'Toward an ecological understanding of the myth of Venice' in John Martin and Dennis Romano (eds), *Venice reconsidered. The history and civilisation of an Italian city-state 1297–1797* (London: Johns Hopkins University Press, 2000), pp. 39–64.

————, 'Venice between Jerusalem, Byzantium and Divine Retribution: the origins of the Ghetto', *Mediterranean Historical Review*, 6 (1991), 163–79.

————, *'Sopra le acque salse': espaces, pouvoir et société à Venise à la fin du Moyen Âge* (2 vols, Rome: Istituto storico italiano per il Medio Evo, 1992).

————, 'Venice and Torcello: history and oblivion', *Renaissance studies*, 8 (1994), 416–27.

————, *Torcello: storia di una città scomparsa* (Rome: Jouvence, 2001).

Crovato, Giorgio and Maurizio Crovato, *Isole abbandonate della laguna: com'erano e come sono* (Venice: Patrocinio Associazione Settemari, 1978).

Cunningham, Andrew and Ole P. Grell (eds), *Medicine and the Reformation* (London: Routledge, 1993).

———— (eds), *Health care and poor relief in Protestant Europe 1500–1700* (London: Routledge, 1997).

———— (eds), with Jon Arrizabalaga, *Health care and poor relief in Counter-Reformation Europe* (London: Routledge, 1999).

————, *Charity and medicine in southern Europe* (London: Routledge, 1999).

————, *The four horsemen of the Apocalypse: religion, war, famine and death in Reformation Europe* (Cambridge: Cambridge University Press, 2000).

d'Aversa, Arnaldo, *Medici, epidemie e ospedali a Brescia* (Brescia: Fondazione Civiltà Bresciana, 1990).

da Mosto, Andrea, *L'archivio di stato di Venezia* (Rome: Biblioteca d'Arte, 1937–40).

————, *I Dogi di Venezia nella vita pubblica e privata* (Florence: Giunti-Martello, 1983).

dal Borgo, Michela (ed.), *Giustizia penale veneta: documenti d'archivio* (Venice: Archivio di Stato, 2006).

dal Fiume, Antonio, 'Medici, medicina e peste nel Veneto durante il sec XVI', *Archivio Veneto*, 5th series, 116 (1981), 33–58.

Davies, Paul and David Hemsoll, *Michele Sanmicheli* (Milan: Electa, 2004).

Davis, James C. (ed.), *Pursuit of power; Venetian ambassadors' reports on Spain, Turkey, and France in the age of Philip II, 1560–1600* (New York: Harper & Row, 1970).

———, *The decline of the Venetian nobility as a ruling class* (Baltimore MD: Johns Hopkins University Press, 1962).

Davis, Natalie Z., *Women on the margins: three seventeenth-century lives* (Cambridge MA: Harvard University Press, 1995).

Davis, Robert C., *Shipbuilders of the Venetian Arsenal: workers and workplace in the pre-industrial city* (Baltimore MD: Johns Hopkins University Press, 1991).

———, *The war of the fists: popular culture and public violence in late Renaissance Venice* (Oxford: Oxford University Press, 1994).

———, 'Venetian shipbuilders and the fountain of wine' *Past and Present*, 156 (1997), 55–87.

———, 'Pilgrim-Tourism in late Medieval Venice' in Paula Findlen, Michelle M. Fontaine and Duane J. Osheim (eds), *Beyond Florence: the contours of medieval and early modern Italy* (Stanford CA: Stanford University Press, 2003), pp. 119–32.

Davis, Robert C. and Benjamin Ravid (eds), *The Jews of early modern Venice* (London: Johns Hopkins University Press, 2001).

Dean, Trevor and Kate J.P. Lowe (eds), *Crime, society and the law in Renaissance Italy* (Cambridge: Cambridge University Press, 1994).

——— (eds), *Marriage in Italy, 1300–1650* (Cambridge: Cambridge University Press, 1998).

de Vivo, Filippo, *Information and communication in Venice: rethinking early modern politics* (Oxford: Oxford University Press, 2007).

del Torre, Giuseppe, *Venezia e la terraferma dopo la guerra di Cambrai. Fiscalità e amministrazione 1515–1530* (Milan: F. Angeli, 1986).

Delumeau, Jean, *Vie economique et sociale de Rome dans la seconde moitié du XVI siècle* (2 vols, Paris: Boccard, 1957–9).

Dinges, Martin, 'Sud-Nord-Gefälle in der Pestbekämpfung Italien, Deutschland und England im Vergleich' in Wolfgang U. Eckart and Robert Jütte (eds), *Das europaische Gesundheitssystem Gemeinsamkeiten und Unterschiede in historisches Perspektive* (Stuttgart: F. Steiner, 1994), pp. 19–53.

Dizionario di erudizione storico-ecclesiastico (Venice, 1852).

Dobson, Mary, *Contours of death and disease in early modern England* (Cambridge: Cambridge University Press, 1997).

Dols, Michael W., 'The comparative communal responses to the Black Death in Muslim and Christian societies', *Viator*, 5 (1974), 269–87.

Douglas, Mary, *Purity and danger: an analysis of concepts of pollution and taboo* (London: Routledge, 2002).

Duden, Barbara, *The woman beneath the skin: a doctor's patients in eighteenth-century Germany* (London: Harvard University Press, 1991).

Dunn, Marilyn, 'Spaces shaped for spiritual perfection: convent architecture and nuns in early modern Rome' in Helen Hills (ed.), *Architecture and the politics of gender in early modern Europe* (Aldershot: Ashgate, 2003) pp. 151–76.

Durey, Michael, *The return of plague. British society and the cholera 1831–2* (Dublin: Macmillan, 1979).

Eamon, William, 'Pharmaceutical self-fashioning or How to get rich and famous in the Renaissance medical marketplace', *Pharmacy in history* 45:3 (2003), 123–29.

———, 'Books of secrets in medieval and early modern science', *Sudhoffs Archiv: zeitschrift fur Wissenschaftsgeschichte*, 69 (1985), 26–49.

———, '"With the rules of life and an enema": Leonardo Fioravanti's medical primitivism' in Judith V. Field and Frank A.J.L. James (eds), *Renaissance and revolution: humanists, scholars, craftsmen and natural philosophers in early modern Europe* (Cambridge: Cambridge University Press, 1993), pp. 29–45.

———, 'Science as a hunt', *Physis*, 31 (1994), 393–432.

———, *Science and the secrets of nature: books of secrets in medieval and early modern culture* (Princeton NJ: Princeton University Press, 1994).

———, 'Plagues, healers and patients in early modern Europe', *Renaissance quarterly*, 52 (1999), 474–86.

Eckstein, Nicholas A., *The district of the green dragon: neighbourhood life and social change in Renaissance Florence* (Florence: L.S. Olschki, 1995).

Elias, Norbert and John L. Scotson, *The established and the outsiders: a sociological enquiry into community problems* (London: F. Cass, 1965).

Ell, Stephen R., 'Venetian plague of 1630–1', *Janus*, 73 (1986–90), 85–104.

———, 'Three days in October 1630', *Review of infectious diseases*, 11 (1989), 128–39.

Ellero, Giuseppe, *L'archivio IRE: inventario dei fondi antichi degli ospedali e luoghi pii di Venezia* (Venice: IRE, 1987).

Epstein, Steven, *Wills and wealth in medieval Genoa, 1150–1250* (London, Cambridge MA: Harvard University Press, 1984).

Faccini, S., 'L'ospedale dei Santi Giacomo e Lazzaro alla Tomba in età moderna' in Alessandro Pastore, Gian Maria Varanini, Paola Marini and Giorgio Marini (eds), *L'ospedale e la città: cinquecento anni d'arte a Verona* (Verona: Cierre, 1996), pp. 63–67.

Farr, James R., *Artisans in Europe 1300–1914* (Cambridge: Cambridge University Press, 2000).

Farrell, William J., 'The role of Mandeville's bee analogy in "the grumbling hive"', *Studies in English Literature 1500–1900*, 25:3 (1985), 511–27.

Fazzini, Gerolamo (ed.), *Venezia: isola del lazzaretto nuovo* (Venice: [s.n.], 2004).

———, 'Il sale di Venezia', *ArcheoVenezia,* 16 (2006) p. 4.

Ferrari, Ciro, 'L'ufficio di sanità di Padova nella prima metà del sec. XVII', *Miscellanea di storia veneta* 3:1(1910), 1–267.

Ferraro, Joanne, *Family and public life in Brescia, 1580–1650* (Cambridge: Cambridge University Press, 1992).

Findlen, Paula, Michelle M. Fontaine and Duane J. Osheim (eds), *Beyond Florence: the contours of medieval and early modern Italy* (Stanford CA: Stanford University Press, 2003).

Finlay, Robert, *Politics in Renaissance Venice* (London: Ernest Benn, 1980).

———, 'Crisis and crusade in the Mediterranean: Venice, Portugal and the Cape Route to India (1498–1509)', *Studi veneziani*, n.s. 28 (1994), 45–91.

———, 'The Immortal Republic: the myth of Venice during the Italian Wars (1494–1530)', *Sixteenth century journal*, 30 (1999), 931–44.

Finzsch, Norbert and Robert Jütte (eds), *Institutions of confinement: hospitals, asylums and prisons in Western Europe and North America 1500–1950* (Cambridge: Cambridge University Press, 1996).

Flinn, Michael W., 'Plague in Europe and the Mediterranean Countries', *Journal of European Economic History*, 8 (1979), 131–48.

———, *The European Demographic system 1500–1820* (Brighton: Harvester, 1981).

Flood, John L., '"Safer on the battlefield than in the city": England, the "sweating sickness" and the continent', *Renaissance studies* 17:2 (2003), 147–77.

Foligno, Cesare, *The story of Padua* (London: Dent, 1910).

Foucault, Michel, *The birth of the clinic: an archaeology of medical perception* (London: Routledge, 2000).

Frari, Angelo A., *Cenni storici sull'isola di Poveglia e sulla sua importanza sotto l'aspetto sanitario* (Venice, 1837).

Gaier, Martin, *Facciate sacre a scopo profano: Venezia e la politica dei monumenti dal Quattrocento al Settecento* (Venice: Istituto veneto di scienze, lettere ed arti, 2002).

Gaimster, David and Roberta Gilchrist, *The archaeology of Reformation, 1480–1580* (Leeds: Maney, 2003).

Garbellotti, Marina, 'Ospedali e storia nell'Italia moderna: percorsi di ricerca', *Medicina e storia*, 6 (2003), 115–31.

Garcia Ballester, Luis, Roger French, Jon Arrizabalaga and Andrew Cunningham, (eds), *Practical medicine from Salerno to the Black Death* (Cambridge: Cambridge University Press, 1994).

Gazzola, Piero (ed.), *Michele Sanmicheli* (Venice: N. Pozza, 1960).

Geary, Patrick J., *Furta sacra: thefts of relics in the central Middle Ages* (Princeton NJ: Princeton University Press, 1990).

Geltner, Guy, *The medieval prison: a social history* (Princeton NJ: Princeton University Press, 2008).

Gentilcore, David, *From Bishop to Witch: the system of the sacred in early modern Terra d'Otranto* (Manchester: Manchester University Press, 1992).

————, 'All that pertains to medicine: protomedici and protomedicati in early modern Italy', *Medical history*, 38 (1994), 121–42.

————, 'The fear of disease and the disease of fear' in William G. Naphy and Penny Roberts (eds), *Fear in early modern society* (Manchester: Manchester University Press, 1997) pp. 184–208.

————, *Healers and healing in early modern Italy* (Manchester: Manchester University Press, 1998).

————, 'Cradle of saints and useful institutions: health care and poor relief in the Kingdom of Naples' in Andrew Cunningham and Ole P. Grell with Jon Arrizabalaga (eds), *Health care and poor relief in Counter-Reformation Europe* (London: Routledge, 1999), pp. 132–50.

————, 'The Protomedicato tribunals and health in Italian cities 1600–1800: a comparison' in Eugenio Sonnino (ed.), *Living in the city (14th–20th centuries)* (Rome: Casa editrice La Sapienza, 2004), pp. 407–30.

————, 'Charlatans, the regulated marketplace and the treatment of venereal disease in Italy' in Kevin Siena (ed.), *Sins of the flesh: responding to sexual disease in early modern Europe* (Toronto: Centre for Reformation and Renaissance Studies, 2005), pp. 57–80.

————, *Medical charlatanism in early modern Italy* (Oxford: Oxford University Press, 2006).

Gianighian, Giorgio and Paola Pavarini, *Dietro i palazzi: tre secoli di architettura minore a Venezia 1492–1803* (Venice: Arsenale, 1984).

Gilbert, Felix, 'Venice in the League of Cambrai' in John R. Hale (ed.), *Renaissance Venice* (London: Faber and Faber, 1973), pp. 274–92.

Gilman, Sander L., *Disease and representation: images of illness from madness to AIDS* (London: Cornell University Press, 1988).

————, *Health and illness: images of difference* (London: Reaktion Books, 1995).

Girardi, Elisabetta, 'La peste del 1630–1 nell'altopiano dei Sette Comuni', *Archivio Veneto,* 205 (2008), 59–91.

Goldin, Grace, *Works of mercy: a picture history of hospitals* (Ontario: Boston Mills Press 1994).

Gordon, Bruce and Peter Marshall (eds), *The place of the dead: death and remembrance in late medieval and early modern Europe* (Cambridge: Cambridge University Press, 2000).

Gottardi, Michele, 'La situazione socio-sanitaria nel Friuli occidentale durante la peste del 1630', *Studi veneziani*, 6 (1982), 161–93.

Goy, Richard, *Chioggia and the villages of the Venetian lagoon: studies in urban history* (Cambridge: Cambridge University Press, 1985).

————, *Venetian vernacular architecture: traditional housing in the Venetian lagoon* (Cambridge: Cambridge University Press, 1989).

————, *Venice: the city and its architecture* (London: Phaidon, 1999).

Granshaw, Lindsay and Roy Porter (eds), *The hospital in history* (London: Routledge, 1989).

Gray, Louise, 'Petitioning for survival: medical care and welfare provision in early modern German towns', *Medicina e storia*, 6 (2003), 73–91.

Grell, Ole P., 'Plague in Elizabethan and Stuart London: the Dutch response', *Medical history*, 34 (1990), 424–39.

————, 'Conflicting duties: plague and the obligations of early modern physicians towards patients and commonwealth in England and the Netherlands' in Andrew Wear, Johanna Geyer-Kordesch and Roger French (eds), *Doctors and ethics: the earlier historical setting of professional ethics* (Amsterdam: Rodopi, 1993), pp. 131–53.

————, 'Review: The religious duty of care and the social need for control in early modern Europe', *The Historical Journal*, 39 (1996), 257–63.

———— (ed.), *Paracelsus: the man and his reputation, his ideas and their transformation* (Leiden: Brill, 1998).

Grendler, Paul F., 'Francesco Sansovino and Italian popular history 1560–1600', *Studies in the Renaissance*, 16 (1969), 139–80.

Grieco, Allen J., 'Il vitto di un ospedale: pratica, distizioni sociali e teorie mediche alla metà del Quattrocento' in Lucia Sandri (ed.), *Gli Innocenti e Firenze nei secoli: un ospedale, un archivio, una città* (Florence: S.P.E.S., 1996) pp. 85–92.

Groebner, Valentin, *Who are you? Identification, deception and surveillance in early modern Europe* (New York: Zone books, 2007).

Grubb, James S., 'When myths lose power: four decades of Venetian historiography', *Journal of modern history*, 58 (1986), 43–94.

————, *Firstborn of Venice: Vicenza in the early Renaissance state* (London: Johns Hopkins University Press, 1988).

————, *Provincial families of the Renaissance: private and public life in the Veneto* (Baltimore MD: Johns Hopkins University Press, 1996).

Hacke, Daniela, *Women, sex and marriage in early modern Venice* (Aldershot: Ashgate, 2004).

Haitsma Mulier, Eco O.G., *The myth of Venice and Dutch Republican thought in the seventeenth century* (Assen: Van Gorcum, 1980).

Hale, John R. (ed.), *Renaissance Venice* (London: Faber and Faber, 1973).

————, *Renaissance fortification: art or engineering?* (London: Thames and Hudson, 1977).

Hallam, Elizabeth, Jenny Hockey and Glennys Howarth, *Beyond the body: death and social identity* (London: Routledge, 1999).

Harding, Vanessa, 'Burial of the plague dead in early modern London' in Justin A.I. Champion (ed.), *Epidemic disease in London* (London: Centre for Metropolitan History, 1993), pp. 53–64.

————, *The dead and the living in Paris and London 1500–1670* (Cambridge: Cambridge University Press, 2002).

Harris, Jonathan Gil, *Foreign bodies and the body politic: discourses of social pathology in early modern England* (Cambridge: Cambridge University Press, 1998).

————, *Sick economies: drama, mercantilism and disease in Shakespeare's England* (Philadelphia PA: University of Pennsylvania Press, 2004).

Harris, Lawrence E., 'Land drainage and reclamation' in Salvatore Ciriacono (ed.), *Land drainage and irrigation* (Aldershot: Ashgate, 1998), pp. 135–58.

Hatcher, John, *Plague, population and the English economy 1348–1530* (Basingstoke: Macmillan, 1977).

————, 'Understanding the population history of England 1450–1750', *Past and Present*, 180 (2003), 83–130.

————, *The Black Death: an intimate history* (London: Weidenfeld and Nicolson, 2008).

Hayum, Andrée, *The Isenheim altarpiece: God's medicine and the painter's vision* (Princeton NJ: Princeton University Press, 1989).

Healy, Margaret, 'Discourses of the plague in early modern London' in Justin A.I. Champion (ed.) *Epidemic disease in London* (London: Centre for Metropolitan History, 1993), pp. 19–34.

————, *Fictions of disease in early modern England: bodies, plagues and politics* (Basingstoke: Palgrave, 2001).

Henderson, John, *Piety and charity in late medieval Florence* (Oxford: Clarendon Press, 1994).

————, 'Healing the body and saving the soul: hospitals in Renaissance Florence', *Renaissance studies*, 15 (2001), 188–216.

————, '"La schifezza, madre di corruzione": Peste e società a Firenze nella prima epoca moderna', *Medicina e storia*, 2 (2001), 23–56.

————, 'Historians and plagues in pre-industrial Italy over the longue durée', *History and philosophy of the life sciences,* 25 (2003), 481–99.

————, *The Renaissance hospital: healing the body and healing the soul* (London: Yale University Press, 2006).

Henderson, John and Katherine P. Park, '"The first hospital among Christians": the ospedale di Santa Maria Nuova in early sixteenth-century Florence', *Medical history*, 35 (1991), 164–88.

Henderson, John and Richard Wall (eds), *Poor women and children in the European past* (London: Routledge, 1994).

Herlihy, David, 'The population of Verona in the first century of Venetian rule' in John R. Hale (ed.), *Renaissance Venice* (London: Faber and Faber, 1973), pp. 91–121.

————, *The Black Death and the transformation of the West* (Cambridge MA: Harvard University Press, 1997).

Herlihy, David and Christine Klapisch-Zuber, *Tuscans and their families: a study of the Florentine catasto of 1427* (London: Yale University Press, 1985).

Hillman, David and Carla Mazzio (eds), *The body in parts: fantasies of corporeality in early modern Europe* (London: Routledge, 1997).

Hills, Helen, *Invisible city: the architecture of devotion in seventeenth-century Neapolitan convents* (Oxford: Oxford University Press, 2004).

Hindle, Steve, *On the parish? The micropolitics of poor relief in rural England c.1550–1750* (Oxford: Clarendon, 2004).

Hinnells, John R. and Roy Porter (eds), *Religion, health and suffering* (London: Kegan Paul International, 1999).

Hirst, Leonard F., *The conquest of plague* (Oxford: Clarendon Press, 1953).

Hocquet, Jean-Claude, *Il sale e la fortuna di Venezia* (Rome: Jouvence, 1996).

Honeybourne, Marjorie B., 'The leper hospitals of the London area', *Transactions of the London and Middlesex archaeological society*, 21 (1967), 1–61.

Hopkins, Andrew, 'Architecture and "infirmitas": Doge Andrea Gritti and the chancel of San Marco', *Journal of the society of architectural historians*, 57 (1998), 182–97.

———, *Santa Maria della Salute: architecture and ceremony in Baroque Venice* (Cambridge: Cambridge University Press, 2000).

Horrox, Rosemary (ed.), *The Black Death* (Manchester: Manchester University Press, 1994).

Howard, Deborah, *Jacopo Sansovino: architecture and patronage in Renaissance Venice* (London: Yale University Press, 1975).

———, *Venice and the East: the impact of the Islamic world on Venetian architecture 1100–1500* (London: Yale University Press, 2000).

———, *The architectural history of Venice* (London: Yale University Press, 2002).

Howe, Eunice, 'The architecture of institutionalisation: women's space in Renaissance hospitals' in Helen Hills (ed.), *Architecture and the politics of gender in early modern Europe* (Aldershot: Ashgate, 2003) pp. 63–82.

Huguet-Termes, Teresa, 'Carità e sanità per una nuova capitale: Madrid asburgica (1561–1700)', *Medicina e storia*, 6 (2003), 93–113.

———, 'Madrid hospitals and welfare in the context of the Habsburg empire' in Teresa Huguet-Termes, Jon Arrizabalaga and Harold J. Cook (eds), *Health and medicine in Habsburg Spain: agents, practices, representations* (London: Wellcome Trust Centre for the History of Medicine at UCL, 2009), pp. 64–88.

Hurlburt, Holly S., *The Dogaressa of Venice, 1200–1500: wife and icon* (Basingstoke: Palgrave Macmillan, 2006).

Ingold, Tim, *The perception of the environment: essays on livelihood, dwelling and skill* (London: Routledge, 2000).

Jardine, Lisa, *Wordly goods: a new history of the Renaissance* (London: Macmillan, 1996).

Jenner, Mark S., 'The great dog massacre' in William G. Naphy and Penny Roberts (eds), *Fear in early modern society* (Manchester: Manchester University Press, 1997), pp. 44–61.

———, 'Underground, overground: pollution and place in urban history', *Journal of urban history*, 24 (1997), 97–110.

———, 'Civilization and deodorization? Smell in early modern English culture' in Peter Burke, Brian Harrison and Paul Slack (eds), *Civil histories: essays presented to Sir Keith Thomas* (Oxford: Oxford University Press, 2000), pp. 127–44.

Jenner, Mark S.R. and Patrick Wallis, *Medicine and the market in England and its colonies, c.1450–c.1850* (Basingstoke: Palgrave Macmillan, 2007).

Jones, Colin, 'The construction of the hospital patient in early modern France' in Norbert Finzsch and Robert Jütte (eds), *Institutions of confinement: hospitals, asylums and prisons in Western Europe and North America 1500–1950* (Cambridge: Cambridge University Press, 1996), pp. 55–75.

———, 'Languages of plague in early modern France' in Sally Sheard and Helen J. Power (eds), *Body and city: histories of urban public health* (Aldershot: Ashgate, 2000), pp. 41–9.

Jütte, Robert, *Poverty and deviance in early modern Europe* (Cambridge: Cambridge University Press, 1994).

Kinzelbach, Anne-Marie, 'Hospitals, medicine and society: southern German imperial towns in the sixteenth century', *Renaissance studies*, 15 (2001), 217–28.

———, 'Infection, contagion and public health in late medieval and early modern German Imperial towns', *Journal of the history of medicine and allied sciences*, 61 (2006), 369–89.

Kohl, Benjamin G., *Culture and politics in early Renaissance Padua* (Aldershot: Ashgate, 2001).

Konstantinidou, Katerina, 'Gli Uffici di Sanità delle isole ionie durante il seicento e il settecento', *Studi veneziani*, 49 (2005), 379–91.

Koslofsky, Craig, *The Reformation of the dead: death and ritual in early modern Germany, 1450–1700* (Basingstoke: Palgrave, 2000).

Kovesi Killerby, Catherine, *Sumptuary law in Italy, 1200–1500* (Oxford: Clarendon Press, 2002).

Krekić, Bariša, *Dubrovnik in the fourteenth and fifteenth centuries: a city between East and West* (Norman OK: University of Oklahoma Press, 1972).

Kromm, Jane, 'Domestic spatial economies and Dutch charitable institutions in the late sixteenth and early seventeenth centuries' in Sandra Cavallo and Silvia Evangelisti (eds), *Domestic Institutional Interiors in Early Modern Europe* (Aldershot: Ashgate, 2009), pp. 109–11.

La Cava, A. Francesco, *La peste di S Carlo: note storico-mediche sulla peste 1576* (Milan: U. Hoepli, 1945).

Lanaro, Paola, '"Essere famiglia di consiglio": social closure and economic change in the Veronese patriciate of the sixteenth century', *Renaissance studies*, 8 (1994), 428–38.

———, 'Carità e assistenza, paure e segregazione: le istituzioni ospedaliere veronesi nel cinque e seicento verso la specializzazione' in Alessandro Pastore, Gian Maria Varanini, Paola Marini and Giorgio Marini (eds), *L'ospedale e la città: cinquecento anni d'arte a Verona* (Verona: Cierre, 1996), pp. 43–57.

——— (ed.), *At the centre of the old world: trade and manufacturing in Venice and the Venetian mainland 1400–1800* (Toronto: Centre for Reformation and Renaissance Studies, 2006).

Lanaro Sartori, Paola, 'L'attività di prestito dei monti di pietà in terraferma veneta: legalità e illeciti tra quattrocento e primo seicento', *Studi storici Luigi Simeoni*, 33 (1983), 161–77.

———, 'Patrizi e poveri. Assistenza controllo sociale e carità nella Verona rinescimentale' in Amelio Tagliaferri (ed.), *I ceti dirigenti in Italia in età moderna e contemporanea* (Udine: Del Bianco, 1984), pp. 131–49.

———, *Un'oligarchia urbana nel Cinquecento veneto: istituzioni, economia, società* (Turin: G. Giappichelli, 1992).

Lane, Frederic C., *Venice and history: the collected papers of Frederic C. Lane* (Baltimore MD: Johns Hopkins University Press, 1966).

Lanfranchi, Luigi (ed.), *S Giorgio Maggiore* (Venice: Il Comitato Editore, 1968).

Langenskiöld, Eric, *Michele Sanmicheli: the architect of Verona* (Uppsala: Almquist & Wiksells, 1938).

Laven, David, *Venice and Venetia under the Habsburgs, 1815–1835* (Oxford: Oxford University Press, 2002).

Laven, Mary, *Virgins of Venice: broken vows and cloistered lives in the Renaissance convent* (Harmondsworth: Penguin, 2003).

Laven, Peter, 'The Venetian rivers in the sixteenth century' in Jean-François Bergier (ed.), *Montagnes, fleuves, forêts dans l'histoire: barrières, ou lignes de convergence?* (St Katharinen: Scripta Mercaturae, 1989), pp. 198–217.

———, 'Venice and her Dominions, 1381–1797', *The Historical Journal*, 37 (1994), 447–55.

———, 'Banditry and lawlessness on the Venetian terraferma in the later Cinquecento' in Trevor Dean and Kate J.P. Lowe (eds), *Crime, society and the law in Renaissance Italy* (Cambridge: Cambridge University Press, 1994), pp. 221–48.

Law, John E., 'Venice and the "closing" of the Veronese constitution in 1405', *Studi veneziani*, n.s. 1 (1977), 69–103.

———, 'The cittadella of Verona' in David S. Chambers, Cecil H. Clough and Michael E. Mallett, *War, culture and society in Renaissance Venice* (London: Hambledon Press, 1993), pp. 9–27.

———, *Venice and the Veneto in the early Renaissance* (Aldershot: Ashgate, 2000).

Le Goff, Jacques, 'Head or heart? The political use of body metaphors in the Middle Ages' in Michael Feher, Ramona Naddaff and Nadia Tazi (eds), *Fragments for a history of the human body* (3 vols, New York: Zone, 1989), volume three, pp. 13–26.

———, *The birth of Purgatory*, Arthur Goldhammer (trans.) (Aldershot: Ashgate, 1990).

Lindemann, Mary, *Health and healing in eighteenth-century Germany* (London: Johns Hopkins University Press, 1996).

———, *Medicine and society in early modern Europe* (Cambridge: Cambridge University Press, 1999).

Livi Bacci, Massimo, *Population and nutrition: an essay on European demographic history* (Cambridge: Cambridge University Press, 1991).

McCray Beier, Lucinda, 'In sickness and in health: a seventeenth-century family's experience' in Roy Porter (ed.), *Patients and practitioners: lay perceptions of medicine in pre-industrial society* (Cambridge: Cambridge University Press, 1985), pp. 101–28.

McGough, Laura, 'Quarantining beauty: the French disease in early modern Venice', in Kevin Siena (ed.), *Sins of the flesh: responding to the French disease in early modern Europe* (Toronto: Centre for Reformation and Renaissance Studies, 2005), pp. 212–37.

———, *Gender, sexuality and syphilis in early modern Venice: the disease that came to stay* (London: Palgrave Macmillan, 2011).

McHugh, Tim J., 'Establishing medical men at the Paris Hotel-Dieu, 1500–1715', *Social history of medicine*, 19:2 (2006), 209–24.

McVaugh, Michael R., *Medicine before the plague: practitioners and their patients in the Crown of Aragon 1285–1345* (Cambridge: Cambridge University Press, 1993).

Mackenney, Richard, *Tradesmen and traders: the world of the guilds in Venice and Europe c.1250–c.1650* (London: Croom Helm, 1987).

———, 'Letters from the Venetian archive', in Brian Pullan and Susan Reynolds (eds), *Towns and townspeople in Medieval and Renaissance Europe: essays in memory of J.K. Hyde, Bulletin of the John Rylands University Library of Manchester* 72:3 (1990), 133–44.

———, 'Continuity and change in the *scuole piccole*', *Renaissance studies*, 8 (1994), 388–404.

———, 'Public and private in Renaissance Venice', *Renaissance studies*, 12 (1998), 109–131.

Mallett, Michael E., 'Ambassadors and their audiences in Renaissance Italy', *Renaissance studies*, 8 (1994), 229–43.

Mallett, Michael E. and John R. Hale *The military organisation of a Renaissance state: Venice c.1400–1617* (Cambridge: Cambridge University Press, 1984).

Manconi, Francesco, *Castigo de Dios: la grande peste barocca nella Sardegna di Filippo IV* (Rome: Donzelli, 1994).

Marchi, Gian Paolo, *'Il gran contagio di Verona' di Francesco Pona* (Verona: Centro per la formazione professionale grafica, 1972).

Marino, John, *Early modern Italy* (Oxford: Oxford University Press, 2002).

Marshall, Louise, 'Manipulating the sacred: image and plague in Renaissance Italy', *Renaissance quarterly*, 47 (1994), 485–532.

Martin, A. Lynn, *Plague? Jesuit accounts of epidemic disease in the sixteenth century* (Kirksville MO: Sixteenth Century Journal Publishers, 1996).

Martin, John J., *Venice's hidden enemies: Italian heretics in a Renaissance city* (Berkeley CA: University of California Press, 1993).

Martin, John and Dennis Romano (eds), *Venice reconsidered. The history and civilisation of an Italian city-state 1297–1797* (London: Johns Hopkins University Press, 2000).

Martin, Ruth, *Witchcraft and the Inquisition in Venice, 1550–1650* (Oxford: Blackwell, 1989).

Martz, Linda, *Poverty and welfare in Habsburg Spain: the example of Toledo* (Cambridge: Cambridge University Press, 1983).

Masiero, Franco, *Le isole delle lagune venete: natura, storia, arte, turismo* (Milan: Mursia, 1981).

Meneghini, Gino, *La peste del 1576 a Padova* (Padua: Officine grafiche Stediv, 1956).

Mezzetti, Carlo, Giorgio Bucciarelli and Fausto Pugnaloni, *Il lazzaretto di Ancona: un'opera dimenticata* (Ancona: Cassa di risparmio di Ancona, 1978).

Molà, Luca, *The silk industry of Renaissance Venice* (London: Johns Hopkins University Press, 2000).

Molmenti, Pompeo, *La storia di Venezia nella vita privata dalle origini alla caduta della Repubblica* (3 vols, Bergamo: Istituto italiano d'arti grafiche, 1906), *parte seconda: lo splendore*.

Monahan, Patrick, 'Sanudo and the Venetian villa surburbana', *Annali di architettura*, 21 (2009), 151–67.

Mooney, Graham and Jonathan Reinarz (eds), *Permeable walls: historical perspectives on hospital and asylum visiting* (Amsterdam: Rodopi, 2009).

Morman, Edward T., 'Guarding against alien impurities: the Philadelphia lazaretto, 1854–93', *The Pennsylvania magazine of history and biography*, 108:2 (1984), 131–52.

Morpurgo, Emilio, 'Lo studio di Padova, le epidemie e i contagi durante il governo dell Repubblica veneta' in *Memorie e documenti per la storia della Università di Padova* (Padua: La Garangola, 1922), pp. 107–240.

Mozzato, Andrea, *La Mariegola dell'Arte della Lana di Venezia 1244–1594* (Venice: Comitato per la pubblicazione delle fonti relative alla storia di Venezia, 2002).

Mueller, Reinhold C., 'Charitable institutions, Jewish communities and Venetian society', *Studi veneziani*, 14 (1972), 37–83.

———, *The Procuratori di San Marco and the Venetian credit market* (New York: Arno Press, 1977).

———, 'Aspetti sociali ed economici della peste a Venezia nel Medioevo' in *Venezia e la peste 1348–1797* (Venice, 1980), pp. 71–92.

———, *Money and banking in Renaissance Venice,* volume two, 'The Venetian money market: Banks, panics, and the public debt, 1200–1500' (London: Johns Hopkins University Press, 1997).

Muir, Edward, 'Images of power: art and pageantry in Renaissance Venice', *American historical review*, 84 (1979), 16–52.

———, *Civic ritual in Renaissance Venice* (Princeton NJ: Princeton University Press, 1981).

————, 'Mad blood stirring': vendetta and factions in Friuli during the Renaissance (London: Johns Hopkins University Press, 1993).

————, Ritual in early modern Europe (Cambridge: Cambridge University Press, 1997).

————, 'The Virgin on the street corner' in Steven Ozment (ed.), Religion and culture in the Renaissance and the Reformation (Kirksville MO: Sixteenth Century Journal Publishers, 1998), pp. 25–42.

————, 'Was there Republicanism in the Renaissance republics? Venice after Agnadello' in John Martin and Dennis Romano (eds), Venice reconsidered. The history and civilisation of an Italian city-state 1297–1797 (London: Johns Hopkins University Press, 2000), pp. 137–67.

Muir, Edward and Ronald F.E. Weissman, 'Social and symbolic places in Renaissance Venice and Florence' in John A. Agnew and James S. Duncan (eds), The power of place: bringing together geographical and social imaginations (London: Unwin Hyman, 1989), pp. 81–103.

Muldrew, Craig, The economy of obligation: the culture of credit and social relations in early modern England (Basingstoke: Macmillan, 1998).

Mullett, Charles F., 'Plague policy in Scotland 16th–17th Centuries', Osiris, 9 (1950), 435–56.

Munkhoff, Richelle, 'Searchers of the dead: authority, marginality and the interpretation of plague in England (1574–1665)', Gender and history 11 (1999), 1–29.

Najemy, John, Italy in the age of the Renaissance (Oxford: Oxford University Press, 2004).

Naphy, William G., Plagues, poisons and potions: plague-spreading conspiracies in the western alps c.1530–1640 (Manchester: Manchester University Press, 2003).

Naphy, William G. and Penny Roberts (eds), Fear in early modern society (Manchester: Manchester University Press, 1997).

Nichols, Charlotte, 'Plague and politics in early modern Naples: the relics of San Gennaro' in Laurinda S. Dixon, In sickness and in health: disease as metaphor in art and popular wisdom (Newark NJ: University of Delaware Press, 2004), pp. 21–45.

Nockels Fabbri, Christiane, 'Treating medieval plague: the wonderful virtues of theriac', Early science and medicine 12 (2007), 247–83.

Nutton, Vivian, 'The seeds of disease: an explanation of contagion and infection from the Greeks to the Renaissance' in Vivian Nutton (ed.), From Democedes to Harvey: studies in the history of medicine (London: Variorum Reprints, 1983), pp. 1–34.

————, 'Humanist surgery' in Andrew Wear, Roger K. French and Iain M. Lonie (eds), The medical Renaissance of the sixteenth century (Cambridge, 1985), pp. 75–100.

———— (ed.), Medicine at the courts of Europe 1500–1837 (London: Routledge, 1990).

————, *Ancient medicine* (New York: Taylor & Francis, 2004).

———— (ed.), *Pestilential complexities: understanding medieval plague* (London: Wellcome Trust Centre for the History of Medicine at UCL, 2008).

Olivieri, A., 'Il medico ebreo nella Venezia del Quattrocento e Cinquecento' in Gaetano Cozzi (ed.), *Gli ebrei a Venezia sec XIV–XVIII* (Milan: Edizioni Comunità, 1987), pp. 449–68.

O'Malley, Michelle and Evelyn Welch (eds), *The material Renaissance* (Manchester: Manchester University Press, 2007).

Origo, Iris, *The world of San Bernardino* (London: Jonathan Cape, 1963).

Pagel, Walter, *Paracelsus: an introduction to philosophical medicine in the era of the Renaissance* (New York: Kargel, 1958).

Palmer, Richard J, 'Physicians and surgeons in sixteenth-century Venice', *Medical history*, 23 (1979), 451–60.

————, 'Nicolo Massa: his family and his fortune', *Medical history*, 25 (1981), 385–410.

————, 'Physicians and the state in post-medieval Italy' in Andrew W. Russell (ed.), *The town and state physicians in Europe from the Middle Ages to the Enlightenment* (Wolfenbüttel: Herzog August Bibliothek, 1981), pp. 47–61.

————, 'The Church, leprosy and plague in medieval and early modern Europe', *Studies in Church History*, 19 (1982), 79–101.

————, *The studio of Venice and its graduates in the sixteenth century* (Padua: Edizioni LINT, 1983).

————, 'Pharmacy in the Republic of Venice in the sixteenth century' in Andrew Wear, Roger K. French and Iain M. Lonie (eds), *The medical Renaissance of the sixteenth century* (Cambridge: Cambridge University Press, 1985), pp. 100–18.

————, 'Medical botany in northern Italy in the Renaissance', *Journal of the Royal Society of Medicine*, 78 (1985), 149–57.

————, 'Health, hygiene and longevity in medieval and Renaissance Europe' in Yosio Kawakita, Shizu Sakai and Yasuo Otsuka (eds), *History of hygiene* (Toyko: Ishiyaku EuroAmerica Inc., 1987), pp. 75–98.

————, 'Physicians and the Inquisition in sixteenth-century Venice: the case of Girolamo Donzellini' in Andrew Cunningham and Ole P. Grell (eds), *Medicine and the Reformation* (London: Routledge, 1993), pp. 118–34.

————, '"Ad una sancta perfettione": health care and poor relief in the Republic of Venice in the era of the Counter-Reformation' in Andrew Cunningham, Ole P. Grell with Jon Arrizabalaga (eds), *Health care and poor relief in Counter Reformation Europe* (London: Routledge, 1999), pp. 87–102.

————, *Catalogue of western manuscripts in the Wellcome library for the Understanding and History of Medicine 5120–6244* (London: Wellcome Trust, 2000).

————, 'In bad odour: smell and its significance in medicine from antiquity to the seventeenth century' in William F. Bynum and Roy Porter (eds), *Medicine and the five senses* (Cambridge: Cambridge University Press, 2005), pp. 61–9.

Panzac, Daniel, *Quarantaines et lazarets: l'Europe et la peste d'Orient (XVIIe–XXe siècles)* (Aix-en-Provence: Édisud, 1986).

Pastore, Alessandro, *Crimine e giustizia in tempo di peste dell'Europa moderna* (Rome: Laterza, 1991).

———, 'L'organizzazione sanitaria nella Repubblica di Venezia al tempo di William Harvey' in Giuseppe Ongaro, Maurizio Rippa Bonati and Gaetano Thiene (eds), *Harvey e Padova* (Treviso: Antilia, 2006), pp. 201–17.

Pastore, Alessandro, Gian Maria Varanini, Paola Marini and Giorgio Marini (eds), *L'ospedale e la città: cinquecento anni d'arte a Verona* (Verona: Cierre, 1996).

Pellegrini, Francesco, *Un consulto di Gerolamo Fracastoro per Giovanni Matteo Giberti vescovo di Verona* (Verona: R. Cabianca, 1934).

———, 'Frammento inedito di Gerolamo Fracastoro riguardante la pestilenza del 1534–35', *Rivista di storia della scienze, mediche e naturali*, 26 (1935), 11–12.

———, 'L'epidemia di "morbus peticularis" del 1546–47 e il medico del concilio di Trento', *Rivista Castalla*, 2:5 (1946), 1–8.

———, 'Il lazzaretto di Verona', *Studi storici veronese*, 2 (1949–50), 143–93.

Pelling, Margaret, 'Medicine and the environment in Shakespeare's England' in *The common lot: sickness, medicine and the urban poor in early modern England* (London: Longman, 1998), pp. 19–38.

Pelling, Margaret with Frances White, *Medical conflicts in early modern London: patronage, physicians and irregular practitioners, 1550–1640* (Oxford: Clarendon Press, 2003).

Perry, Mary Elizabeth, 'Finding Fatima, a slave woman of early modern Spain', *Journal of Women's History*, 20:1 (2008), 151–67.

Pesce, Luigi, 'Gli statuti (1486) del Lazzaretto di Treviso composti dal Rolandello', *Archivio Veneto*, quinta serie, CXII (1979), 33–71.

Pettegree, Andrew (ed.), *The Reformation World* (London: Routledge, 200).

Pezzolo, Luciano, *L'oro dello stato: società, finanza e fisco nella Repubblica veneta del secondo '500* (Venice: Il cardo, 1990).

Pighi, Giovanni Battista et al. (eds), *Verona e il suo territorio* (6 vols, Verona: Istituto per gli studi storici veronesi, 1995).

Piva, Luigi, *Le pestilenze nel Veneto* (Camposanpiero: Edizioni del noce, 1991).

Po-chia Hsia, Ronnie, 'Civic wills as sources for the study of piety in Muenster 1530–1618', *Sixteenth century journal*, 14 (1983), 321–48.

Polecritti, Cynthia L., 'In the shop of the Lord: Bernardino of Siena and popular devotion' in Paula Findlen, Michelle M. Fontaine and Duane J. Osheim (eds), *Beyond Florence: the contours of medieval and early modern Italy* (Stanford CA: Stanford University Press, 2003), pp. 147–59.

Politi, Giorgio, Mario Rosa and Franco della Peruta (eds), *Timore e carità: i poveri nell'Italia moderna: atti del convegno 'Pauperismo e assistenza negli antichi stati italiani'* (Cremona: Biblioteca statale e librería civica di Cremona, 1982).

Pomata, Gianna, *Contracting a cure: patients, healers and the law in early modern Bologna* (London: Johns Hopkins University Press, 1998).

Porter, Roy, 'History of the body' in Peter Burke (ed.), *New perspectives on historical writing* (Cambridge: Polity Press, 1991), pp. 206–32.

———, 'Howard's beginnings: prisons, disease, hygiene' in Richard Creese, William F. Bynum and Joe Bearn (eds), *The health of prisoners: historical essays* (Amsterdam: Rodolpi, 1995), pp. 5–26.

——— (ed.), *Cambridge illustrated history of medicine* (Cambridge: Cambridge University Press, 1996).

Porter, Roy and George S. Rousseau, *Gout: the patrician malady* (London: Yale University Press, 1998).

Porter, Roy and Andrew Wear (eds), *Problems and methods in the history of medicine* (London: Croom Helm, 1987).

Povolo, Claudio, 'Centro e perifera nella Repubblica di Venezia: un profilo' in Giorgio Chittolini, Anthony Molho and Pierangelo Shiera (eds), *Origini dello stato processi di formazione statale Italia fra medioevo ed età moderna* (Bologna: Il Mulino, 1994), pp. 207–25.

Preto, Paolo, *Peste e società a Venezia nel 1576* (Vicenza: N. Pozza, 1978).

———, *Epidemia, paura e politica nell'Italia moderna* (Bari: Laterza, 1987).

———, 'Gli Emarginati' in Giuseppe Galasso (ed.), *Mentalità, comportamenti e istituzioni tra Rinascimento e decadenza 1550–1700* (Milan: Electa, 1988), pp. 158–77.

———, 'Le grandi paure di Venezia nel secondo '500: le paure naturali (peste, carestie, incendi, terremoti)' in Vittore Branca and Carlo Ossola (eds), *Crisi e rinnovamenti nell'autunno del rinascimento a Venezia* (Florence: Leo S. Olschki, 1991), pp. 177–92.

———, *I servizi segreti di Venezia* (Milan: Il Saggiatore, 1994).

Prodi, Paolo, *Disciplina dell'anima, disciplina del corpo e disciplina della società tra medioevo ed età moderna* (Bologna: Società editrice il Mulino, 1994).

Pullan, Brian (ed.), *Crisis and change in the Venetian economy in the sixteenth and seventeenth centuries* (London: Methuen, 1968).

———, *Rich and poor in Renaissance Venice: the social institutions of a Catholic state, to 1620* (Oxford: Blackwell, 1971).

———, 'The old Catholicism, the new Catholicism and the poor' in Giorgio Politi, Rosa, Mario and della Peruta, Franco (eds), *Timore e carità: i poveri nell'Italia moderna: atti del convegno 'Pauperismo e assistenza negli antichi stati italiani'* (Cremona: Biblioteca statale e librería civica di Cremona, 1982), pp. 13–25.

———, 'Support and redeem: charity and poor relief in Italian cities from the fourteenth to the seventeenth century', *Continuity and Change*, 3 (1988), 177–208.

———, 'Plague and perceptions of the poor' in Paul Slack and Terence Ranger (eds), *Epidemics and ideas: essays on the historical perception of pestilence* (Cambridge: Cambridge University Press, 1992), pp. 101–25.

———, 'Orphans and foundlings in early modern Europe', *Poverty and charity: Europe, Italy, Venice, 1400–1700* (Aldershot: Ashgate, 1994) III, pp. 5–18.

————, 'The Counter Reformation, medical care and poor relief' in Ole P. Grell, Andrew Cunningham and Jon Arrizabalaga (eds), *Health care and poor relief in Counter Reformation Europe* (London: Routledge, 1999), pp. 18–40.

————, 'Catholics, Protestants and the poor in early modern Europe', *Journal of interdisciplinary history*, 35:3 (2005), 441–56.

Puppi, Lionello (ed.), *Ritratto di Verona: lineamenti di una storia urbanistica* (Verona: Banca popolare di Verona, 1978).

———— (ed.), *Alvise Cornaro e il suo tempo: catalogo di una mostra* (Padua: Comune di Padova, 1980).

————, *Palladio e Venezia* (Florence: Sansoni, 1982).

————, *Michele Sanmicheli architetto: opera completa* (Rome: Caliban Editrice, 1986).

Puppi, Lionello, Giandomenico Romanelli and Susanna Biadene (eds), *Longhena* (Milan: Electa, 1982).

Puppi, Lionello and Mario Universo, *Padova* (Rome: Laterza, 1982).

Rankin, Alisha, 'Becoming an expert practitioner: court experimentalism and the medical skills of Anna of Saxony (1532–1585)', *Isis* 98 (2007), 23–53.

Rapp, Richard T., *Industry and economic decline in seventeenth-century Venice* (Cambridge MA: Harvard University Press, 1976).

Ravid, Benjamin, 'The religious, economic and social background and context of the establishment of the Ghetti of Venice' in Gaetano Cozzi (ed.), *Gli ebrei e Venezia secoli XIV–XVIII* (Milan: Edizioni Comunità, 1987), pp. 211–59.

Rawcliffe, Carole, *Medicine for the soul: the life, death and resurrection of an English Medieval hospital* (Stroud: Sutton, 1999).

————, 'The seventh comfortable work: charity and mortality in the Medieval hospital', *Medicina e storia*, 3 (2003), pp. 11–35.

————, *Leprosy in Medieval England* (Woodbridge: Boydell Press, 2006).

————, 'Delectable sightes and fragrant smelles: gardens and health in late medieval and early modern England', *Garden History*, 36:1 (2008), 3–22.

————, 'A marginal occupation? The medieval laundress and her work', *Gender and history* 21:1 (2009), 147–69.

Relazioni dei rettori veneti in terraferma vol IV: Podestaria e capitanato di Padova (Milan: Giuffrè, 1975).

Relazioni dei rettori veneti in terraferma vol IX: Podestaria e capitanato di Verona (Milan: Giuffrè, 1977).

Reynolds, Barbara (ed.), *Cambridge Italian dictionary* (2 vols, Cambridge: Cambridge University Press, 1981).

Rigoli, Paolo, 'Il virtuoso in gabbia: musicisti in quarantena al lazzaretto di Verona (1655–1740)' in Francesco Passadore and Franco Rossi (eds), *Musica, scienza e idee nella Serenissima durante il Seicento* (Venice: Fondazione Levi, 1996), pp. 139–50.

Riis, Thomas (ed.), *Aspects of poverty in early modern Europe* (Alphen aan den Rijn: Sijthoff, 1981).

Rinne, Katherine W., *The waters of Rome: aqueducts, fountains and the birth of the Baroque city* (London: Yale University Press, 2010).

Risse, Günter B., *Mending bodies, saving souls: a history of hospitals* (Oxford: Oxford University Press, 1999).

Rizzi, Alberto, *Vere da pozzo di Venezia: i puteali pubblici di Venezia e della sua laguna* (Venice: Stamperia di Venezia editrice, 1981).

———, *Scultura esterna a Venezia: corpus delle sculture erratiche all'aperto di Venezia della sua laguna* (Venice: Stamperia di Venezia editrice, 1987).

———, *I leoni di San Marco: il simbolo della Repubblica veneta nella scultura e nella pittura* (2 vols, Venice: Arsenale, 2001).

Roberts, Penny, 'Agencies human and divine fire in French cities, 1520–1720' in William G. Naphy and Penny Roberts (eds), *Fear in early modern society* (Manchester: Manchester University Press, 1997), pp. 9–27.

Rodenwaldt, Ernst, *Pest in Venedig 1575–7: ein Beitrag zur Frage der Infektkette bei den Pestepidemien West-Europas* (Heidelberg: Springer, 1953).

Rösch, Gerhard, *Venedig und das Reich: Handels- und verkehrspolitische Beziehungen in der deutschen Kaiserzeit* (Tübingen: Niemeyer, 1982).

Romano, Dennis, 'Gender and the urban geography of Renaissance Venice', *Journal of social history*, 23 (1989), 339–55.

———, 'Aspects of patronage in fifteenth- and sixteenth-century Venice', *Renaissance quarterly*, 46 (1993), 712–33.

———, *Housecraft and statecraft: domestic service in Renaissance Venice, 1400–1600* (London: Johns Hopkins University Press, 1996).

Roper, Lyndal, *Witch craze: terror and fantasy in Baroque Germany* (London: Yale University Press, 2004).

Rosand, Ellen, 'Music in the myth of Venice', *Renaissance quarterly*, 30 (1977), 511–37.

Rossetto, Luca (ed.), *La giustizia penale delegata a Padova (sec XVI–XVIII) Aspetti storici e documentari* (Venice: Archivio di Stato, 2006).

Rousseau, George S. (ed.), *Framing and imagining disease in cultural history* (Basingstoke: Palgrave Macmillan, 2003).

Rublack, Ulinka, 'Fluxes: the early modern body and the emotions', *History Workshop Journal* 53 (2002), 1–16.

———, *Dressing up: cultural identity in Renaissance Europe* (Oxford: Oxford University Press, 2010).

Rubinstein, Nicolai, *The palazzo vecchio, 1298–1532: government, architecture and imagery in the civic palace of the Florentine Republic* (Oxford: Clarendon Press, 1995).

Rudmann, Valnea, 'Lettera della canzone per la peste di Venezia di Maffio Venier', *Atti dell'Istituto veneto di scienze, lettere ed arti,* 121 (1962–3), 600–41.

Rushton, Neil S., 'Monastic charitable provision in Tudor England: quantifying and qualifying poor relief in the early sixteenth century', *Continuity and Change*, 16 (2001), 9–44.

Russell, Andrew W. (ed.), *The town and state physicians in Europe from the Middle Ages to the Enlightenment* (Wolfenbüttel: Herzog August Bibliothek, 1981).

Rütten, Thomas, 'Cholera in Thomas Mann's Death in Venice', *Gesnerus* 66:2 (2009), pp. 256–87.

Sahlins, Peter, *Boundaries: the making of France and Spain in the Pyrenees* (Berkeley CA: University of California Press, 1989).

Sancassini, Giulio, 'Le lettere dell'archivio della Sanità di Verona', *Notizie degli Archivi di Stato*, 8 (1948), 182–85.

———, 'Il lazzaretto di Verona è del Sanmicheli?' *Atti e memorie della Accademia di agricoltura, scienze e lettere di Verona*, VI (1958–9), 365–77.

Sarti, Raffaella, *Europe at home: family and material culture, 1500–1800* (London: Yale University Press, 2002).

Savelli, R., 'Dalle confraternite allo stato: il sistema assistenziale Genovese nel Cinquecento', *Atti della società ligure di storia patria*, nuova serie XXIV (1984), 171–216.

Savona–Ventura, Charles, *Knight hospitaller medicine in Malta 1530–1798* (Malta: PEG, 2004).

Sawday, Jonathan, *The body emblazoned: dissection and the human body in Renaissance culture* (London: Routledge, 1995).

Scarpa, Tiziano, *Venezia è un pesce: una guida* (Milan: Feltrinelli, 2005).

Schama, Simon, *Embarrassment of riches: an interpretation of Dutch culture in the golden age* (London: Fontana, 1991).

———, *Landscape and memory* (New York: Vintage Books, 1995).

Schmidt, Ariadne, 'Managing a large household. The gender division of work in orphanages in Dutch towns in the early modern period, 1580–1800', *History of the family* 13 (2008), 42–57.

Šćitaroci, Mladen O., 'The Renaissance gardens of the Dubrovnik area, Croatia', *Garden History* 24:3 (1996), 184–200.

Schneider, Robert A., 'Crown and capitoulat: municipal government in Toulouse 1500–1789' in Philip Benedict (ed.), *Cities and social change in early modern France* (London: Unwin Hyman, 1989), pp. 195–220.

Schulz, Jürgen, *The printed plans and panoramic views of Venice (1486–1797)* (Florence: L.S. Olschki, 1970).

Schupbach, William M., 'A Venetian plague miracle in 1464 and 1576', *Medical history*, 20 (1976), 312–16.

Sciolla, Gianni Carlo (ed.), *La città ideale nel Rinascimento* (Turin: UTET, 1995).

Screpanti, Ernesto, *L'angelo della liberazione nel tumult dei Ciompi: Firenze, giugno-agosto 1378* (Siena: Protagon, 2008).

Sennett, Richard, *Flesh and stone: the body and the city in Western civilization* (London: Faber and Faber, 1994).

Shaw, James E., *The justice of Venice: authorities and liberties in the urban economy, 1550–1700* (Oxford: Oxford University Press, 2006).

Shaw, James E. and Evelyn Welch, *Making and Marketing Medicine in Renaissance Florence* (Amsterdam: Rodolfi, 2011).

Shefer-Mossensohn, Miri, *Ottoman medicine: healing and medical institutions, 1500–1700* (New York: Albany, 2009).

Shrewsbury, John F.D., *A history of bubonic plague in the British Isles* (Cambridge: Cambridge University Press, 1970).

Siena, Kevin (ed.), *Sins of the flesh: responding to the French disease in early modern Europe* (Toronto: Centre for Reformation and Renaissance Studies, 2005).

———, 'Searchers of the dead in long eighteenth-century London' in Kim Kippen and Lori Woods (eds), *Worth and repute: valuing gender in late medieval and early modern Europe. Essays in honour of Barbara Todd* (Toronto: CRRS, 2011), pp. 123–52.

Siraisi, Nancy G., *Medieval and early Renaissance medicine: an introduction to knowledge and practice* (London: University of Chicago Press, 1990).

Slack, Paul, 'Social policy and the constraints of Government 1547–48' in Jennifer Loach and Robert Tittler (eds), *The mid-Tudor polity c. 1540–60* (London: Macmillan, 1980), pp. 94–116.

———, 'The disappearance of plague: an alternative view', *The economic history review*, 34 (1981), 469–76.

———, *Impact of plague in Tudor and Stuart England* (London: Routledge & Kegan Paul, 1985).

———, *Poverty and policy in Tudor and Stuart England* (London: Longman, 1988).

———, 'Responses to plague in early modern England: public policies and their consequences' in John Walter and Roger Schofield (eds), *Famine, disease and the social order in early modern society* (Cambridge: Cambridge University Press, 1989), pp. 167–88.

Smith, Alison A., 'Gender, ownership and domestic space: inventories and family archives in Renaissance Verona', *Renaissance studies*, 12 (1998), 375–91.

Snodin, Michael and Nigel Llewellyn, *Baroque: style in the age of magnificence 1620–1800* (London: V&A Publishing, 2009).

Spada, Nicolò, 'Leggi veneziane sulle industrie chimiche a tutela della salute pubblica dal secolo XIII al XVIII', *Archivio Veneto*, 5th series, 7 (1930), 126–56.

Sperling, Jutta, 'The paradox of perfection: reproducing the body politic in late Renaissance Venice', *Comparative studies in society and history*, 41 (1999), 3–32.

———, *Convents and the body politic in late Renaissance Venice* (London: University of Chicago Press, 1999).

Spicciani, Amleto, 'The "poveri vergognosi" in fifteenth-century Florence' in Thomas Riis (ed.), *Aspects of poverty in early modern Europe* (Alphen aan den Rijn: Sijthoff, 1981), pp. 119–82.

Spufford, Margaret, *Figures in the landscape: rural society in England 1500–1700* (Aldershot: Ashgate, 2000).

Stein, Claudia, *Negotiating the French pox in early modern Germany* (Aldershot: Ashgate, 2008).

Stevens Crawshaw, Jane L., 'The beasts of burial: pizzigamorti and public health for the plague in early modern Venice', *Social history of medicine* 24:3 (2011), 570–87.

Strasser, Ulrike, *State of virginity: gender, religion and politics in an early modern Catholic state* (Ann Arbor MI: University of Michigan Press, 2004).

Stuard, Susan M., 'A communal program of medical care: medieval Ragusa/ Dubrovnik', *Journal of the history of Medicine and Allied Sciences*, 28 (1973), 126–42.

Stuart, Kathy, *Defiled trades and social outcasts: honor and ritual pollution in early modern Germany* (Cambridge: Cambridge University Press, 1999).

Styles, John, 'Product innovation in early modern London', *Past and Present*, 168 (2000), 124–69.

Tafuri, Manfredo, 'Alvise Cornaro, Palladio e Leonardo Donà: un dibattito sul bacino marciano' in Lionello Puppi (ed.), *Palladio e Venezia* (Florence: Sansoni, 1982), pp. 9–27.

——— (ed.), *'Renovatio urbis': Venezia nell'età di Andrea Gritti* (1523–1538) (Rome: Officina, 1984).

———, *Ricerca dei Rinascimento: principi, città, architetti* (Turin: Einaudi, 1992).

Tagliaferri, Amelio (ed.), *Atti del convegno: 'Venezia e la Terraferma attraverso le relazioni dei rettori'* (Milan: Giuffrè, 1981).

Tenenti, Alberto and Ugo Tucci et al. (eds), *Storia di Venezia dalle origini alla caduta della Serenissima* (12 vols, Rome: Istituto della Enciclopedia italiana, 1991–).

Terpstra, Nicholas, *Abandoned children of the Italian Renaissance: orphan care in Florence and Bologna* (London: Johns Hopkins University Press, 2005).

Thomas, Keith, *Man and the natural world: changing attitudes in England 1500– 1800* (London: Penguin, 1983).

Tilly, Charles and Wim P. Blockmans, *Cities and the rise of states in Europe AD1000–1800* (Boulder CO: Westview Press, 1994).

Torno, Armando (ed.), *La peste di Milano del 1630: la cronica e le testimonianze del tempo del Cardinale Federico Borromeo* (Milan: Rusconi, 1998).

Trexler, Richard, 'Charity and the defence of urban elites in Italian communes' in Frederic C. Jaher (ed.), *The rich, the wellborn and the powerful: elites and upper classes in history* (Secaucus NJ: Citadel, 1973), pp. 64–110.

Twigg, Graham, *The Black Death: a biological reappraisal* (London: Batsford Academic and Educational, 1984).

Ulvioni, Paolo, *Il gran castigo di Dio: carestia ed epidemie a Venezia e nella terraferma 1628–32* (Milan: Franco Angeli, 1982).

van Andel, Martinus A., 'Plague regulations in the Netherlands', *Janus*, 21 (1916), 410–44.

Van Gelder, Martje, *Trading places: the Netherlandish merchants in early modern Venice* (Leiden: Brill, 2009).

Vanzan Marchini, Nelli-Elena, *La memoria della salute: Venezia e il suo ospedale dal XVI al XX secolo* (Venice: Arsenale, 1985).

———, *L'ospedali di Veneziani: storia, patrimonio, progetto* (Venice: Comune di Venezia, 1986).

———, *I mali e i rimedi della Serenissima* (Vicenza: N. Pozza, 1995).

———, *Le leggi di sanità della Repubblica di Venezia* (Treviso: Canova, 2000).

———, *Rotte mediterranee e baluardi di sanità: Venezia e i lazzaretti mediterranei: catalogo di una mostra* (Milan: Skira, 2004).

———, *Venezia: luoghi di paure e voluttà* (Venice: Edizioni della Laguna, 2005).

Varanini, Gian Maria, 'Per la storia delle istituzioni ospedaliere nelle città della terraferma veneta nel Quattrocento' in Allen J. Grieco and Lucia Sandri (eds), *Ospedali e città: L'Italia del centro-nord XIII–XVI sec* (Florence: Le Lettere, 1997), pp. 107–55.

Vené, Armando, 'Il lazzaretto vecchio di Verona', *Dedalo*, 12 (1932), 253–59.

Venezia e la peste 1348–1797 (Venice: Comune di Venezia, 1980).

Ventura, Angelo, *Nobiltà e popolo nella società veneta del '400 e '500* (Bari: Laterza, 1964).

Viggiano, Alfredo, *Governanti e governati: legittimità del potere ed esercizio dell'autorità sovrana nello stato veneto della prima età moderna* (Treviso: Edizioni Canova, 1993).

Visconti, Alessandro, 'Il magistrato di sanità nello stato di Lombardia', *Archivio storico lombardo*, 15 (1911), 261–84.

Waldis, Vera, 'Hospitalisation und Absonderung in Pestzeiten – die Schweiz im Vergleich zu Oberitalien', *Gesnerus*, 39 (1982), 71–8.

Wallis, Patrick, 'Plagues, morality and the place of medicine in early modern England', *English Historical Review*, 121 (2006), 1–24.

———, 'A dreadful heritage: interpreting epidemic disease at Eyam, 1666–2000', *History Workshop Journal* 61:1 (2006), 31–56.

Watson, Gilbert, *Theriac and mithridatium: a study in therapeutics* (London: Wellcome Historical Medical Library, 1966).

Wear, Andrew (ed.), *Medicine in society: historical essays* (Cambridge: Cambridge University Press, 1992).

———, 'Making sense of health and the environment in early modern England' in *Health and healing in early modern England: studies in social and intellectual history* (Aldershot: Ashgate, 1998), chapter four.

———, 'Fear, anxiety and the plague in early modern England' in John R. Hinnells and Roy Porter (eds), *Religion, health and suffering* (London: Kegan Paul International, 1999), pp. 339–63.

———, *Knowledge and practice in English medicine, 1550–1680* (Cambridge: Cambridge University Press, 2000).

Webster, Charles (ed.), *Health, medicine and mortality in the sixteenth century* (Cambridge: Cambridge University Press, 1979).

Weddle, Saundra, '"Women in wolves' mouths": nun's reputations, enclosure and architecture at the convent of Le Murate in Florence' in Helen Hills (ed.), *Architecture and the politics of gender in early modern Europe* (Aldershot: Ashgate, 2003) pp. 115–29.

Wheeler, Jo, 'Stench in sixteenth-century Venice' in Alexander Cowan and Jill Steward (eds), *The city and the senses: urban culture since 1500* (Aldershot: Ashgate, 2007), pp. 25–38.

Wiel, Alethea, *The story of Verona* (London: J.M. Dent, 1902).

Wiesner Hanks, *Merry, Christianity and sexuality in the early modern world: regulating desire, reforming practice* (London: Routledge, 2010).

Wiesner, Merry, *Working women in Renaissance Germany* (New Brunswick NJ: Rutgers University Press, 1986).

Wilson, Adrian, 'The ceremony of childbirth and its interpretation' in Valerie Fides (ed.), *Women as mothers in pre-industrial England. Essays in memory of Dorothy McLaren* (London: Routledge, 1990), pp. 68–107.

Wilson, Bronwen, *The world in Venice: print, the city and early modern identity* (London: University of Toronto Press, 2005).

Wilson, Bee, *The hive: the story of the honeybee and us* (London: John Murray, 2004).

Wilson Bowers, Kirsty, 'Balancing individual and communal needs: plague and public health in early modern Seville', *Bulletin of the history of medicine,* 81 (2007), 335–358.

Wolters, Wolfgang, *Storia e politica nei dipinti di Palazzo Ducale* (Venice: Arsenale, 1987).

Woolf, Stuart J., 'Venice and the terraferma: problems of the change from commercial to landed activities' in Brian Pullan (ed.), *Crisis and change in the Venetian economy in the sixteenth and seventeenth centuries* (London: Methuen, 1968), pp. 175–203.

Wootton, David, 'Ulysses Bound? Venice and the idea of liberty from Howell to Hume' in David Wootton (ed.), *Republicanism, Liberty, and Commercial Society, 1649–1776* (Stanford CA: Stanford University Press, 1994), pp. 341–67.

Worcester, Thomas, 'Plague as spiritual medicine and medicine as spiritual metaphor: three treatises by Etienne Binet S.J. (1569–1639)' in Franco Mormando and Thomas Worcester (eds), *Piety and Plague: from Byzantium to the Baroque* (Kirksville MI: Truman State University Press, 2007) pp. 224–36.

Wray, Shona K., *Communities and crisis: Bologna during the Black Death* (Leiden: Brill, 2009).

Wright, Diana, 'Bartolomeo Minio: Venetian administration in fifteenth-century Nauplion', *Electronic Journal of Oriental Studies*, 3:5 (2000), 1–235.

Zorzi, Alvise, *Venezia scomparsa* (Milan: Electa, 1972).

UNPUBLISHED SOURCES

Allerston, Patricia, 'The market in secondhand clothes and furnishings in Venice c.1500–c.1650' (unpublished PhD. thesis, European University Institute, 1996).

Bamji, Alexandra, 'Religion and disease in Venice c.1620–1700' (unpublished PhD. thesis, University of Cambridge, 2007).

Benyovsky, Irena, 'Plague and urban policy of medieval Dubrovnik' (unpublished conference paper, Sixth International Conference on urban history, Edinburgh, 2002).

Bonastra, Joaquim, 'Ciencia, sociedad y planificación territorial en la institución del lazareto' (unpublished PhD thesis, 2006, University of Barcelona).

Christensen, Daniel E. 'Politics and the plague: efforts to combat health epidemics in seventeenth-century Braunschweig-Wolfenbuttel, Germany' (unpublished PhD thesis, 2004, University of California Riverside).

Fusaro, Maria, 'The English mercantile communities in Venice and in the Ionian islands 1570–1670' (unpublished PhD. thesis, University of Cambridge, 2002).

Henderson, John, 'Plague, putrefaction and the poor in early modern Florence' (unpublished seminar paper, Institute of Historical Research, 19 January 2006).

Laughran, Michelle, 'The body, public health and social control in sixteenth-century Venice' (unpublished PhD. thesis, University of Connecticut, 1998).

Oakes, Simon P., 'The presence, patronage and artistic importance of the German community in early Cinquecento Venice' (unpublished PhD. thesis, University of Cambridge, 2006).

Palmer, Richard J., 'The control of plague in Venice and northern Italy 1348–1600' (unpublished PhD. thesis, University of Kent, 1978).

Index